T0259522

Fibromyalgia

Guest Editor

PHILIP J. MEASE, MD

RHEUMATIC DISEASE CLINICS OF NORTH AMERICA

www.rheumatic.theclinics.com

May 2009 • Volume 35 • Number 2

SAUNDERS an imprint of ELSEVIER, Inc.

W.B. SAUNDERS COMPANY

A Division of Elsevier Inc.

1600 John F. Kennedy Blvd., Suite 1800 • Philadelphia, PA 19103-2899

http://www.theclinics.com

RHEUMATIC DISEASE CLINICS OF NORTH AMERICA Volume 35, Number 2
May 2009 ISSN 0889-857X, ISBN 13: 978-1-4377-0539-3, ISBN 10: 1-4377-0539-1

Editor: Rachel Glover
Developmental Editor: Donald Mumford

Rheumatic Disease Clinics of North America (ISSN 0889-857X) is published quarterly by Elsevier Inc., 360 Park Avenue South, New York, NY 10010-1710. Months of issue are February, May, August, and November. Business and editorial offices: 1600 John F. Kennedy Boulevard, Suite 1800, Philadelphia, PA 19103-2899. Customer Service offices: 11830 Westline Industrial Drive, St. Louis, MO 63146. Periodicals postage paid at New York, NY and additional mailing offices. Subscription prices are USD 244.00 per year for US individuals, USD 414.00 per year for US institutions, USD 122.00 per year for US students and residents, USD 288.00 per year for Canadian individuals, USD 512.00 per year for Canadian institutions, USD 342.00 per year for international individuals, USD 512.00 per year for international institutions, and USD 171.00 per year for Canadian and foreign students/residents. To receive student/resident rate, orders must be accompanied by name of affiliated institution, date of term, and the *signature* of program/residency coordinator on institution letterhead. Orders will be billed at individual rate until proof of status received. Foreign air speed delivery is included in all *Clinics* subscription prices. All prices are subject to change without notice. **POSTMASTER:** Send address changes to *Rheumatic Disease Clinics of North America,* Elsevier Journals Customer Service, 11830 Westline Industrial Drive, St. Louis, MO 63146. **Customer Service: 1-800-654-2452 (US and Canada). From outside of the US and Canada: 314-453-7041. Fax: 314-453-5170. For print support, e-mail: JournalsCustomerService-usa@elsevier. com. For online support, e-mail: JournalsOnlineSupport-usa@elsevier.com.**

Reprints. For copies of 100 or more of articles in this publication, please contact the Commercial Reprints Department, Elsevier Inc., 360 Park Avenue South, New York, New York, 10010-1710; Tel.: (+1) 212-633-3813, Fax: (+1) 212-462-1935, and E-mail: reprints@elsevier.com.

Rheumatic Disease Clinics of North America is covered in *MEDLINE/PubMed (Index Medicus), Current Contents/Clinical Medicine, Science Citation Index, ISI/BIOMED,* and *EMBASE/Excerpta Medica.*

Printed and bound by CPI Group (UK) Ltd, Croydon, CR0 4YY

Transferred to Digital Print 2011

Contributors

GUEST EDITOR

PHILIP J. MEASE, MD
Seattle Rheumatology Associates; Chief, Rheumatology Clinical Research, Swedish Hospital Medical Center; and Clinical Professor, University of Washington School of Medicine, Seattle, Washington

AUTHORS

KOBBY ABLIN, MD
Institute of Rheumatology, Tel Aviv Medical Center, Tel Aviv, Israel

ROBERT M. BENNETT, MD, FRCP, MACR
Professor of Medicine and Nursing, Oregon Health & Science University, Portland, Oregon

DAN BUSKILA, MD
Professor of Medicine, Division of Internal Medicine, Head of Department of Medicine H, Soroka Medical Center, Faculty of Health Sciences, Ben Gurion University, Beer Sheva, Israel

ERNEST H. CHOY, MD, FRCP
Director, Sir Alfred Baring Garrod Clinical Trials Unit, Academic Department Rheumatology, Weston Education Centre, King's College London, London, United Kingdom

DANIEL J. CLAUW, MD
Department of Anesthesiology and Medicine, University of Michigan, Ann Arbor, Michigan

RICHARD N. GEVIRTZ, PhD
Distinguished Professor of Psychology, California School of Professional Psychology, Alliant International University, San Diego, California

JENNIFER M. GLASS, PhD
Research Assistant Professor, Department of Psychiatry; and Assistant Research Scientist, Institute for Social Research, University of Michigan, Ann Arbor, Michigan

RICHARD H. GRACELY, PhD
Center for Neurosensory Disorders, University of North Carolina, Chapel Hill, North Carolina

AFTON L. HASSETT, PsyD
Assistant Professor, Department of Medicine, Division of Rheumatology, University of Medicine and Dentistry of New Jersey–Robert Wood Johnson Medical School, New Brunswick, New Jersey

KATHLEEN F. HOLTON, MPH
Research Associate, Department of Orthopaedics and Rehabilitation, Oregon Health & Science University, Portland, Oregon; and PhD Candidate, Department of Nutritional Sciences, University of Arizona, Tucson, Arizona

KIM D. JONES, PhD, RN, FNP
Associate Professor, Office of Research and Development, School of Nursing, Oregon Health & Science University, Portland, Oregon

LINDSAY L. KINDLER, RN, PhD
Clinical Nurse Specialist, Kaiser Permanente, West Interstate Medical Office, Portland, Oregon; and Post-doctoral Fellow, University of Florida, Comprehensive Center for Pain Research, Gainesville, Florida

ALICE A. LARSON, PhD
Professor, Department of Veterinary Pathobiology, University of Minnesota, St. Paul, Minnesota

GINEVRA L. LIPTAN, MD
Assistant Adjunct Clinical Faculty, Division of Arthritis and Rheumatic Diseases, Oregon Health & Science University; and Legacy Good Samaritan Pain Management Center, Portland, Oregon

MANUEL MARTINEZ-LAVIN, MD
Chief, Rheumatology Department, National Cardiology Institute, Mexico City, Mexico

PHILIP J. MEASE, MD
Seattle Rheumatology Associates; Chief, Rheumatology Clinical Research, Swedish Hospital Medical Center; and Clinical Professor, University of Washington School of Medicine, Seattle, Washington

HARVEY MOLDOFSKY, MD, FRCPC
Professor Emeritus, Faculty of Medicine, University of Toronto; and President and Medical Director, Sleep Disorders Clinics of the Centre for Sleep & Chronobiology, Toronto, Ontario, Canada

MARY B. NEBEL, BSE
Center for Neurosensory Disorders, University of North Carolina, Chapel Hill, North Carolina

I. JON RUSSELL, MD, PhD
Associate Professor, Department of Medicine, Division of Clinical Immunology and Rheumatology; and Director, University Clinical Research Center, The University of Texas Health Science Center at San Antonio, San Antonio, Texas

STEPHEN SCHILLING, PhD
Senior Psychometrician, English Language Institute Testing, University of Michigan, Ann Arbor, Michigan

ROLAND STAUD, MD
Professor, Department of Medicine, University of Florida, Gainesville, Florida

ANGELICA VARGAS, MD
Staff Physician, Rheumatology Department, National Cardiology Institute, Mexico City, Mexico

DAVID A. WILLIAMS, PhD
Professor of Anesthesiology, Department of Anesthesiology, Psychiatry and Psychology; and Associate Director, Chronic Pain & Fatigue Research Center, University of Michigan, Ann Arbor, Michigan

Contents

Since the publication of the American College of Rheumatology Classification Criteria for Fibromyalgia 18 years ago, there have been an ever-
increasing number of research articles and reviews. From the National
Library of Medicine alone there are more than 10,000 articles related to
fibromyalgia. The major clinical manifestations of fibromyalgia have not
changed, but their prevalence, associations, relative importance to the patient, and scientific underpinnings are increasingly better understood. This
article provides an update on fibromyalgia symptomatology and looks at
issues that need to be considered in the development of updated diagnostic guidelines. There is still no gold standard for making a diagnosis of
fibromyalgia, but there is an increasing consensus for the development
of new guidelines for diagnosis that modifies the currently proscribed
tender point evaluation.

This article attempts to demonstrate insight into understanding the evolving spectrum of functional somatic syndromes. It will become evident that
in understanding these highly complex disorders, neither the Cartesian
dichotomy regarding body-mind distinction nor the pure reductionist
approach to disease (which attempts to explain clinical phenomena on
the basis of underlying structural derangement) can be strictly adhered
to. Only use of a truly integrative framework of thinking can allow us to
both recognize and accept the overlapping basic similarity between these
conditions and, in turn, teach us about nearly any medical condition characterized by pain or sensory symptoms.

Fibromyalgia is an idiopathic chronic pain syndrome defined by widespread nonarticular musculoskeletal pain and generalized tender points.
The syndrome is associated with a constellation of symptoms, including
fatigue, nonrefreshing sleep, irritable bowel, and more. Central nervous
system sensitization is a major pathophysiologic aspect of fibromyalgia;
in addition, various external stimuli such as trauma and stress may

Clinical and laboratory evidence confirm that dyscognition is a real and
troubling symptom in fibromyalgia (FM), and that the cognitive mechanisms most affected in FM are working memory, episodic memory, and
semantic memory. Recent evidence provides further convergence on
specific difficulty with attentional control. Dyscognition in FM cannot be attributed solely to concomitant psychiatric conditions such as depression
and poor sleep, but does seem to be related to the level of pain. This article
presents recent contributions regarding the etiology of the cognitive
dysfunction, its impact on patients, and highlights the need for further
research on this facet of FM.

Functional MRI blood oxygenation level dependent activation studies on
patients who have fibromyalgia have demonstrated augmented sensitivity
to painful pressure and the association of this augmentation with variables
such as depression and catastrophizing and have also been used to evaluate the symptoms of cognitive dysfunction. Using a wide array of techniques, these studies have found differences in opioid receptor binding,
in the concentration of metabolites associated with neural processing in
pain-related regions, in functional brain networks, and in regional brain
volume and white matter tracks. A common theme of all of these methods
is that they provide information that may be pertinent to the otherwise
unobservable and poorly treated symptoms of persistent widespread
chronic pain.

This article discusses the key symptom domains to be assessed in fibromyalgia. Development of a consensus on a core set of outcome measures
that should be assessed and reported in all clinical trials is needed to facilitate interpretation, pooling, and comparison of results. This aligns with the
key objective of the Outcome Measures in Rheumatoid Arthritis Clinical
Trials initiative to improve outcome measurement in rheumatic diseases
through a data-driven interactive consensus process.

Fibromyalgia (FM) has historically been considered a chronic pain condition. Recent clinical studies, however, reveal that while pain may be the
cardinal symptom of FM, there are many other symptoms and

consequences of having FM that have an impact on the lives of individuals with this condition. As such, an area of intense clinical research has focused upon improving approaches to assessment for FM. This article provides an overview of how the art of assessing FM has evolved over time, current methods of assessment, the value of patients' perspectives in assessment, and emerging advancements representing the future of for FM.

RELATED INTEREST
Medical Clinics of North America
Pain Management Parts I and II
Howard S. Smith, MD, *Guest Editor*

THE CLINICS ARE NOW AVAILABLE ONLINE!

Access your subscription at:
www.theclinics.com

Preface

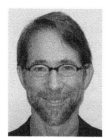

Philip J. Mease, MD
Guest Editor

Since the previous fibromyalgia (FM) issue of *Rheumatic Diseases Clinics of North America*, published in 2002, there has been a steady increase of understanding and awareness of this condition and its inter-relatedness with other disorders of central sensitization, as well as other chronic illness conditions. The current issue is timely in its ability to provide a comprehensive update of our knowledge of the basic and clinical science of FM to accompany the first approvals by the Food and Drug Administration of pharmacotherapy directed at known pathophysiologic mechanisms of FM.

It is appropriate that Bennett, a pioneer of FM research and education, is author the first article of this issue, which documents the multidimensional symptom domains of FM, along with current approaches to diagnosis and classification of the disorder. Ablin and Clauw proceed to place FM in the context of the family of Central Sensitization Syndromes, integrating our growing understanding of the neuropathophysiologic and genetic underpinnings of a variety of conditions characterized by pain and other symptoms caused by central sensory dysregulation. That FM can exist in the pediatric age population is under-appreciated. Clinical cohorts of children and adolescents with FM are discussed by Buskila.

The evidence for the neurobiologic pathophysiology of FM, with emphasis on excessive nociceptive input and deficient function of inhibitory pain pathways, is reviewed by Staud. Research into the role of sleep pathology in FM, first pursued by Moldofsky in the 1970s, is updated by him in this issue. Martinez-Lavin and Vargas discuss the complex subject of autonomic dysfunction in FM and proposes a conceptual approach to understanding the various symptom domains of FM based on these findings. FM patients frequently complain of a state of cognitive dysfunction, often called "fibro-fog." The evidence for cognitive impairment is reviewed by Glass. Emerging neuroimaging techniques have contributed significantly to our understanding of FM, as described by Nebel and Gracely.

In order for us to assess the various symptom domains of FM, and measure response to treatment, a variety of outcome measures have been used in clinical trials. What are the key symptom domains that should be measured? A working group of the Outcome Measures of Rheumatology Clinical Trials research consortia has conducted focus groups of FM patients and Delphi exercises among patients and clinicians, as

Rheum Dis Clin N Am 35 (2009) xiii–xiv
doi:10.1016/j.rdc.2009.07.001
0889-857X/09/$ – see front matter

well as analyzing data from clinical trials, to address this question. Choy and Mease review the outcome of this process and Williams and Schilling review the measures used in clinical trials, as well as proposals for future refinement of our ability to measure disease activity and response to therapy.

Treatment of FM optimally utilizes a multimodal approach of pharmacologic and nonpharmacologic therapies. Mease and Choy review the medications that have commonly been used for the treatment of FM and have been studied in controlled trials. Focus is placed on the therapies that target known pathophysiologic mechanisms in FM and the safety and efficacy data that support the recent approvals of agents that diminish nociceptive input, such as pregabalin, and augment inhibitory sensory mechanisms, such as duloxetine and milnacipran. The basis for rational combination pharmacotherapy is discussed. Jones and Liptan review the evidence for the benefits of exercise therapy. Hassett and Gevirtz discuss other modalities, such as cognitive behavioral therapy, and Holton and colleagues review the evidence for dietary interventions in FM.

Providing a perspective on the bridging of what we know about mechanisms with practical approaches to management, Jon Russell provides an integrated summary of the basic and clinical science reviewed in this issue.

It is our intent to provide a comprehensive review and bibliographic reference to the important advances in the field of FM—since this was last addressed by *Rheumatic Disease Clinics of North America*—that is both in-depth enough for the researcher with special interest in this field of medicine and practical enough for the practicing clinician to apply the insights that are addressed. Ultimately, it is our intent to improve the daily experience of the patient with FM through broadening the understanding and improving the management of this difficult and complex condition.

Philip J. Mease, MD
Seattle Rheumatology Associates
1101 Madison Street
Suite 1000
Seattle, WA 98104, USA

E-mail address:
hpmease@nwlink.com (P.J. Mease)

Clinical Manifestations and Diagnosis of Fibromyalgia

Robert M. Bennett, MD, FRCP, MACR

KEYWORDS

- Fibromyalgia • Symptoms • Diagnosis • Pain • Fatigue
- Stiffness

The basic clinical manifestations of fibromyalgia (FM), in terms of pain, fatigue, dysfunctional sleep, and tenderness were described by Smythe and Moldofsky[1] in 1977 and elaborated by Yunus and colleagues[2] in 1981. The 1990 American College of Rheumatology (ACR) fibromyalgia classification paper listed many other symptoms that were commonly reported by FM patients (paresthesia, anxiety, headaches, irritable bowel, urinary urgency, sicca symptoms, noise and cold intolerance, dysmenorrhea, depression, low back pain, neck pain, Raynaud phenomenon, and weather-related effects).[3] An Internet survey conducted by the National Fibromyalgia Association (NFA) on 2569 people who have diagnosed fibromyalgia reported the rank order of symptoms as: morning stiffness, fatigue, nonrestorative sleep, pain, forgetfulness, poor concentration, difficulty falling asleep, muscle spasms, anxiety, and depression (**Table 1**).[4] A similar questionnaire from the German Fibromyalgia Association (DFV) was mailed to 3996 patients and was completed by 699 patients; the rank order of the most frequent symptoms was: muscle pain, morning stiffness, nonrestorative sleep, poor concentration, lack of energy, low productivity, and forgetfulness.[5] Since that time, many of these symptoms have been subject to further study and the patients' perspective has been more rigorously evaluated as part of the OMERACT (Outcome Measures in Rheumatology Clinical Trials) process.[6]

PAIN

The core symptom of FM, according to the 1990 ACR classification criteria, is chronic widespread pain (WSP).[3] FM patients usually describe their pain as arising from muscle and joints,[5] and the majority of FM patients also have tender skin.[1,7] Fibromyalgia pain typically waxes and wanes in intensity; flares are associated with unaccustomed exertion, prolonged inactivity, soft tissue injuries, surgery, poor sleep, cold exposure, long car trips, and psychological stressors. Many FM patients describe

Oregon Health & Science University, 3455 SW Veterans Road, Portland, OR 97239, USA
E-mail address: bennetrob1@comcast.net

Rheum Dis Clin N Am 35 (2009) 215–232
doi:10.1016/j.rdc.2009.05.009
0889-857X/09/$ – see front matter

Table 1
A comparison of the major patient-perceived manifestations of fibromyalgia

OMERACT 7 Patient Delphi	NFA Survey	DFV Survey
Pain or physical discomfort	Morning stiffness	Pain
Joint pain or aching	Fatigue	Fatigue
Fatigue or lack of energy	Nonrestorative sleep	Nonrestorative sleep
Poor sleep	Pain	Morning stiffness
Fibro-fog	Forgetfulness	Poor concentration
Stiffness	Poor concentration	Lack of energy
Disorganized thinking	Difficulty falling asleep	Low productivity
Difficulty with moving	Muscle spasms	Forgetfulness
Having to push yourself to accomplish things	Anxiety	Irritability
Problems with setting goals and completing tasks	Depression	Weather sensitivity
Tenderness to touch	Headaches	Feeling hands are swollen
Depression	Anger	Dizziness
Limitations in normal daily activities	Restless legs	Headaches
Poor memory	Abdominal pain	Visual disturbances

increased pain with cold, damp weather and low barometric pressure.[4] FM pain is predominantly axial in distribution, but pain in the hands and feet is not uncommon and may lead to a misdiagnosis of early rheumatoid arthritis (RA).[8] Staud and colleagues[9] has surmised that "peripheral factors account for most of the variance of overall clinical FM pain, suggesting that the input of pain by the peripheral tissues is clinically relevant." Many patients describe a feeling of swelling in their soft tissues; this is often localized to the area of joints, which may lead to self-diagnosis of arthritis and referral to a rheumatologist. Martinez-Lavin and colleagues[7] reported that many FM symptoms are similar to those experienced by patients with neuropathic pain syndromes; these neuropathic symptoms refer mainly to changes in skin sensation. Fibromyalgia pain and stiffness typically have a diurnal variation, with a nadir from about 11:00 AM to 3:00 PM.[10] Fibromyalgia often occurs in the setting of other pain syndromes, such as RA, systemic lupus erythematosus (SLE), osteoarthritis, and so forth. There has been a profusion of sophisticated psychoneurophysiological and imaging studies indicating that FM pain is a result of disordered sensory processing.[11]

FATIGUE

Fatigue is one of the most common symptoms encountered in patients seeking medical care, with a prevalence of 24% in one report.[12] The association of fatigue and pain has a long history and was a prominent feature of neurasthenia as described in the late nineteenth century.[13] The differential diagnosis of fatigue includes many medical illnesses, but a well-defined diagnosis is only found in about 5% of fatigued patients presenting in primary care.[14] The OMERACT 8 patient Delphi rated fatigue as the third most important symptom after two pain-related items; it was endorsed by 96% of participants. In the NFA and DFV surveys, it was rated as the second most troublesome symptom (see **Table 1**). The Fibromyalgia Impact Questionnaire (FIQ) includes "How tired have you been?" with anchors of "No tiredness" and

"Very tired" on a 0–10 visual analog scale (VAS); it is often used a surrogate measure of fatigue. However, exactly what is meant by "fatigue" must be considered. Sleepiness and fatigue are interrelated-but-distinct phenomena that are often reported in the context of medical disorders, psychiatric disorders, and primary sleep disorders. Sleepiness and fatigue usually have different implications in terms of diagnosis and treatment; however, they are often used interchangeably or merged under the more general lay term of "feeling tired." Most FM patients describe their fatigue as a weariness of mind and body that impairs their productivity and enjoyment of life.

A careful analysis is required in the evaluation of the fatigued patient to determine the possible cause of the symptoms and the patient's reaction to being fatigued. Wessely[15] conceptualized four components of fatigue: behavior (effects of fatigue), feeling (subjective experience), mechanisms, and context (environment, attitudes). He stresses that even when a discrete cause for fatigue is identified, such as chronic infection or multiple sclerosis, the social, behavioral, and psychological variables are still important in the comprehensive evaluation of a patient's fatigue. Arnold[16] emphasized the wide range of symptoms that can masquerade as fatigue; she divides fatigue into three major domains: (1) *Physical* (eg, reduced activity, low energy, tiredness, decreased physical endurance, increased effort with physical tasks and with overcoming inactivity, general weakness, heaviness, slowness or sluggishness, nonrestorative sleep, and sleepiness); (2) *Cognitive* (eg, decreased concentration, decreased attention, decreased mental endurance, and slowed thinking); and (3) *Emotional* (eg, decreased motivation or initiative, decreased interest, feeling overwhelmed, feeling bored, aversion to effort, and feeling low). In FM patients, the two most obvious contributors to fatigue are depression and nonrestorative sleep. However, although antidepressant therapy often results in a modest improvement in fatigue scales, they are seldom curative of this symptom.[17–19] Furthermore, improvements in nonrestorative sleep do not necessarily translate into absence of fatigue. In the 2009 sodium oxybate study, the overall improvement of sleep was about 30% (Jenkins sleep questionnaire) and tiredness (FIQ) was reduced by about 25%.[20]

Chronic pain itself appears to have a fatiguing effect.[21] This is probably the result of comorbidities such as insomnia, deconditioning, and depression. However, there is increasing interest in the notion that the fatigue/pain association may be a direct result of chronic pain modulating the release of inflammatory cytokines from pain-activated astrocytes and microglia within the brain, inducing a "sickness syndrome."[22]

STIFFNESS

Stiffness is a prominent condition in many musculoskeletal disorders. Patients in the NFA online survey rated morning stiffness as their most troublesome symptom; German FM patients rated it as their fourth most important symptom (see **Table 1**). In the OMERACT 8 Delphi, stiffness was reported by 91% of participants and was rated the sixth most important symptom. The combination of stiffness with the common FM experience of joint pain raises questions about a diagnosis of an early inflammatory arthritis; many patients who have early FM request to be seen by a rheumatologist. Stiffness is an item on the FIQ,[23] and thus an indication of its relevance can be found in the many studies that have used the FIQ.[24] There have not been any physiologic studies of stiffness in FM. Muscle stiffness is a combination of the intrinsic properties of muscle tissue (mainly nonelastic connective tissue) and resting muscle tone. There is an increase in this nonelastic tissue with aging,[25] and muscle tissue displays thixotropic properties (ie, it stiffens with increasing rest and vice versa);[26] this may be relevant to the benefits of exercise in FM. On the other hand, exercise-induced muscle damage increases muscle stiffness,[27] thus the need for restraint in the prescription of vigorous exercise in FM patients.[28] Muscle stiffness may be a prominent early symptom of several disorders; for instance, stiffness is a feature of severe hypothyroidism (Hoffman's syndrome)[29] and is often an early symptom of Parkinson disease.[30] It is quite evident that a greater understanding of stiffness in FM patients should yield important clues as to clinically relevant changes in muscle composition, muscle tone, and deconditioning.

DISORDERED SLEEP

Fibromyalgia patients usually report disturbed sleep.[31,32] They often have problems with sleep initiation and maintenance; the most notable feature is feeling tired upon awakening. This is usually referred to as nonrestorative sleep (NRS) and typically causes greater daytime impairment than does difficulty initiating or maintaining sleep.[33,34] There is no definitive classification of NRS; Stone and colleagues[35] suggested this definition: "a report of persistently feeling unrefreshed upon awakening in the presence of normal sleep duration, occurring in the absence of a sleep disorder." This is partly captured in the FIQ question on sleep: "How have you felt when you get up in the morning?" with the 0–10 VAS ranging between "Awoke well rested" and "Awoke very tired." NRS has been associated with certain EEG changes. In the 1970s, alpha intrusion into the delta rhythm of non–rapid eye movement (NREM) sleep was initially described in psychiatric subjects,[36] and shortly thereafter Moldofsky and colleagues[37] described a similar abnormality in "fibrositis" subjects. It is now apparent that alpha–delta sleep is not always found in FM subjects and does not always correlate with the symptom of NRS.[38] More recently, other abnormal EEG patterns have been found in FM subjects. Rizzi and colleagues[39] reported that a cyclic alternating pattern of sleep correlated with FM symptoms, and Roizenblatt and associates[40] reported that alpha intrusion had several different patterns, with a phasic pattern correlating most closely with FM symptoms. Landis and colleagues[41] reported that female FM subjects had fewer spindles during NREM stage 2 sleep and a lower spindle time per epoch of NREM stage 2 sleep.

In the clinical evaluation of disturbed sleep in FM subjects, the most important issue is the determination as to whether a patient has a primary sleep disorder. By far the most common is restless leg syndrome (RLS), which is associated with periodic limb movement disorder in most cases.[42] A 2008 study found a 64% prevalence of RLS in 3302 women who have fibromyalgia and noted that these subjects experienced more sleep disturbances and pronounced daytime sleepiness.[43] The history and response to a dopamine agonist are so typical that a formal sleep study is often unnecessary to diagnose RLS unless comorbid sleep apnea is suspected. However, it is suggested that patients who have RLS have a ferritin level, as there is a relationship of RLS with iron deficiency.[44] This iron deficiency seems similar to the iron deficiency of chronic disease and is often unresponsive to oral iron supplements. Interestingly, patients who have RLS have been reported to have low levels of iron in the substantia nigra and putamen;[45] neuropathological studies have led to the notion that RLS may be a functional disorder resulting from impaired iron acquisition by the neuromelanin cells.[46] There are no large studies of sleep apnea prevalence in FM; one study of 50 subjects attending a sleep clinic found the prevalence of FM was 10 times higher in subjects who have sleep apnea/hypopnea compared with the reported prevalence of FM in the general population.[47] Upper-airway resistance syndrome (UARS) is increasingly being diagnosed in patients who have dysfunctional sleep; this diagnosis will be missed unless additional channels are incorporated into the polysomnography testing.[48] UARS was found in 26 out of 28 female FM subjects attending a sleep clinic; only one subject had obstructive sleep apnea. A continuous positive airway pressure machine resulted in an improvement in functional symptoms ranging from 23% to 47%.[49] If these results were confirmed in a larger sample, there would be a good rationale for including polysomnography in the routine evaluation of FM patients.

TENDERNESS

FM patients typically report that they are more sensitive to touch, and experience pain on relatively minor contact (see **Table 1**). Skin roll tenderness (from the interscapular area) was incorporated into an early diagnostic definition of FM.[1] Some 95% of FM subjects endorsed the Leeds neuropathic pain question, "Does your pain make the affected skin abnormally sensitive to touch?"[7] Superficial pressure pain thresholds using von Frey hairs were found to be less in FM than in healthy controls, as were deep pressure pain thresholds and tourniquet test tolerance.[50] Another feature of some FM patients that suggests cutaneous sensitization is dermatographia, which is reactive hyperemia, that is, increased local blood flow and edema that occur on mechanical or chemical stimulation of the skin. It results from the local release of histamine from mast cells and the antidromic release of substance P, neurokinin A, and calcitonin gene-related peptide from the peripheral endings.[51] Dermatographia was one of the six clinical features used in FM diagnosis in the 1976 paper reporting on NREM sleep changes in subjects who had "fibrositis syndrome."[37] Littlejohn and colleagues[52] subsequently reported that FM subjects had an exaggerated skin flare response to both mechanical and chemical (capsaicin) stimulation and a positive correlation between the size of the flare and the number of tender points. It was suggested that the exaggerated skin response reflected increased activity of polymodal nociceptors of afferent nerves and that this may play a role in FM-related skin tenderness. These observations were largely forgotten until Salemi and colleagues[53] found that the skin biopsies of about 30% of FM subjects had demonstrable amounts of messenger RNA coding for IL-1βb, IL-6, and TNF-α, whereas no cytokine-coding mRNA was found in skin biopsies from healthy controls. This finding was surmised to be a result of neurogenic inflammation. Supportive of this explanation was the finding of dermal deposits of IgG and increased numbers of mast cells in FM compared with controls.[54] Interestingly, there is one report of experimental slow-wave sleep disruption being related to an exaggerated skin response and a reduced pain threshold.[55] This is a currently neglected area of FM research that may be of relevance in relation to the initiation and maintenance of central sensitization.[56]

COGNITIVE DYSFUNCTION

Difficulties with memory, concentration, and dual tasking are major problems of many fibromyalgia patients, according to self-reports.[57] On three self-rating surveys (see **Table 1**), dyscognition was the fifth most distressing symptom. Patients commonly describe difficulties with short-term memory, concentration, logical analysis, and motivation. This decrease in cognitive performance has been estimated to be equivalent to 20 years of aging.[58] Defects have been described in terms of working memory, episodic memory, and verbal fluency. Short-term memory problems have been linked to a disproportionate interference from distraction influences.[59] Some investigators have noted that cognitive defects in FM may be a result of associated fatigue, pain, and depression,[60,61] and others have failed to find significant defects using automated neuropsychological assessment.[62] Newer imaging technology may provide some explanation for these deficits. For instance, a proton magnetic resonance spectroscopy study showed lower levels of *N*-acetylaspartate in the hippocampus of FM subjects.[63] The hippocampus is important in the formation of new memories; thus, its dysfunction may be implicated in short-term memory loss.[64] There are several recent studies reporting a reduction in hippocampal volume in chronically stressed subjects.[65–67] Using the relatively new technique of magnetic resonance diffusion-tensor imaging and MR imaging of voxel-based morphometry, defects in neuronal circuitry were noted in FM subjects along with decreases in gray matter volume in the postcentral gyri, amygdalae, hippocampi, superior frontal gyri, and anterior cingulate gyri.[68] Luerding and colleagues[69] reported that cognitive deficits in nonverbal working memory were positively correlated with gray matter values in the left dorsolateral prefrontal cortex, whereas working memory was positively correlated with gray matter values in the supplementary motor cortex.

DYSESTHESIA

FM patients commonly report numbness and tingling in the extremities without any obvious cause coming to light upon further testing. In some patients this may be due to restless leg syndrome and in others an early peripheral neuropathy. Symptoms mimicking a neurologic disorder were first reported some 20 years ago.[70] More recently, Martinez-Lavin[71] postulated that fibromyalgia is a neuropathic pain syndrome and that dysesthetic sensations are evidence for this notion. To test this hypothesis, the Leeds neuropathic pain questionnaire was given to 20 FM subjects and 20 RA subjects. Sensory symptoms were more common in the FM cohort: dysesthetic (95% versus 30%), evoked (95% versus 35%), paroxysmal (90% versus 15%), and thermal (90% versus 20%).[7] Another explanation for the experience of these neurologic-sounding symptoms is a conflict between sensory–motor central nervous processing[72] and central sensitization syndrome.[73]

POOR BALANCE

Poor balance is increasingly being recognized as a manifestation of fibromyalgia. In the NFA survey, balance problems were reported by 45% of participants.[4] Jones and colleagues[74] studied 32 FM subjects and 32 controls regarding number of falls, confidence about balance, and a clinical evaluation of physiologic dysfunctions (stability limits, anticipatory postural adjustments, reactive postural responses, sensory orientation, and stability in gait) relating to balancing. Over a 6-month period, FM subjects had 37 falls compared with six falls in the controls. FM subjects lacked confidence in their ability to do specific tasks with an increased fear of falling compared with controls. The reasons for this imbalance in FM is unclear at this time; relevant issues may include poor proprioception, vestibular dysfunction, disturbed spatiovisual orientation, lower limb weakness, concentration/distraction deficits, and orthostatic hypotension.

RAYNAUD PHENOMENON

FM patients often report being cold in situations whereas others are not; this phenomenon is often associated with changes in the color of their fingers. Symptoms suggestive of primary Raynaud's have been reported in FM patients for the last 25 years, with a prevalence ranging from 8.8% to 53.3%.[75–77] One study of nail-fold capillaroscopy in FM did not find any of the morphologic changes that have been described in connective tissue disorders, but did note sluggish circulation in those subjects who have Raynaud's.[78] Bennett and colleagues[79] reported on quantitative evaluation of cold-induced vasospasm in 29 FM subjects using the Nielsen test; 41% had an abnormal test and 38% had elevated levels of platelet α2-adrenergic receptors. There was a positive correlation between the percentage of change in finger systolic pressure on cooling (Nielsen test) and the number of α2-adrenergic receptors. Digital photoplethysmography did not reveal any changes suggestive of organic disease in the digital vessels. Thermosensory testing has uniformly found a reduced threshold for cold-induced pain.[50,80,81] The relationship of cold intolerance and Raynaud phenomenon to the dysautonomia of FM and reduced perfusion of muscle warrants further research.[82,83]

ORAL AND OCULAR SYMPTOMS

Dry mouth is a common symptom of FM patients, with estimates ranging from 18% to 71%.[76,84] In some cases, this may be a result of side effects from tricyclic antidepressants,[85] coexistent hepatitis C infection,[86] or dysautonomia;[87] but in the majority of cases, no obvious cause can be found.[84] However, FM does appear to have a common association with Sjogren's syndrome, with a 22% prevalence in one study,[88] and is often the only diagnosis that can be made in patients who have keratoconjunctivitis sicca.[89] On the other hand, a diagnosis of biopsy-proven Sjogren's syndrome was only found in 7% of 72 FM patients.[90] In a study of 67 FM subjects, a high prevalence of oral symptoms were recorded: xerostomia 70.9%, glossodynia 32.8%, dysphagia 37.3%, and dysgeusia, 34.2%.[91] Blurred vision that cannot be corrected by prescription lenses is also a common phenomenon (R.M. Bennett, MD, unpublished data).

IMPAIRED FUNCTION

Most FM patients report some limitations of function. Item 1 of the FIQ consists of 11 questions relating to function with an average value of between 40 and 50 (on a 0–100 VAS) in several recent pharmaceutical studies.[18,92] Difficulty with moving and low productivity are prominent conditions (see **Table 1**). An analysis of the NFA survey data found that over 25% of female FM subjects reported difficulties in taking care of personal needs and the majority reported problems with light housework and negotiating one flight of stairs.[93] The average FM patient in this sample was assessed as having less functional ability than a typical woman in her 80s. In general, reduced function was associated with higher levels of pain, fatigue, depression, balance problems, irritable bladder, restless legs, and muscle spasms. FM patients' reports of reduced functioning have been correlated to reduced activity on electronic ambulatory monitoring.[94] There is some evidence that depression plays a role in reduced daytime activity.[95] Problems with physical function and cognitive defects may result in difficulties in sustained employment.[96,97]

SEXUALITY

It is not surprising that chronic pain and fatigue have an adverse effect on sexuality. This is an area of clinical manifestations that has only recently been explored.[98] Orellana and colleagues[99] gave the Changes in Sexual Functioning Questionnaire to 31 FM subjects along with 20 healthy controls and 26 subjects who had RA. Sexual dysfunction was more frequent among FM subjects (97%) and RA subjects (84%) compared with controls. There was a major correlation of sexual dysfunction with intensity of depression. A similar association with depression was reported by Aydin and colleagues.[100] On the other hand, a study using the Female Sexual Function Index compared sexual dysfunction in 40 subjects who had FM only, 27 who had FM plus major depression, and 33 healthy controls found no association with depression.[101] One prevalence study of vulvodynia reported that FM subjects have an increased odds ratio of 3.84 for having this problem.[102] Pelvic pain syndrome is also common according to one study;[103] its relationship to endometriosis in FM subjects needs further investigation.

HEADACHES

Headaches were prominently ranked in the NFA and DFV surveys, but not in the OMERACT Delphi (see **Table 1**). The prevalence of International Headache Society diagnoses in one study of FM subjects was: migraine without aura. 20%; migraine with aura, 23%; tension alone, 24%; combined tension and migraine, 22%; posttraumatic, 5%; and probable analgesic overuse syndrome, 8% alone ($n = 15$ with aura, $n = 17$ without aura); tension-type alone ($n = 18$); combined migraine and tension-type ($n = 16$); posttraumatic ($n = 4$); and probable analgesic overuse headache ($n = 6$).[104] It was reported that FM/migraine subjects have more disabling headaches and have higher cerebrospinal fluid glutamate levels than migraine alone.[105] Other investigators have also opined that migraine, daily chronic headache, and fibromyalgia are an expression of abnormal pain processing.[106] Questions regarding headache should be part of the comprehensive evaluation of all FM patients.

PSYCHOLOGICAL DISTRESS

Self-reported depression is a common symptom in FM patients (see **Table 1**). As FM was once considered to be a psychiatric diagnosis, there have been numerous studies evaluating the psychological profiles of FM subjects. For instance, early studies noted elevations of certain scales on the Minnesota Multiphasic Personality Inventory (MMPI), especially the hypochondriasis, hysteria, and depression scales.[107] Smythe[108] noted that any patient who had chronic pain would give positive answers on the MMPI to questions relating to pain and somatic symptoms, and concluded that there was a 40% bias of labeling such a patient as being neurotic. There is a general consensus that depression, anxiety disorders, and PTSD are common in FM patients.[109] Arnold and colleagues[110] reported that the odds ratios for psychiatric diagnoses in individuals who have fibromyalgia versus individuals who have RA are: bipolar disorder, 153; major depressive disorder, 2.7; any anxiety disorder, 6.7; any eating disorder, 2.4; and any substance use disorder, 3.3. Contrary to popular misconceptions, personality disorders are not especially common in the FM population. Thieme and colleagues[111] found a prevalence of 8.7% and Fietta and associates[112] found a prevalence of 7%. The coexistence of anxiety and depression with FM generally has a negative influence on the expression of FM symptoms and functionality, but this association can be quite variable.[113]

ASSOCIATED DISORDERS

In addition to the numerous clinical manifestations of FM described here, many FM patients have an associated clinical syndrome such as irritable bowel, overactive bladder, restless legs, multiple chemical sensitivity, chronic fatigue syndrome, vulvodynia, and so forth. The association of these disorders with FM and between themselves is now considered to be a manifestation of widespread central sensitization and are increasingly being referred to as "central sensitivity syndromes."[73] (See the article by Dr. Clauw elsewhere in this issue for further exploration of these associated syndromes.)

DIAGNOSIS OF FIBROMYALGIA

The diagnosis of FM is usually based on the ACR's classification criteria.[3] This is certainly true for the entry of FM subjects into scientific research protocols. Although these criteria were intended for purposes of epidemiologic classification, the discussion section of the 1990 criteria paper noted that "the sensitivity of the criteria suggests that they may be useful for diagnosis as well as classification."

These exact criteria are seldom used in the primary care setting, however, and are only used by about 50% of rheumatologists in their routine practice. The problem lies in performing the ACR-designated tender point evaluation, which requires training and experience that is lacking in most primary care settings and probably underestimates a diagnosis of FM in males.[114] Thus, the question has arisen as to whether an office-based clinical diagnosis of FM can be made more simply.

Using a History of Widespread Pain as a Diagnostic Criterion

There are many epidemiologic studies of WSP reporting that most of the surveyed subjects have ACR-defined FM.[115] Subjects who have WSP and FM are generally more symptomatic, dysfunctional, and depressed than those who have WSP without FM.[116,117] On the other hand, there are several studies indicating that the finding of widespread allodynia is predictive of WSP.[118,119] In general, there is a relationship between the number of tender points and changes in nociceptive processing in subjects who have WSP not fulfilling a diagnosis of FM.[50,120] This has given rise to the concept that ACR-defined FM is at one end of a continuous spectrum of pain complaints.[121]

Any new office-friendly definition of FM probably ought to be based on more than a history of WSP. A Swedish epidemiologic study of 9952 subjects found WSP without widespread allodynia in 4.5% of the population and ACR-defined FM in 2.5%.[116] However, 50% of subjects who had WSP without FM had other diagnoses, such as inflammatory rheumatic disorders, stroke, whiplash-associated disorders, diabetic neuropathy, myopathy, herniated discs, and osteoarthritis. Conditions that may masquerade as WSP are given in **Box 1**.

As with any patient, the evaluation of a patient who has WSP must always consider the differential diagnosis, but the finding of another disorder or investigational abnormality does not necessarily rule out a diagnosis of FM. Indeed, it is very common for FM patients to have associated disorders such as rheumatoid arthritis, SLE, and other pain-related states. Considering these factors, diagnosing FM solely on the basis of WSP, though being valid in the majority of cases and a useful surrogate in epidemiologic studies, will lead to diagnostic errors that are unacceptable in the clinical setting.

Using a Combination of Symptoms as Diagnostic Criteria

FM patients have so many symptoms that, for years, many physicians were skeptical of FM as a distinct clinical disorder.[122] However, it is now generally accepted that widespread central sensitization generates a wide array of symptoms.[123–125] Unless a patient has another central sensitization syndrome, the wide range of seemingly unrelated FM symptoms could be useful in diagnosis, especially if combined with the history of WSP. In fact, such combinations were proposed by Yunus and colleagues[2] in the 1980s and tested in the 1990 ACR criteria study.[3] The 1990 ACR

Box 1
A list of disorders that need to be considered in the differential diagnosis of widespread pain

Disorder

Polymyalgia rheumatica

Viral infections

Early stages of RA and SLE

Sjogren's syndrome

Polyarticular osteoarthritis

Early stages of a spondyloarthropathy

Severe vitamin D deficiency

Hypothyroidism

Statin therapy

Inflammatory myopathies

Metabolic myopathies

Joint hypermobility syndromes

Metastatic malignancies

Myotonic dystrophy type 2

---

criteria had a sensitivity of 88%, specificity of 81%, and accuracy of 85%, whereas the combination of WSP sine tender points and five or more of Yunus's minor criteria (fatigue, aggravation of symptoms by physical activity, modulation of symptoms by weather changes, anxiety, chronic headaches, irritable bowel symptoms, subjective swelling, and numbness) had a sensitivity of 77%, a specificity of 76%, and an accuracy of 77%. Reducing the number of symptoms to just three (sleep disturbance, fatigue, and morning stiffness), resulted in a sensitivity of 81%, a specificity of 61%, and an accuracy of 72%. Hauser and colleagues[126] suggested that a symptom-based diagnosis of FM without tender point examination is helpful for primary medical care, after exclusion of inflammatory rheumatoid, endocrinological, and neurologic diseases. From a cluster analysis of common symptoms in 533 German FM subjects compared with a representative population sample, the symptoms of limb pain and chronic fatigue were the most discriminatory symptoms. The authors concluded that "the survey method has the advantage that it does not require physical examination." In a similar vein, Katz and colleagues[127] have evaluated a combination of a fatigue VAS (0–10) and the regional pain score (0–19) as a possible simplified method for arriving at a diagnosis of FM. They evaluated 120 subjects with a clinical diagnosis of FM (clinician's impression irrespective of ACR criteria) and found that clinical and survey criteria were concordant in 74.8% of cases, clinical criteria and ACR criteria were concordant in 75.2% of cases, and survey criteria and ACR criteria were concordant in 72.3% of cases.

Using Tenderness as Diagnostic Criterion

The ACR criteria use the combination of WSP and 11 or more out of 18 tender points, but the question arises as to whether it is possible to replace the ACR-defined tender point examination with a more simple test of widespread allodynia.[128] There is now ample evidence that the 18 ACR tender points are not "special," because FM subjects

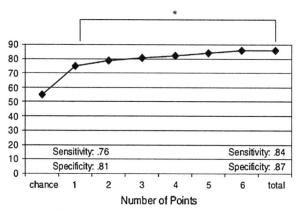

Fig. 1. The worse-case classification accuracy (y-axis) for a diagnosis of fibromyalgia as a function of the number of tender points used (x-axis). * P < .05 greater than chance prediction. *From* Harden RN, Revivo G, Song S, et al. A critical analysis of the tender points in fibromyalgia. Pain Med 2007;8(2):147–56; with permission.

have been shown to have widespread sensitivity to a number of neurophysiologic tests.[129,130] In general, subjective reporting of tenderness to palpation has correlated with abnormal neurophysiological testing, but there is a variable component of psychological distress that colors the reporting of tenderness to palpation.[131,132] A more limited evaluation of tenderness would probably suffice in the diagnosis of FM. For instance, Harden and colleagues[119] found that, whereas an algometer-based scoring of ACR tender points differentiated FM from normals with 85.7% accuracy, a single point had an accuracy of between 75% and 89%. Furthermore, it was reported that tenderness at three "sham" points (the glabella, the middle of the biceps, and the middle of the hamstring) differentiated FM from normals with 85.7% classification accuracy. Using hierarchical cluster analysis, it was found that three points provided the same classification accuracy as all 18 points (**Fig. 1**). Vargas reported that 69% of FM subjects had sphygmomanometry-evoked allodynia in contrast to 10% of subjects who had osteoarthritis, 5% who had rheumatoid arthritis, and 2% of healthy subjects. The mean systolic blood pressure value for allodynia in FM was 143+/−40 mm Hg, whereas in the three other groups it was 176+/−11 mm Hg.[133] Petzke and colleagues[134] compared the diagnostic utility of dolorimetry-based pain thresholds at all 18 ACR tender points with a limited number of tender points. It was found that pain thresholds at two sets of three paired tender points (supraspinatus, epicondyle, occiput; and thumbnail, midtrapezius, epicondyle), had a diagnostic accuracy similar to all 18 tender points. Thus, it appears that a more simplified methodology for determining if a patient has widespread allodynia could be developed.

SUMMARY

Since the publication of the 1990 ACR Classification Criteria for Fibromyalgia, there has been an impressive advancement in our understanding of FM symptoms and their psychoneurologic underpinnings in terms of central sensitization and genetic influences. However, the roles of peripheral pain states, sleep disorders, psychopathology, and cytokines in initiating and perpetuating disordered sensory processing are less clear. There is now a general agreement that FM is a common disorder that causes much distress and dysfunction, but there is a need for a simplified office-based diagnostic evaluation. In this author's opinion, a combination of a few key symptoms along with a simplified assessment of widespread allodynia, such as sphygmoma-nometer-induced tenderness, would be a reasonable point to start.

REFERENCES

1. Smythe HA, Moldofsky H. Two contributions to understanding of the "fibrositis" syndrome. Bull Rheum Dis 1977;28:928–31.
2. Yunus M, Masi AT, Calabro JJ, et al. Primary fibromyalgia (fibrositis): clinical study of 50 patients with matched normal controls. Semin Arthritis Rheum 1981;11:151–71.
3. Wolfe F, Smythe HA, Yunus MB, et al. The American College of Rheumatology 1990 criteria for the classification of fibromyalgia: report of the Multicenter Criteria Committee. Arthritis Rheum 1990;33(2):160–72.
4. Bennett RM, Jones J, Turk DC, et al. An internet survey of 2,596 people with fibromyalgia. BMC Musculoskelet Disord 2007;8:27.
5. Hauser W, Zimmer C, Felde E, et al. What are the key symptoms of fibromyalgia? Results of a survey of the German Fibromyalgia Association. Schmerz 2008; 22(2):176–83.
6. Mease PJ, Arnold LM, Crofford LJ, et al. Identifying the clinical domains of fibro-myalgia: contributions from clinician and patient delphi exercises. Arthritis Rheum 2008;59(7):952–60.
7. Martinez-Lavin M, Lopez S, Medina M, et al. Use of the leeds assessment of neuropathic symptoms and signs questionnaire in patients with fibromyalgia. Semin Arthritis Rheum 2003;32(6):407–11.
8. Reilly PA, Littlejohn GO. Peripheral arthralgic presentation of fibrositis/fibromyal-gia syndrome. J Rheumatol 1992;19:281–3.
9. Staud R, Vierck CJ, Robinson ME, et al. Overall fibromyalgia pain is predicted by ratings of local pain and pain-related negative affect–possible role of peripheral tissues. Rheumatology (Oxford) 2006;45(11):1409–15.
10. Moldofsky H. Chronobiological influences on fibromyalgia syndrome: theoretical and therapeutic implications. Baillieres Clin Rheumatol 1994;8:801–10.
11. Marchand S. The physiology of pain mechanisms: from the periphery to the brain. Rheum Dis Clin North Am 2008;34(2):285–309.
12. Kroenke K, Price RK. Symptoms in the community. Prevalence, classification, and psychiatric comorbidity. Arch Intern Med 1993;153(21):2474–80.
13. Beard GM. Neurasthenia, or nervous exhaustion. Boston Med Surg J 1869;80: 217–21.
14. Kroenke K, Wood DR, Mangelsdorff D, et al. Chronic fatigue in primary care: prevalence, patient characteristics, and outcome. JAMA 1988;260:929–34.
15. Wessely S. Chronic fatigue: symptom and syndrome. Ann Intern Med 2001; 134(9 Pt 2):838–43.
16. Arnold LM. Understanding fatigue in major depressive disorder and other medical disorders. Psychosomatics 2008;49(3):185–90.
17. Arnold LM. Duloxetine and other antidepressants in the treatment of patients with fibromyalgia. Pain Med 2007;8(2):S63–74.
18. Mease PJ, Russell IJ, Arnold LM, et al. A randomized, double-blind, placebo-controlled, phase III trial of pregabalin in the treatment of patients with fibromyal-gia. J Rheumatol 2008;35(3):502–14.

19. Crofford LJ, Rowbotham MC, Mease PJ, et al. Pregabalin for the treatment of fibromyalgia syndrome: results of a randomized, double-blind, placebo-controlled trial. Arthritis Rheum 2005;52(4):1264–73.
20. Russell IJ, Perkins AT, Michalek JE. Sodium oxybate relieves pain and improves function in fibromyalgia syndrome: a randomized, double-blind, placebo-controlled, multicenter clinical trial. Arthritis Rheum 2009;60(1):299–309.
21. Fishbain DA, Lewis J, Cole B, et al. Multidisciplinary pain facility treatment outcome for pain-associated fatigue. Pain Med 2005;6(4):299–304.
22. Maier SF, Watkins LR. Cytokines for psychologists: implications of bidirectional immune-to- brain communication for understanding behavior, mood, and cognition. Psychol Rev 1998;105(1):83–107.
23. Burckhardt CS, Clark SR, Bennett RM. The fibromyalgia impact questionnaire: development and validation. J Rheumatol 1991;18:728–33.
24. Bennett R. The Fibromyalgia Impact Questionnaire (FIQ): a review of its development, current version, operating characteristics and uses. Clin Exp Rheumatol 2005;23(5 Suppl 39):S154–62.
25. Wolfarth S, Lorenc-Koci E, Schulze G, et al. Age-related muscle stiffness: predominance of non-reflex factors. Neuroscience 1997;79(2):617–28.
26. Lakie M, Robson LG. Thixotropy: stiffness recovery rate in relaxed frog muscle. Q J Exp Physiol 1988;73(2):237–9.
27. McHugh MP, Connolly DA, Eston RG, et al. The role of passive muscle stiffness in symptoms of exercise-induced muscle damage. Am J Sports Med 1999; 27(5):594–9.
28. Jones KD, Clark SR. Individualizing the exercise prescription for persons with fibromyalgia. Rheum Dis Clin North Am 2002;28(2):419–36.
29. Deepak S, Harikrishnan, Jayakumar B. Hypothyroidism presenting as Hoffman's syndrome. J Indian Med Assoc 2004;102(1):41–2.
30. de Lau LM, Koudstaal PJ, Hofman A, et al. Subjective complaints precede Parkinson disease: the rotterdam study. Arch Neurol 2006;63(3):362–5.
31. Moldofsky H. The significance of the sleeping-waking brain for the understanding of widespread musculoskeletal pain and fatigue in fibromyalgia syndrome and allied syndromes. Joint Bone Spine 2008;75(4):397–402.
32. Harding SM. Sleep in fibromyalgia patients: subjective and objective findings. Am J Med Sci 1998;315(6):367–76.
33. Ohayon MM. Prevalence and correlates of nonrestorative sleep complaints. Arch Intern Med 2005;165(1):35–41.
34. Moldofsky H. The significance, assessment, and management of nonrestorative sleep in fibromyalgia syndrome. CNS Spectr 2008;13(3 Suppl 5):22–6.
35. Stone KC, Taylor DJ, McCrae CS, et al. Nonrestorative sleep. Sleep Med Rev 2008;12(4):275–88.
36. Hauri P, Hawkins DR. Alpha-delta sleep. Electroencephalogr Clin Neurophysiol 1973;34:233–7.
37. Moldofsky H, Scarisbrick P, England R, et al. Musculosketal symptoms and non-REM sleep disturbance in patients with "fibrositis syndrome" and healthy subjects. Psychosom Med 1975;37:341–51.
38. Mahowald ML, Mahowald MW. Nighttime sleep and daytime functioning (sleepiness and fatigue) in less well-defined chronic rheumatic diseases with particular reference to the 'alpha-delta NREM sleep anomaly'. Sleep Med 2000;1(3): 195–207.
39. Rizzi M, Sarzi-Puttini P, Atzeni F, et al. Cyclic alternating pattern: a new marker of sleep alteration in patients with fibromyalgia? J Rheumatol 2004;31(6):1193–9.

40. Roizenblatt S, Moldofsky H, Benedito-Silva AA, et al. Alpha sleep characteristics in fibromyalgia. Arthritis Rheum 2001;44(1):222–30.
41. Landis CA, Lentz MJ, Rothermel J, et al. Decreased sleep spindles and spindle activity in midlife women with fibromyalgia and pain. Sleep 2004;27(4):741–50.
42. Mahowald MW. Restless leg syndrome and periodic limb movements of sleep. Curr Treat Options Neurol 2003;5(3):251–60.
43. Stehlik R, Arvidsson L, Ulfberg J. Restless legs syndrome is common among female patients with fibromyalgia. Eur Neurol 2008;61(2):107–11.
44. Allen RP, Earley CJ. Restless legs syndrome: a review of clinical and pathophysiologic features. J Clin Neurophysiol 2001;18(2):128–47.
45. Allen RP, Barker PB, Wehrl F, et al. MRI measurement of brain iron in patients with restless legs syndrome. Neurology 2001;56(2):263–5.
46. Connor JR, Boyer PJ, Menzies SL, et al. Neuropathological examination suggests impaired brain iron acquisition in restless legs syndrome. Neurology 2003;61(3):304–9.
47. Germanowicz D, Lumertz MS, Martinez D, et al. Sleep disordered breathing concomitant with fibromyalgia syndrome. J Bras Pneumol 2006;32(4):333–8.
48. Bao G, Guilleminault C. Upper airway resistance syndrome—one decade later. Curr Opin Pulm Med 2004;10(6):461–7.
49. Gold AR, Dipalo F, Gold MS, et al. Inspiratory airflow dynamics during sleep in women with fibromyalgia. Sleep 2004;27(3):459–66.
50. Carli G, Suman AL, Biasi G, et al. Reactivity to superficial and deep stimuli in patients with chronic musculoskeletal pain. Pain 2002;100(3):259–69.
51. Sann H, Pierau FK. Efferent functions of C-fiber nociceptors. Z Rheumatol 1998; 57(2):8–13.
52. Littlejohn GO, Weinstein C, Helme RD. Increased neurogenic inflammation in fibrositis syndrome. J Rheumatol 1987;14:1022–5.
53. Salemi S, Rethage J, Wollina U, et al. Detection of interleukin 1beta (IL-1beta), IL-6, and tumor necrosis factor-alpha in skin of patients with fibromyalgia. J Rheumatol 2003;30(1):146–50.
54. Enestrom S, Bengtsson A, Frodin T. Dermal IgG deposits and increase of mast cells in patients with fibromyalgia—relevant findings or epiphenomena? Scand J Rheumatol 1997;26(4):308–13.
55. Lentz MJ, Landis CA, Rothermel J, et al. Effects of selective slow wave sleep disruption on musculoskeletal pain and fatigue in middle aged women. J Rheumatol 1999;26(7):1586–92.
56. Bennett R. Fibromyalgia: present to future. Curr Rheumatol Rep 2005;7(5):371–6.
57. Glass JM. Fibromyalgia and cognition. J Clin Psychiatry 2008;69(2):20–4.
58. Park DC, Glass JM, Minear M, et al. Cognitive function in fibromyalgia patients. Arthritis Rheum 2001;44(9):2125–33.
59. Leavitt F, Katz RS. Distraction as a key determinant of impaired memory in patients with fibromyalgia. J Rheumatol 2006;33(1):127–32.
60. Suhr JA. Neuropsychological impairment in fibromyalgia. Relation to depression, fatigue, and pain. J Psychosom Res 2003;55(4):321–9.
61. Grisart J, Van der LM, Masquelier E. Controlled processes and automaticity in memory functioning in fibromyalgia patients: relation with emotional distress and hypervigilance. J Clin Exp Neuropsychol 2002;24(8):994–1009.
62. Walitt B, Roebuck-Spencer T, Bleiberg J, et al. Automated neuropsychiatric measurements of information processing in fibromyalgia. Rheumatol Int 2008; 28(6):561–6.

63. Emad Y, Ragab Y, Zeinhom F, et al. Hippocampus dysfunction may explain symptoms of fibromyalgia syndrome. A study with single-voxel magnetic resonance spectroscopy. J Rheumatol 2008;35(7):1371–7.
64. Parkin AJ. Human memory: the hippocampus is the key. Curr Biol 1996;6(12): 1583–5.
65. Tischler L, Brand SR, Stavitsky K, et al. The relationship between hippocampal volume and declarative memory in a population of combat veterans with and without PTSD. Ann N Y Acad Sci 2006;1071:405–9, 405–409.
66. Kim JJ, Diamond DM. The stressed hippocampus, synaptic plasticity and lost memories. Nat Rev Neurosci 2002;3(6):453–62.
67. McEwen BS. Plasticity of the hippocampus: adaptation to chronic stress and allostatic load. Ann N Y Acad Sci 2001;933:265–77.
68. Lutz J, Jager L, de QD, et al. White and gray matter abnormalities in the brain of patients with fibromyalgia: a diffusion-tensor and volumetric imaging study. Arthritis Rheum 2008;58(12):3960–9.
69. Luerding R, Weigand T, Bogdahn U, et al. Working memory performance is correlated with local brain morphology in the medial frontal and anterior cingulate cortex in fibromyalgia patients: structural correlates of pain-cognition interaction. Brain 2008;131(Pt 12):3222–31.
70. Simms RW, Goldenberg DL. Symptoms mimicking neurologic disorders in fibromyalgia syndrome. J Rheumatol 1988;15:1271–3.
71. Martinez-Lavin M. Fibromyalgia as a sympathetically maintained pain syndrome. Curr Pain Headache Rep 2004;8(5):385–9.
72. McCabe CS, Cohen H, Blake DR. Somaesthetic disturbances in fibromyalgia are exaggerated by sensory motor conflict: implications for chronicity of the disease? Rheumatology (Oxford) 2007;46(10):1587–92.
73. Yunus MB. Central sensitivity syndromes: a new paradigm and group nosology for fibromyalgia and overlapping conditions, and the related issue of disease versus illness. Semin Arthritis Rheum 2008;37(6):339–52.
74. Jones KD, Horak FB, Winters-Stone K, et al. Fibromyalgia is associated with impaired balance and falls. J Clin Rheumatol 2009;15(1):16–21.
75. Vaeroy H, Helle R, Forre O, et al. Elevated CSF levels of substance P and high incidence of Raynaud phenomenon in patients with fibromyalgia: new features for diagnosis. Pain 1988;32:21–6.
76. Dinerman H, Goldenberg DL, Felson DT. A prospective evaluation of 118 patients with the fibromyalgia syndrome: prevalence of Raynaud's phenomenon, sicca symptoms, ANA, low complement, and Ig deposition at the dermal-epidermal junction. J Rheumatol 1986;13:368–73.
77. Yunus MB, Hussey FX, Aldag JC. Antinuclear antibodies and connective disease features in fibromyalgia syndrome: a controlled study. J Rheumatol 1993;20:1557–60.
78. Frodin T, Bengtsson A, Skogh M. Nail fold capillaroscopy findings in patients with primary fibromyalgia. Clin Rheumatol 1988;73:84–8.
79. Bennett RM, Clark SR, Campbell SM, et al. Symptoms of Raynaud's syndrome in patients with fibromyalgia. A study utilizing the Nielsen test, digital photoplethysmography, and measurements of platelet alpha 2-adrenergic receptors. Arthritis Rheum 1991;34:264–9.
80. Hurtig IM, Raak RI, Kendall SA, et al. Quantitative sensory testing in fibromyalgia patients and in healthy subjects: identification of subgroups. Clin J Pain 2001; 17(4):316–22.

81. Berglund B, Harju EL, Kosek E, et al. Quantitative and qualitative perceptual analysis of cold dysesthesia and hyperalgesia in fibromyalgia. Pain 2002; 96(1–2):177–87.

82. Elvin A, Siosteen AK, Nilsson A, et al. Decreased muscle blood flow in fibromyalgia patients during standardised muscle exercise: a contrast media enhanced colour Doppler study. Eur J Pain 2006;10(2):137–44.

83. Katz DL, Greene L, Ali A, et al. The pain of fibromyalgia syndrome is due to muscle hypoperfusion induced by regional vasomotor dysregulation. Med Hypotheses 2007;69(3):517–25.

84. Gunaydin I, Terhorst T, Eckstein A, et al. Assessment of keratoconjunctivitis sicca in patients with fibromyalgia: results of a prospective study. Rheumatol Int 1999;19(1–2):7–9.

85. Keene JJ Jr, Galasko GT, Land MF. Antidepressant use in psychiatry and medicine: importance for dental practice. J Am Dent Assoc 2003;134(1):71–9.

86. Ramos-Casals M, Munoz S, Zeron PB. Hepatitis C virus and Sjogren's syndrome: trigger or mimic? Rheum Dis Clin North Am 2008;34(4):869–84, vii.

87. Klein CM, Vernino S, Lennon VA, et al. The spectrum of autoimmune autonomic neuropathies. Ann Neurol 2003;53(6):752–8.

88. Ostuni P, Botsios C, Sfriso P, et al. Fibromyalgia in Italian patients with primary Sjogren's syndrome. Joint Bone Spine 2002;69(1):51–7.

89. Price EJ, Venables PJ. Dry eyes and mouth syndrome–a subgroup of patients presenting with sicca symptoms. Rheumatology (Oxford) 2002; 41(4):416–22.

90. Bonafede RP, Downey DC, Bennett RM. An association of fibromyalgia with primary Sjogren's syndrome: a prospective study of 72 patients. J Rheumatol 1995;22:133–6.

91. Rhodus NL, Fricton J, Carlson P, et al. Oral symptoms associated with fibromyalgia syndrome. J Rheumatol 2003;30(8):1841–5.

92. Bennett RM, Kamin M, Karim R, et al. Tramadol and acetaminophen combination tablets in the treatment of fibromyalgia pain: a double-blind, randomized, placebo-controlled study. Am J Med 2003;114(7):537–45.

93. Jones J, Rutledge DN, Jones KD, et al. Self-assessed physical function levels of women with fibromyalgia: a national survey. Womens Health Issues 2008;18(5): 406–12.

94. Kop WJ, Lyden A, Berlin AA, et al. Ambulatory monitoring of physical activity and symptoms in fibromyalgia and chronic fatigue syndrome. Arthritis Rheum 2005; 52(1):296–303.

95. Korszun A, Young EA, Engleberg NC, et al. Use of actigraphy for monitoring sleep and activity levels in patients with fibromyalgia and depression. J Psychosom Res 2002;52(6):439–43.

96. Gerdle B, Bjork J, Coster L, et al. Prevalence of widespread pain and associations with work status: a population study. BMC Musculoskelet Disord 2008;9: 102.

97. White LA, Birnbaum HG, Kaltenboeck A, et al. Employees with fibromyalgia: medical comorbidity, healthcare costs, and work loss. J Occup Environ Med 2008;50(1):13–24.

98. Ryan S, Hill J, Thwaites C, et al. Assessing the effect of fibromyalgia on patients' sexual activity. Nurs Stand 2008;23(2):35–41.

99. Orellana C, Casado E, Masip M, et al. Sexual dysfunction in fibromyalgia patients. Clin Exp Rheumatol 2008;26(4):663–6.

100. Aydin G, Basar MM, Keles I, et al. Relationship between sexual dysfunction and psychiatric status in premenopausal women with fibromyalgia. Urology 2006; 67(1):156–61.
101. Tikiz C, Muezzinoglu T, Pirildar T, et al. Sexual dysfunction in female subjects with fibromyalgia. J Urol 2005;174(2):620–3.
102. Arnold LD, Bachmann GA, Rosen R, et al. Vulvodynia: characteristics and associations with comorbidities and quality of life. Obstet Gynecol 2006;107(3): 617–24.
103. Hughes L. Physical and psychological variables that influence pain in patients with fibromyalgia. Orthop Nurs 2006;25(2):112–9.
104. Marcus DA, Bernstein C, Rudy TE. Fibromyalgia and headache: an epidemiological study supporting migraine as part of the fibromyalgia syndrome. Clin Rheumatol 2005;24(6):595–601.
105. Peres MF, Zukerman E, Senne Soares CA, et al. Cerebrospinal fluid glutamate levels in chronic migraine. Cephalalgia 2004;24(9):735–9.
106. Centonze V, Bassi A, Cassiano MA, et al. Migraine, daily chronic headache and fibromyalgia in the same patient: an evolutive "continuum" of non organic chronic pain? About 100 clinical cases. Neurol Sci 2004;25(3):S291–2.
107. Ahles TA, Yunus MB, Gaulier B, et al. The use of contemporary MMPI norms in the study of chronic pain patients. Pain 1986;24:159–63.
108. Smythe HA. Problems with the MMPI. J Rheumatol 1984;11:417–8.
109. Buskila D, Cohen H. Comorbidity of fibromyalgia and psychiatric disorders. Curr Pain Headache Rep 2007;11(5):333–8.
110. Arnold LM, Hudson JI, Keck PE, et al. Comorbidity of fibromyalgia and psychiatric disorders. J Clin Psychiatry 2006;67(8):1219–25.
111. Thieme K, Turk DC, Flor H. Comorbid depression and anxiety in fibromyalgia syndrome: relationship to somatic and psychosocial variables. Psychosom Med 2004;66(6):837–44.
112. Fietta P, Fietta P, Manganelli P. Fibromyalgia and psychiatric disorders. Acta Biomed 2007;78(2):88–95.
113. Giesecke T, Williams DA, Harris RE, et al. Subgrouping of fibromyalgia patients on the basis of pressure-pain thresholds and psychological factors. Arthritis Rheum 2003;48(10):2916–22.
114. Chesterton LS, Barlas P, Foster NE, et al. Gender differences in pressure pain threshold in healthy humans. Pain 2003;101(3):259–66.
115. Rohrbeck J, Jordan K, Croft P. The frequency and characteristics of chronic widespread pain in general practice: a case-control study. Br J Gen Pract 2007;57(535):109–15.
116. Coster L, Kendall S, Gerdle B, et al. Chronic widespread musculoskeletal pain - a comparison of those who meet criteria for fibromyalgia and those who do not. Eur J Pain 2008;12(5):600–10.
117. Pamuk ON, Yethornil AY, Cakir N. Factors that affect the number of tender points in fibromyalgia and chronic widespread pain patients who did not meet the ACR 1990 criteria for fibromyalgia: are tender points a reflection of neuropathic pain? Semin Arthritis Rheum 2006;36(2):130–4.
118. Gupta A, McBeth J, MacFarlane GJ, et al. Pressure pain thresholds and tender point counts as predictors of new chronic widespread pain in somatising subjects. Ann Rheum Dis 2007;66(4):517–21.
119. Harden RN, Revivo G, Song S, et al. A critical analysis of the tender points in fibromyalgia. Pain Med 2007;8(2):147–56.

120. Laursen BS, Bajaj P, Olesen AS, et al. Health related quality of life and quantitative pain measurement in females with chronic non-malignant pain. Eur J Pain 2005;9(3):267–75.
121. Croft P, Burt J, Schollum J, et al. More pain, more tender points: is fibromyalgia just one end of a continuous spectrum? Ann Rheum Dis 1996;55:482–5.
122. Hadler NM. A critical reappraisal of the fibrositis concept. Am J Med 1986;81: 26–30.
123. Bennett RM. Emerging concepts in the neurobiology of chronic pain: evidence of abnormal sensory processing in fibromyalgia. Mayo Clin Proc 1999;74(4): 385–98.
124. Yunus MB. Fibromyalgia and overlapping disorders: the unifying concept of central sensitivity syndromes. Semin Arthritis Rheum 2007;36(6):339–56.
125. Clauw DJ. Elusive syndromes: treating the biologic basis of fibromyalgia and related syndromes. Cleve Clin J Med 2001;68(10):830, 832–830, 834.
126. Hauser W, Akritidou I, Felde E, et al. Steps towards a symptom-based diagnosis of fibromyalgia syndrome. Symptom profiles of patients from different clinical settings. Z Rheumatol 2008;67(6):511–5.
127. Katz RS, Wolfe F, Michaud K. Fibromyalgia diagnosis: a comparison of clinical, survey, and American College of Rheumatology criteria. Arthritis Rheum 2006; 54(1):169–76.
128. Harth M, Nielson WR. The fibromyalgia tender points: use them or lose them? A brief review of the controversy. J Rheumatol 2007;34(5):914–22.
129. Price DD, Staud R. Neurobiology of fibromyalgia syndrome. J Rheumatol Suppl 2005;75:22–8.
130. Dadabhoy D, Crofford LJ, Spaeth M, et al. Biology and therapy of fibromyalgia. Evidence-based biomarkers for fibromyalgia syndrome. Arthritis Res Ther 2008; 10(4):211.
131. Croft P, Schollum J, Silman A. Population study of tender point counts and pain as evidence of fibromyalgia. BMJ 1994;309(6956):696–9.
132. Gracely RH. A pain psychologist's view of tenderness in fibromyalgia. J Rheumatol 2007;34(5):912–3.
133. Vargas A, Vargas A, Hernandez-Paz R, et al. Sphygmomanometry-evoked allodynia—a simple bedside test indicative of fibromyalgia: a multicenter developmental study. J Clin Rheumatol 2006;12(6):272–4.
134. Petzke F, Khine A, Williams D, et al. Dolorimetry performed at 3 paired tender points highly predicts overall tenderness. J Rheumatol 2001;28(11):2568–9.

From Fibrositis to Functional Somatic Syndromes to a Bell-Shaped Curve of Pain and Sensory Sensitivity: Evolution of a Clinical Construct

Kobby Ablin, MD[a], Daniel J. Clauw, MD[b],*

KEYWORDS

• Pain • Fibromyalgia • Somatic • Functional • Fatigue

In his classical 1972 article entitled "More is Different," Anderson attempted to demonstrate some of the limitations of reductionist thinking in science.[1] Anderson argued that although reductionism can legitimately organize scientific disciplines into a hierarchical order (eg, particle physics, many body physics, chemistry, molecular biology, cellular biology, physiology, psychology and social sciences), "this does not imply that one science is just an applied version of the science that precedes it.... At each stage, entirely new laws, concepts and generalizations are necessary, requiring inspiration and creativity to just as great a degree as in the previous one."

This article attempts to demonstrate how this insight may be applied to understanding of the evolving spectrum of the functional somatic syndromes. It will become evident that in understanding these highly complex disorders, neither the Cartesian dichotomy regarding body-mind distinction nor the pure reductionist approach to disease (which attempts to explain clinical phenomena on the basis of underlying structural derangement) can be strictly adhered to. Only use of a truly integrative framework of thinking (one might hazard using the term *holistic* had it not been over-exploited to the verge of a cliché) can allow us to both recognize and accept the overlapping basic similarity between these conditions and, in turn, teach us about nearly any medical condition characterized by pain or sensory symptoms.

[a] Institute of Rheumatology, Tel Aviv Medical Center, Tel Aviv, Israel
[b] Division of Rheumatology, Department of Medicine, University of Michigan, 24 Frank Lloyd Wright Drive, PO Box 385, Ann Arbor, MI 48105, USA
* Corresponding author.
E-mail address: dclauw@umich.edu (D.J. Clauw).

Rheum Dis Clin N Am 35 (2009) 233–251
doi:10.1016/j.rdc.2009.06.006
0889-857X/09/$ – see front matter © 2009 Elsevier Inc. All rights reserved.

THE BEGINNING OF FIBROMYALGIA

Although there are clear descriptions of individuals with what we now call fibromyalgia dating back centuries in the medical literature, we begin this treatise at around the turn of the twentieth century. While describing the attributes of lumbago pain, Sir William Gowers coined the term "fibrositis," which was considered a form of muscular rheumatism caused by inflammation of fibrous tissue overlying muscles.[2]

Although other terms such as "psychogenic rheumatism" were proposed and used in the mid-twentieth century, the term fibrositis remained the most widely used term to describe individuals with chronic widespread pain and no alternative explanation. Several investigators began to suggest that this term was a misnomer because there was not inflammation of the muscles. Moldofsky[3–6] performed seminal studies showing that individuals with fibrositis sustained objective sleep disturbances and showed that these same symptoms could be induced in healthy individuals deprived of sleep. Hudson and colleagues[7,8] were arguably the first to note the strong familial tendency to develop fibromyalgia and proposed that this was a variant of depression, coining the term "affective spectrum disorder." In parallel during this same period of time, Yunus and colleagues[9] similarly began to note the high frequency of associated functional somatic syndromes such as irritable bowel syndrome and headache with fibromyalgia, again steering the focus away from skeletal muscle. Nonetheless, the theories regarding skeletal muscle having a pathophysiologic role took some time to fade, persisting into the mid-1990s.[10–12]

Just as spastic colitis became irritable bowel syndrome, temporomandibular joint syndrome became temporomandibular disorder (when it was recognized that the problem was not in the joint), chronic Epstein-Barr virus syndrome became chronic fatigue syndrome (when it was realized that this syndrome occurs commonly after many viral illnesses and without infection with this pathogen), fibrositis became fibromyalgia.

It had also become clear that fibromyalgia was not just fibromyalgia. There is now significant evidence that fibromyalgia is part of a much larger continuum that has been called many things, including functional somatic syndromes, medically unexplained symptoms, chronic multisymptom illnesses, somatoform disorders, and, perhaps most appropriately, central sensitivity syndromes (CSS). Yunus and coworkers[9] showed fibromyalgia to be associated with tension type headache, migraine, and irritable bowel syndrome. Together with primary dysmenorrhea, these entities were depicted by Yunus in a Venn diagram in 1984, emphasizing the epidemiologic and clinical overlap between the syndromes.[9] At that point "muscle spasm" was the concept placed in the center of the diagram, being considered to be the unifying element common to the various components of the spectrum depicted. Since then, the Venn diagram has been broadened continuously and currently includes at least 13 separate clinical entities per Yunus.

We present our view of the syndromes that have clearly been established as being part of this continuum in **Box 1** and use the term *central sensitivity syndromes* as proposed by Yunus, because we feel that this represents the best nosologic term at present for these syndromes.[13]

Extensive reviews on the overlap between these syndromes have been published by Aaron and Buchwald[14,15] as well as by Yunus.[13] As noted in these reviews, the actual magnitude of the overlap between fibromyalgia and the other syndromes has been given various estimations. Chronic fatigue syndrome has been described in 22% to 74% of patients who have fibromyalgia.[16–21] The frequency of irritable bowel syndrome among patients with fibromyalgia has been estimated between 32% and

---

Box 1
Clinical entities currently considered parts of the spectrum of central sensitivity syndromes

Fibromyalgia

Chronic fatigue syndrome

Irritable bowel syndrome and other functional gastrointestinal disorders

Temporomandibular joint disorder

Restless leg syndrome and periodic limb movements in sleep

Idiopathic low back pain

Multiple chemical sensitivity

Primary dysmenorrhea

Headache (tension greater than migraine, mixed)

Migraine

Interstitial cystitis/chronic prostatitis/painful bladder syndrome

Chronic pelvic pain and endometriosis

Myofascial pain syndrome/regional soft tissue pain syndrome

70%.[22–30] All of these relationships are bidirectional, that is, individuals with entities such as chronic fatigue syndrome, irritable bowel syndrome, and headache are also much more likely to have fibromyalgia than those in the general population.

There is also a clear overlap between these disorders and a variety of psychiatric disorders that are seen more commonly in individuals with this spectrum of illness. The presence of comorbid psychiatric disturbances is somewhat more common in individuals with these illnesses seen in tertiary care settings than in primary care settings.[31,32] **Fig. 1** shows the overlap among fibromyalgia, chronic fatigue syndrome, and a variety of regional pain syndromes as well as psychiatric disorders and shows that the common underlying pathophysiologic mechanism seen in most individuals with fibromyalgia and large subsets of individuals with these other syndromes is pain or sensory amplification.

The use of research methods such as epidemiologic and twin studies, experimental pain testing, functional imaging, and contemporary genetics has led to substantial advances in understanding several of these conditions, most notably fibromyalgia, irritable bowel syndrome, and temporomandibular joint disorder. This understanding has led to an emerging recognition that chronic central pain itself is a disease, and that many of the underlying mechanisms operative in these heretofore "idiopathic" or "functional" pain syndromes may be similar regardless of whether the pain is present throughout the body (eg, in fibromyalgia) or localized to the low back, the bowel, or the bladder. The more contemporary terms used to describe conditions such as fibromyalgia, irritable bowel syndrome, temporomandibular joint disorder, vulvodynia, and related entities include "central," "neuropathic" or "non-nociceptive" pain.[33,34] Furthermore, most investigators believe that the neurobiologic underpinnings of these conditions undermine the psychiatric construct of "somatization," at least with respect to the notion that these phenomena are the somatic representation of psychologic distress with no "real" pathologic basis. **Fig. 2** shows a suggested schema for classifying pain syndromes based upon their underlying mechanism, but it is important to recognize that even patients with "peripheral" pain syndromes such as osteoarthritis or rheumatoid arthritis often have elements of central pain that need to be

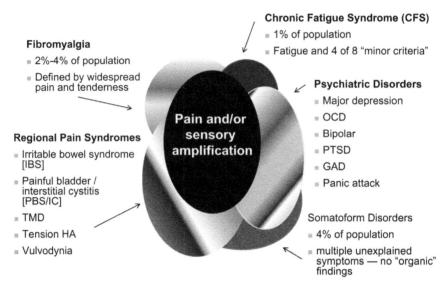

Fig. 1. Overlap between fibromyalgia and related syndromes. GAD, generalized anxiety disorder; HA, headache; OCD, obsessive-compulsive disorder; PTSD, posttraumatic stress disorder.

treated as such, which is why the fibromyalgia construct has moved well beyond simply relevance to functional somatic syndromes.

The current thinking about these overlapping symptoms and syndromes is as follows:

Multifocal pain, fatigue, insomnia, cognitive or memory problems, and in many cases psychologic symptoms are the core symptoms seen in individuals with these illnesses.[35,36] Some individuals in the population only have one of these

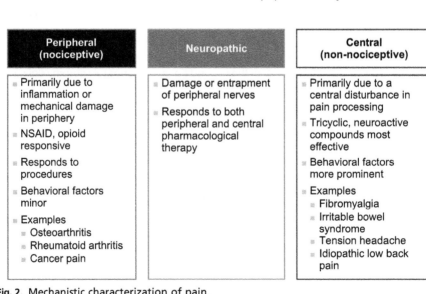

Fig. 2. Mechanistic characterization of pain.

symptoms but more often individuals have many, and the precise location of the pain and predominant symptom at any given point in time change over time.

The presence or absence and the severity of these symptoms occur over a wide continuum in the population. All of our current diagnostic labels are at some level arbitrary because there is no objective tissue pathology or gold standard to anchor "disease" to.

The symptoms and syndromes occur approximately 1.5 to 2 times more commonly in women than men. The sex difference is notably more apparent in clinical samples (especially tertiary care) than in population-based samples.[31,32]

There is a strong familial predisposition to these symptoms and illnesses, and studies clearly show that the somatic symptoms and syndromes are separable from depression and other psychiatric disorders.[37,38]

A variety of biologic stressors seem to be capable of triggering or exacerbating these symptoms and illnesses, including physical trauma, infections, early life trauma, and deployment to war, in addition to some types of psychologic stress (eg, there was no increase in somatic symptoms or worsening of fibromyalgia following the terrorist attacks of 9/11).[39–42]

Groups of individuals with these conditions (eg, fibromyalgia, irritable bowel syndrome, headache, temporomandibular joint disorder) display diffuse hyperalgesia, allodynia, or both.[43,44] Many of these conditions have also been shown to demonstrate more sensitivity to many stimuli other than pain (ie, auditory, visual), and data suggest that these individuals have a fundamental problem with pain or sensory processing rather than an abnormality confined to the specific body region where the pain is being experienced. In fact, the expanded relevance of the fibromyalgia construct is that all individuals (with and without pain) have different "volume control" settings on their pain and sensory processing. Where they sit on this bell-shaped curve of pain or sensory sensitivity determines to a large part whether they will have pain or other sensory symptoms over the course of their lifetime and how severe these symptoms will be (**Fig. 3**).

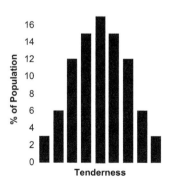

- Like most other physiological processes, we (animals) have a "volume control" setting for how our brain and spinal cord processes pain and other sensory information

- This is likely *set* by the genes that we are born with, and *modified* by environmental influences

- The higher the volume control setting, the more painwe will experience, irresective of periheral nociceptive input

Fig. 3. Pain sensitivity in the general population.

In addition to pain and sensory amplification, other shared underlying mechanisms have been identified in these illnesses that may be partly responsible for symptom expression (but are not reviewed in detail herein), including (1) neurogenic inflammation, especially of mucosal surfaces, leading to increased mast cells and the appearance of a mild inflammatory process; (2) dysfunction of the autonomic nervous system; and (3) hypothalamic pituitary dysfunction.

Similar types of therapies are efficacious for all of these conditions, including pharmacologic (eg, tricyclic compounds such as amitriptyline) and nonpharmacologic treatments (eg, exercise and cognitive behavioral therapy). Conversely, individuals with these conditions typically do not respond to therapies that are effective when pain is due to damage or inflammation of tissues (eg, nonsteroidal anti-inflammatory drugs, opioids, injections, surgical procedures).

EPIDEMIOLOGY AND CLINICAL STUDIES

The large numbers of studies that have directly compared the rate of fibromyalgia in other related CSS and vice versa or the rates of comorbidities between syndromes are not reviewed herein because these have been covered elsewhere. Instead, we focus on describing several lines of research that have better clarified the "big picture" with respect to the interrelationships of these symptoms and syndromes.

Twin Studies

Kato and colleagues[36,45] using a large Swedish twin registry performed a series of studies showing the comorbidities with chronic widespread pain and then later examined a number of functional somatic syndromes and the relationship of these symptoms to those of depression and anxiety. These studies clearly demonstrated that functional somatic syndromes such as fibromyalgia, chronic fatigue syndrome, irritable bowel syndrome, and headache have latent traits that are different than (but overlap somewhat with) psychiatric conditions such as anxiety and depression. Interestingly, the findings are exactly those found in functional neuroimaging studies in which, for example, individuals with fibromyalgia alone primarily have increased activity in the regions of the brain that code for the sensory intensity of stimuli (eg, the primary and secondary somatosensory cortices, posterior insula, thalamus), whereas fibromyalgia patients with comorbid depression also have increased activation in brain regions coding for the affective processing of pain, such as the amygdala and anterior insula.[46] This notion that there are two overlapping sets of traits, one being pain and sensory amplification and the other being mood and affect, is also seen in other genetic studies of idiopathic pain syndromes.[47] Twin studies have been useful in helping tease out potential underlying mechanisms versus "epiphenomena." Buchwald and colleagues[48,49] have compared identical twins with and without symptoms and have found that in many cases the two twins share "abnormalities in sleep or immune function, yet have markedly different symptom profiles." These investigators have likewise suggested that this is evidence of a problem with perceptual amplification in the affected twins.

The Role of Environmental Stressors in Triggering Illness

As with most illnesses that may have a genetic underpinning, environmental factors can have a prominent role in triggering the development of fibromyalgia and related conditions. Environmental "stressors" temporally associated with the development of either fibromyalgia or chronic fatigue syndrome include early life trauma, physical trauma (especially involving the trunk), certain infections such as hepatitis C,

Epstein-Barr virus, parvovirus, and Lyme disease, and emotional stress (**Box 2**). The disorder is also associated with other regional pain conditions or autoimmune disorders.[42,50,51] Of note, each of these stressors only leads to chronic widespread pain or fibromyalgia in approximately 5% to 10% of individuals who are exposed; the overwhelming majority of individuals who experience these same infections or other stressful events regain their baseline state of health.

An excellent recent example of how illnesses such as fibromyalgia might be triggered occurred in the setting of the deployment of troops to liberate Kuwait during the Gulf War in 1990 and 1991. The term *Gulf War illnesses* is now commonly used to refer to a constellation of symptoms developed by approximately 10% to 15% of the 700,000 US troops deployed to the Persian Gulf in the early 1990s. The symptoms, which include headaches, muscle and joint pain, fatigue, memory disorders, and gastrointestinal distress,[35] were seen in troops deployed from the United Kingdom and other countries as well.[52] The panels of experts who examined potential causes for these symptoms and syndromes found that the sickness could not be traced to any single environmental trigger and noted the similarities between these individuals and those diagnosed with fibromyalgia and chronic fatigue. Furthermore, similar syndromes involving multiple somatic symptoms have been noted in veterans of every war the United States or United Kingdom has been involved in during the past century.[53] This observation suggests that war may be an environment where individuals are simultaneously exposed to a multitude of stressors, triggering the development of this type of illness in susceptible individuals.[54]

Wolfe's "Symptom Inventory"

Although an early advocate of the fibromyalgia construct, more recently Wolfe has become critical of the construct, arguing that it is not a discrete illness but rather the end of a continuum.[55] The authors have a difference of opinion. We think it is both a discrete illness (ie, an individual with fibromyalgia) and the end of a continuum of pain processing. Wolfe has performed seminal work in showing that the degree of "fibromyalgia-ness" an individual with any rheumatic disorder has (including individuals with osteoarthritis, rheumatoid arthritis, regional pain syndromes, and so on) as measured by his Symptom Inventory is closely correlated with their level of pain or disability, even if they have a "peripheral" cause for their pain.[56] The Symptom Inventory (or other measures of the current or lifetime level of somatic symptoms or "somatization") is a good measure for whether an individual has a CSS or an element of

---

Box 2
Stressors capable of triggering illness (supported by case-control studies)

Early life stressors

Children born in 1958 experiencing a motor traffic accident or institutionalization 1.5 to 2 times more likely to have chronic widespread pain 42 years later

Peripheral pain syndromes (eg, rheumatoid arthritis, systemic lupus erythematosus, osteoarthritis)[4]

Physical trauma (automobile accidents)[5]

Certain catastrophic events (war but not natural disasters)[6]

Infections

Psychologic stress/distress

central sensitivity, regardless of whether they also have a peripheral cause for their pain. We predict that the genetic factors discussed herein will be shown to be highly predictive of these measures, and that functional imaging (eg, hyperactivity or increases in excitatory neurotransmitters in brain regions such the insula that code for the intensity of all sensory information) and other research methods will similarly show that these self-report measures will have strong biologic underpinnings.[57–60]

GENETIC AND FAMILIAL PREDISPOSITION

Evidence exists for a strong familial component to all of these syndromes, and this observation has arguably been best studied in twin studies comparing a variety of functional somatic syndromes and in fibromyalgia. Regarding the development of fibromyalgia, Arnold and colleagues[38] have shown that the first-degree relatives of individuals with fibromyalgia display an eightfold greater risk of developing fibromyalgia than those in the general population. Family members of individuals with fibromyalgia are more tender than family members of controls, irrespective of the presence of pain, and family members of individuals with fibromyalgia are also much more likely to have other disorders related to fibromyalgia such as irritable bowel syndrome, temporomandibular joint disorder, headaches, and other regional pain syndromes.[61,62] Similarly strong genetic predispositions to chronic pain and to nearly all of the CSS syndromes have been noted, which is congruent with the twin studies that suggest that approximately 50% of the risk of developing one of these disorders is genetic and 50% environmental.[47,63–69]

EVIDENCE OF SENSITIVITY OF PAIN AND SENSORY PROCESSING AS THE MOST REPRODUCIBLE PATHOGENIC FEATURE OF THESE ILLNESSES

As we will subsequently try to demonstrate, central nervous system sensitivity is the most consistent dysfunction common to all of the syndromes previously incorporated under the functional somatic spectrum title. Once fibromyalgia is established, by far the most consistently detected objective abnormalities involve pain and sensory processing systems. Because fibromyalgia is defined in part by tenderness, considerable work has been performed exploring the potential reason for this phenomenon. The results of two decades of psychophysical pressure pain testing in fibromyalgia have been very instructive.[70]

One of the earliest findings in this regard was that the tenderness in fibromyalgia is not confined to tender points but instead extends throughout the entire body.[71,72] Theoretically, such diffuse tenderness could primarily be due to psychologic (eg, hypervigilance, in which individuals are too attentive to their surroundings) or neurobiologic factors (eg, the plethora of factors that can lead to temporary or permanent amplification of sensory input).

Early studies typically used dolorimetry to assess pressure pain threshold and concluded that tenderness was in large part related to psychologic factors, because these measures of pain threshold were correlated with levels of distress.[55,72,73] Also, nuances such as the rate of increase of stimulus pressure, control by the operator versus by the patient, and patient distress have been shown to influence pain threshold when it is measured in this manner.[74,75]

To minimize the biases associated with "ascending" measures of pressure pain threshold (ie, the individual knows that the pressure will be predictably increased), Petzke and colleagues[76–78] performed a series of studies using more sophisticated paradigms of random delivery of pressures. These studies showed that (1) the random measures of pressure pain threshold were not influenced by levels of distress of the individual, whereas tender point count and dolorimetry examinations were; (2) fibromyalgia patients were much more sensitive to pressure even when these more sophisticated paradigms were used; (3) fibromyalgia patients were not any more "expectant" or "hypervigilant" than controls; and (4) pressure pain thresholds at any four points in the body were highly correlated with the average tenderness at all 18 tender points and 4 "control points" (the thumbnail and forehead).

In addition to the heightened sensitivity to pressure noted in fibromyalgia, other types of stimuli applied to the skin are also judged as more painful or noxious by these patients. Fibromyalgia patients also display a decreased threshold to heat,[78–81] cold,[80,82] and electrical stimuli.[83]

Gerster and colleagues[84,85] were the first to demonstrate that fibromyalgia patients display a low noxious threshold to auditory tones, and this finding was subsequently replicated. Because both of these studies used ascending measures of auditory threshold, the findings could theoretically be due to expectancy or hypervigilance. A recent study by Geisser and colleagues[86] used an identical random staircase paradigm to test the threshold of fibromyalgia patient to the loudness of auditory tones and to pressure. This study found that fibromyalgia patients displayed low thresholds to both types of stimuli, and the correlation between the results of auditory and pressure pain threshold testing suggested that some of this was due to shared variance and some unique to one stimulus or the other. The notion that fibromyalgia and related syndromes might represent biologic amplification of all sensory stimuli has significant support from functional imaging studies that suggest that the insula is the most consistently hyperactive region. This region has been noted to have a critical role in sensory integration, with the posterior insula serving a purer sensory role and the anterior insula being associated with the emotional processing of sensations.[59,87,88]

In irritable bowel syndrome, multiple studies have used the technique of rectal balloon inflation to demonstrate central sensitivity[89–92] as well as hyperalgesia produced upon electrical rectal stimulation[93,94] and altered esophageal pain threshold.[95] These and similar findings have been attributed to the presence of "visceral hypersensitivity" in irritable bowel syndrome. Subsequently, it has been shown that patients who have irritable bowel syndrome also posses hyperalgesia/allodynia of the skin to heat,[96] cold,[97] and electrical stimulation.[94] Brain imaging studies have also been reported supporting the existence of central pain augmentation in fibromyalgia, irritable bowel syndrome, low back pain, and several other of these conditions.[98–101]

It is well established that irritable bowel syndrome is characterized by both visceral and somatic central nervous system sensitization. Similarly, patients who have temporomandibular joint disorder have been shown to be hypersensitive to various forms of thermal and ischemic stimulation,[43] and patients with tension type headache have been shown to be hypersensitive to heat and pressure stimulation.[102] It appears as though tension headache patients have greater degrees of hyperalgesia than in migraine headache.[103–105] Similar findings of allodynia or diffuse hyperalgesia in sites not involved by pain have also been noted in idiopathic low back pain, vulvodynia, and interstitial cystitis.[46,106–108]

Diffuse Noxious Inhibitor Control is Altered in Central Sensitivity Syndromes

In addition to all of these syndromes being characterized by diffuse hyperalgesia/allodynia, another finding on experimental pain testing—attenuated diffuse noxious inhibitory control (DNIC)—has been noted in several of these conditions and may contribute to the overall pain sensitivity. When animals or healthy individuals are given an acutely painful stimulus and their pain threshold is subsequently measured, there is an increase in pain threshold (ie, decrease in tenderness).[109–111] This phenomenon has been referred to as DNIC because it involves recruitment of descending analgesic pathways. In both fibromyalgia and irritable bowel syndrome, DNIC has been shown to be attenuated or absent, suggesting a deficiency in descending analgesic systems. Similar deficiencies in DNIC have recently been shown in patients who have temporomandibular joint disorder,[112] and the deficit in pain inhibition in fibromyalgia has been shown to be more pronounced in patients suffering from comorbid depression.[113] A relative deficiency in DNIC appears to be one of the mechanisms of central pain augmentation common to different components of the CSS and may serve to characterize subgroups of patients who may be responsive to particular modes of treatment.

THE ROLE OF SPECIFIC NEUROTRANSMITTERS

Because a review of all of the studies of the roles that different neurotransmitters may have in these syndromes is beyond the scope of this article, we briefly review some of the findings with a specific neurotransmitter (norepinephrine) and then make general comments about all of the neurotransmitters that may have some role in these illnesses. Overall, we believe that the analogy of an increased "volume control" or "gain" setting on pain and sensory processing is supported by studies from a variety of sources. Similar to essential hypertension in which a variety of root causes can lead to elevated systemic blood pressure, we allude to these disorders as being characterized by "essential hypertension of pain and sensory processing pathways." Elevated levels of neurotransmitters that tend to be pro-nociceptive (ie, on the left side of **Fig. 4**) or reduced levels of neurotransmitters that inhibit pain transmission (ie, on the right side of **Fig. 4**) have a tendency to increase the volume control, and drugs that block neurotransmitters on the left or that augment activity of those on the right will typically be found to be effective treatments, at least for a subset of individuals with this spectrum of illness.

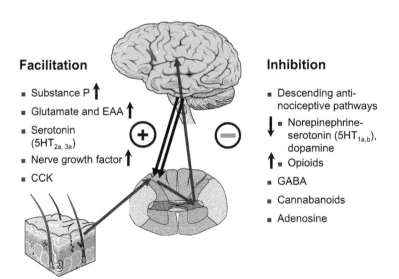

Fig. 4. Supraspinal influences on pain and sensory processing. CCK, cholecystokinin; EAA, excitatory amino acids; GABA, gamma-aminobutyric acid.

Catecholamines

Several groups have described the role of COMT (catecholamine o-methyl transferase), the enzyme responsible for catecholamine degradation, in pain transmission. Zubieta[114] demonstrated that the val158met polymorphism was responsible for differential pain sensitivity in humans, working in part by modulating the opioidergic activity. Diatchenko and Maixner used haplotype analyses to identify three subsets of individuals based on the findings in four single nucleotide polymorphisms termed *low (LPS)*, *average (APS)*, and *high pain sensitive (HPS)* groups. These subgroups are highly predictive of pain sensitivity on a variety of different experimental pain tasks.[115] Moreover, in a prospective study in which 240 pain-free individuals were phenotyped at baseline and followed for 3 years to determine who would develop temporomandibular joint disorder, carriers of the HPS haplotype were three times as likely as others to reach this endpoint.[116] In animal models, the LPS haplotype produced much higher levels of COMT enzymatic activity when compared with the APS or HPS haplotypes, whereas COMT inhibition resulted in a profound increase in pain sensitivity.

COMT also acts through mediating effects on beta-2 and beta-3 adrenergic receptors. Depressed COMT activity results in enhanced mechanical and thermal pain sensitivity in rats, which can be blocked by the nonselective beta-adrenergic antagonist propranolol or by the combined administration of selective beta-2 and beta-3 adrenergic antagonists.[117] These data provide direct evidence that low COMT activity leads to increased pain sensitivity via a beta-2/beta-3 adrenergic mechanism.

These studies of COMT and beta-2 and beta-3 effects suggest that catecholaminergic activity increases pain. In some clinical situations such as sympathetically mediated pain, catecholamine release in the periphery is also thought to cause or exacerbate pain. Nevertheless, in many other conditions, it appears that norepinephrine exerts analgesic effects at several levels. Electrical stimulation of supraspinal origins of noradrenergic descending fibers or direct application of norepinephrine to spinal neurons produces potent analgesia in laboratory animals.[118,119] These systems are also indirectly activated by stimulation of other brain sites involved in descending analgesia, such as the periaqueductal gray, and have a role in opioid-mediated descending pain inhibition.[120,121]

As noted in **Fig. 4**, norepinephrine highlights the complex roles of many neurotransmitters that can increase or decrease pain sensitivity. The arrows in **Fig. 4** highlight the abnormalities in these neurotransmitter levels (in the cerebrospinal fluid [CSF] or brain) that have been identified to date in fibromyalgia. In fibromyalgia, there is evidence for increases in the CSF levels of substance P, glutamate, nerve growth factor, and brain-derived neurotrophic factor, and low levels of the metabolites of serotonin, norepinephrine, and dopamine, any of which could lead to an "increase in the volume control" and augmented pain and sensory processing.[122–125] The only neurotransmitter system that has been studied to data and not found to be out of line in a direction that would cause augmented pain transmission is the endogenous opioid system. Both CSF levels and brain activity by functional neuroimaging appear to be augmented and not reduced (as would cause augmented pain processing) in fibromyalgia, which may be why opioidergic drugs do not work well to treat fibromyalgia and related pain syndromes.[126,127]

Potential Role of Cytokines in These Illnesses

Although these conditions were originally thought to be autoimmune or inflammatory diseases and then later not thought to be, recent findings are leading to a reconsideration of whether subtle inflammatory changes may be responsible for some of the symptoms seen. Immunologic cascades have a role in the maintenance of central sensitivity and chronic pain which is enhanced through release of proinflammatory cytokines by central nervous system glial cells; therefore, the traditional paradigm regarding inflammatory versus noninflammatory pain may gradually become less dichotomic. As may be expected in any complex biologic system, a delicate apparatus of checks and balances is at work in the spinal transmission of pain. Multiple inhibitory transmitters act at the spinal level to reduce the volume of pain transmission. Serotonin, norepinephrine, enkephalins, dopamine, and gamma-aminobutyric acid[128] are among the better known players in this balance.

SIMILAR TREATMENTS WORK FOR MANY OF THE CENTRAL SENSITIVITY SYNDROMES

Several drug and nondrug therapies have been shown to be effective for nearly any of the CSS disorders, further reinforcing that this may be a large overlapping disorder rather than several separate ones. Among the classes of drugs, there are significant data suggesting that tricyclic compounds are effective for treating most of the conditions noted.[129–131] Newer serotonin-norepinephrine reuptake inhibitors such as duloxetine and tramadol have similarly been shown to be effective across a broad range of these conditions,[132] and, interestingly, duloxetine had much earlier been shown to be helpful in treating the pain associated with depression, which is not surprising. The alpha-2-delta ligands such as pregabalin and gabapentin are also being shown to be efficacious in a wide range of these entities.[133] Any one of these classes of drugs will work well in only about a third of patients, which is entirely consistent with the theory that this is a strongly genetic but polygenic disorder requiring different treatments in different individuals. Going back to the "essential hypertension of pain processing pathway" analogy, just as we use eight to ten classes of drugs acting in different body systems and at different molecular targets to control hypertension with individuals responding well to one class of antihypertensive drugs but not to another, the same is true of CSS syndromes. Nonetheless, our current pharmacologic armamentarium is not nearly as developed for central pain as for essential hypertension, which is likely one of the reasons why these syndromes remain difficult to treat.

Just as many pharmacologic therapies work across all or most of these conditions, nonpharmacologic therapies such as education, exercise, and cognitive behavioral therapy have been demonstrated to be effective across nearly all of the CSS conditions.[134–136] Gynecologists, maxillofacial surgeons, gastroenterologists, and rheumatologists alike have come to realize that when central pain or sensitivity is recognized as the salient feature of a particular clinical entity, both commonsense as well as clinical experience dictate a therapeutic approach aimed at influencing pain transmission in the central nervous system.

Only, as Anderson put it, by recognizing "entirely new laws, concepts and generalizations" do we start to understand that what we thought was a discrete rheumatologic condition has in fact become a metaphor to remind us that pain and any other somatic symptom ultimately is experienced in the brain, which is inexorably connected to the mind and body.

REFERENCES

1. Clauw DJ, Katz P. The overlap between fibromyalgia and inflammatory rheumatic diseases: when and why does it occur? J Clin Rheumatol 1995;1:335–41.
2. McBeth J, Jones K. Epidemiology of chronic musculoskeletal pain. Clin Rheumatol 2007;21(3):403–25.

3. Clauw DJ, Engel CC Jr, Aronowitz R, et al. Unexplained symptoms after terrorism and war: an expert consensus statement. J Occup Environ Med 2003;45(10):1040–8.
4. Simms RW. Fibromyalgia is not a muscle disorder. Am J Med Sci 1998;315(6): 346–50.
5. Moldofsky H, Lue FA. The relationship of alpha and delta EEG frequencies to pain and mood in 'fibrositis' patients treated with chlorpromazine and L-tryptophan. Electroencephalogr Clin Neurophysiol 1980;50(1–2):71–80.
6. Moldofsky H, Scarisbrick P, England R, et al. Musculosketal symptoms and non-REM sleep disturbance in patients with "fibrositis syndrome" and healthy subjects. Psychosom Med 1975;37(4):341–51.
7. Hudson JI, Hudson MS, Pliner LF, et al. Fibromyalgia and major affective disorder: a controlled phenomenology and family history study. Am J Psychiatry 1985;142(4):441–6.
8. Hudson JI, Pope HGJ. Fibromyalgia and psychopathology: is fibromyalgia a form of "affective spectrum disorder"? J Rheumatol Suppl 1989;19:15–22.
9. Yunus MB. Primary fibromyalgia syndrome: current concepts. Compr Ther 1984; 10(8):21–8.
10. Bengtsson A, Henriksson KG. The muscle in fibromyalgia: a review of Swedish studies. J Rheumatol Suppl 1989;19:144–9.
11. Bennett RM, Clark SR, Goldberg L, et al. Aerobic fitness in patients with fibrositis: a controlled study of respiratory gas exchange and 133xenon clearance from exercising muscle. Arthritis Rheum 1989;32(4):454–60.
12. Bennett RM. Muscle physiology and cold reactivity in the fibromyalgia syndrome. Rheum Dis Clin North Am 1989;15(1):135–47.
13. Yunus MB. Central sensitivity syndromes: a new paradigm and group nosology for fibromyalgia and overlapping conditions, and the related issue of disease versus illness. Semin Arthritis Rheum 2008;37(6):339–52.
14. Aaron LA, Buchwald D. A review of the evidence for overlap among unexplained clinical conditions. Ann Intern Med 2001;134(9 Pt 2):868–81.
15. Aaron LA, Herrell R, Ashton S, et al. Comorbid clinical conditions in chronic fatigue: a co-twin control study. J Gen Intern Med 2001;16(1):24–31.
16. Wysenbeek AJ, Shapira Y, Leibovici L. Primary fibromyalgia and the chronic fatigue syndrome. Rheumatol Int 1991;10(6):227–9.
17. Hudson JI, Goldenberg DL, Pope HG Jr, et al. Comorbidity of fibromyalgia with medical and psychiatric disorders. Am J Med 1992;92(4):363–7.
18. Buchwald D, Garron DC. Comparison of patients with chronic fatigue syndrome, fibromyalgia, and multiple chemical sensitivities [see comments]. Arch Intern Med 1994;154(18):2049–53.
19. Jason LA, Taylor RR, Kennedy CL. Chronic fatigue syndrome, fibromyalgia, and multiple chemical sensitivities in a community-based sample of persons with chronic fatigue syndrome-like symptoms [in process citation]. Psychosom Med 2000;62(5):655–63.
20. White KP, Speechley M, Harth M, et al. Co-existence of chronic fatigue syndrome with fibromyalgia syndrome in the general population: a controlled study. Scand J Rheumatol 2000;29(1):44–51.
21. Aaron LA, Burke MM, Buchwald D. Overlapping conditions among patients with chronic fatigue syndrome, fibromyalgia, and temporomandibular disorder. Arch Intern Med 2000;160(2):221–7.
22. Yunus M, Masi AT, Calabro JJ, et al. Primary fibromyalgia (fibrositis): clinical study of 50 patients with matched normal controls. Semin Arthritis Rheum 1981;11(1):151–71.

23. Bengtsson A, Henriksson KG, Jorfeldt L, et al. Primary fibromyalgia: a clinical and laboratory study of 55 patients. Scand J Rheumatol 1986;15(3):340–7.
24. Goldenberg DL. Fibromyalgia syndrome: an emerging but controversial condition. J Am Med Assoc 1987;257(20):2782–7.
25. Romano TJ. Coexistence of irritable bowel syndrome and fibromyalgia. W V Med J 1988;84(2):16–8.
26. Yunus MB, Masi AT, Aldag JC. A controlled study of primary fibromyalgia syndrome: clinical features and association with other functional syndromes. J Rheumatol Suppl 1989;19:62–71.
27. Triadafilopoulos G, Simms RW, Goldenberg DL. Bowel dysfunction in fibromyalgia syndrome. Dig Dis Sci 1991;36(1):59–64.
28. Sperber AD, Atzmon Y, Neumann L, et al. Fibromyalgia in the irritable bowel syndrome: studies of prevalence and clinical implications. Am J Gastroenterol 1999;94(12):3541–6.
29. Sivri A, Cindas A, Dincer F, et al. Bowel dysfunction and irritable bowel syndrome in fibromyalgia patients [see comments]. Clin Rheumatol 1996; 15(3):283–6.
30. Wolfe F, Ross K, Anderson J, et al. The prevalence and characteristics of fibromyalgia in the general population. Arthritis Rheum 1995;38(1):19–28.
31. Aaron LA, Bradley LA, Alarcon GS, et al. Psychiatric diagnoses in patients with fibromyalgia are related to health care-seeking behavior rather than to illness [see comments]. Arthritis Rheum 1996;39(3):436–45.
32. Drossman DA, Li ZM, Andruzzi E, et al. US householder survey of functional gastrointestinal disorders: prevalence, sociodemography, and health impact. Dig Dis Sci 1993;38(9):1569–80.
33. Clauw DJ. Fibromyalgia: update on mechanisms and management. J Clin Rheumatol 2007;13(2):102–9.
34. Woolf CJ. Pain: moving from symptom control toward mechanism-specific pharmacologic management. Ann Intern Med 2004;140(6):441–51.
35. Fukuda K, Nisenbaum R, Stewart G, et al. Chronic multisymptom illness affecting Air Force veterans of the Gulf War. J Am Med Assoc 1998;280(11):981–8.
36. Kato K, Sullivan PF, Evengard B, et al. A population-based twin study of functional somatic syndromes. Psychol Med 2008;39:1–9.
37. Buskila D, Sarzi-Puttini P, Ablin JN. The genetics of fibromyalgia syndrome. Pharmacogenomics 2007;8(1):67–74.
38. Arnold LM, Hudson JI, Hess EV, et al. Family study of fibromyalgia. Arthritis Rheum 2004;50(3):944–52.
39. Williams DA, Brown SC, Clauw DJ, et al. Self-reported symptoms before and after September 11 in patients with fibromyalgia. JAMA 2003;289(13):1637–8.
40. Clauw DJ, Mease P, Palmer RH, et al. Milnacipran for the treatment of fibromyalgia in adults: a 15-week, multicenter, randomized, double-blind, placebo-controlled, multiple-dose clinical trial. Clin Ther 2008;30(11):1988–2004.
41. Raphael KG, Natelson BH, Janal MN, et al. A community-based survey of fibromyalgia-like pain complaints following the World Trade Center terrorist attacks. Pain 2002;100(1–2):131–9.
42. Clauw DJ, Chrousos GP. Chronic pain and fatigue syndromes: overlapping clinical and neuroendocrine features and potential pathogenic mechanisms. Neuroimmunomodulation 1997;4(3):134–53.
43. Maixner W, Fillingim R, Booker D, et al. Sensitivity of patients with painful temporomandibular disorders to experimentally evoked pain. Pain 1995;63(3):341–51.

44. Moshiree B, Price DD, Robinson ME, et al. Thermal and visceral hypersensitivity in irritable bowel syndrome patients with and without fibromyalgia. Clin J Pain 2007;23(4):323–30.
45. Kato K, Sullivan PF, Evengard B, et al. Chronic widespread pain and its comorbidities: a population-based study. Arch Intern Med 2006;166(15):1649–54.
46. Giesecke T, Gracely RH, Williams DA, et al. The relationship between depression, clinical pain, and experimental pain in a chronic pain cohort. Arthritis Rheum 2005;52(5):1577–84.
47. Diatchenko L, Nackley AG, Slade GD, et al. Idiopathic pain disorders: pathways of vulnerability. Pain 2006;123(3):226–30.
48. Armitage R, Landis C, Hoffmann R, et al. Power spectral analysis of sleep EEG in twins discordant for chronic fatigue syndrome. J Psychosom Res 2009;66(1):51–7.
49. Sherlin L, Budzynski T, Kogan BH, et al. Low-resolution electromagnetic brain tomography (LORETA) of monozygotic twins discordant for chronic fatigue syndrome. Neuroimage 2007;34(4):1438–42.
50. Buskila D, Neumann L, Vaisberg G, et al. Increased rates of fibromyalgia following cervical spine injury: a controlled study of 161 cases of traumatic injury [see comments]. Arthritis Rheum 1997;40(3):446–52.
51. McLean SA, Clauw DJ. Predicting chronic symptoms after an acute "stressor": lessons learned from 3 medical conditions. Med Hypotheses 2004;63(4):653–8.
52. Unwin C, Blatchley N, Coker W, et al. Health of UK servicemen who served in Persian Gulf War. Lancet 1999;353(9148):169–78.
53. Hyams KC, Wignall FS, Roswell R. War syndromes and their evaluation: from the US Civil War to the Persian Gulf War. Ann Intern Med 1996;125(5):398–405.
54. Clauw DJ. The health consequences of the first Gulf War. Br Med J 2003;327: 1357–8.
55. Wolfe F. The relation between tender points and fibromyalgia symptom variables: evidence that fibromyalgia is not a discrete disorder in the clinic. Ann Rheum Dis 1997;56(4):268–71.
56. Wolfe F, Rasker JJ. The Symptom Intensity Scale, fibromyalgia, and the meaning of fibromyalgia-like symptoms. J Rheumatol 2006;33(11):2291–9.
57. Clauw DJ, Witter J. Pain and rheumatology: thinking outside the joint. Arthritis Rheum 2009;60(2):321–4.
58. Harris RE, Sundgren PC, Pang Y, et al. Dynamic levels of glutamate within the insula are associated with improvements in multiple pain domains in fibromyalgia. Arthritis Rheum 2008;58(3):903–7.
59. Craig AD. Interoception: the sense of the physiological condition of the body. Curr Opin Neurobiol 2003;13(4):500–5.
60. Brooks JC, Tracey I. The insula: a multidimensional integration site for pain. Pain 2007;128(1–2):1–2.
61. Buskila D, Neumann L, Hazanov I, et al. Familial aggregation in the fibromyalgia syndrome. Semin Arthritis Rheum 1996;26(3):605–11.
62. Kato K, Sullivan PF, Evengard B, et al. Importance of genetic influences on chronic widespread pain. Arthritis Rheum 2006;54(5):1682–6.
63. Camilleri M, Atanasova E, Carlson PJ, et al. Serotonin-transporter polymorphism pharmacogenetics in diarrhea-predominant irritable bowel syndrome. Gastroenterology 2002;123(2):425–32.
64. Whitehead WE. Twin studies used to prove that the comorbidity of major depressive disorder with irritable bowel syndrome is NOT influenced by heredity. Am J Gastroenterol 2007;102(10):2230–1.

65. Tietjen GE, Herial NA, Hardgrove J, et al. Migraine comorbidity constellations. Headache 2007;47(6):857–65.
66. Apkarian AV, Bushnell MC, Treede RD, et al. Human brain mechanisms of pain perception and regulation in health and disease. Eur J Pain 2005;9(4):463–84.
67. Bengtsson B, Thorson J. Back pain: a study of twins. Acta Genet Med Gemellol (Roma) 1991;40(1):83–90.
68. Buskila D. Genetics of chronic pain states. Best Pract Res Clin Rheumatol 2007; 21(3):535–47.
69. Mogil JS. The genetic mediation of individual differences in sensitivity to pain and its inhibition. Proc Natl Acad Sci U S A 1999;96(14):7744–51.
70. Staud R, Spaeth M. Psychophysical and neurochemical abnormalities of pain processing in fibromyalgia. CNS Spectr 2008;13(3 Suppl 5):12–7.
71. Granges G, Littlejohn G. Pressure pain threshold in pain-free subjects, in patients with chronic regional pain syndromes, and in patients with fibromyalgia syndrome. Arthritis Rheum 1993;36(5):642–6.
72. Wolfe F, Ross K, Anderson J, et al. Aspects of fibromyalgia in the general population: sex, pain threshold, and fibromyalgia symptoms. J Rheumatol 1995; 22(1):151–6.
73. Gracely RH, Grant MA, Giesecke T. Evoked pain measures in fibromyalgia. Best Pract Res Clin Rheumatol 2003;17(4):593–609.
74. Jensen K, Andersen HO, Olesen J, et al. Pressure-pain threshold in human temporal region: evaluation of a new pressure algometer. Pain 1986;25(3): 313–23.
75. Petzke F, Gracely RH, Park KM, et al. What do tender points measure? Influence of distress on 4 measures of tenderness. J Rheumatol 2003;30(3):567–74.
76. Petzke F, Gracely RH, Khine A, et al. Pain sensitivity in patients with fibromyalgia (fibromyalgia): expectancy effects on pain measurements. Arthritis Rheum 1999; 42(Suppl 9):S342.
77. Petzke F, Khine A, Williams D, et al. Dolorimetry performed at 3 paired tender points highly predicts overall tenderness. J Rheumatol 2001;28(11):2568–9.
78. Petzke F, Clauw DJ, Ambrose K, et al. Increased pain sensitivity in fibromyalgia: effects of stimulus type and mode of presentation. Pain 2003;105(3):403–13.
79. Gibson SJ, Littlejohn GO, Gorman MM, et al. Altered heat pain thresholds and cerebral event-related potentials following painful CO_2 laser stimulation in subjects with fibromyalgia syndrome. Pain 1994;58(2):185–93.
80. Kosek E, Hansson P. Modulatory influence on somatosensory perception from vibration and heterotopic noxious conditioning stimulation (HNCS) in fibromyalgia patients and healthy subjects. Pain 1997;70(1):41–51.
81. Geisser ME, Casey KL, Brucksch CB, et al. Perception of noxious and innocuous heat stimulation among healthy women and women with fibromyalgia: association with mood, somatic focus, and catastrophizing. Pain 2003;102(3): 243–50.
82. Kosek E, Ekholm J, Hansson P. Sensory dysfunction in fibromyalgia patients with implications for pathogenic mechanisms. Pain 1996;68(2–3):375–83.
83. Arroyo JF, Cohen ML. Abnormal responses to electrocutaneous stimulation in fibromyalgia. J Rheumatol 1993;20(11):1925–31.
84. Gerster JC, Hadj-Djilani A. Hearing and vestibular abnormalities in primary fibrositis syndrome. J Rheumatol 1984;11(5):678–80.
85. McDermid AJ, Rollman GB, McCain GA. Generalized hypervigilance in fibromyalgia: evidence of perceptual amplification. Pain 1996;66(2–3):133–44.

86. Geisser ME, Gracely RH, Giesecke T, et al. The association between experimental and clinical pain measures among persons with fibromyalgia and chronic fatigue syndrome. Eur J Pain 2007;11(2):202–7.
87. Tracey I, Mantyh PW. The cerebral signature for pain perception and its modulation. Neuron 2007;55(3):377–91.
88. Craig AD. Human feelings: why are some more aware than others? Trends Cogn Sci 2004;8(6):239–41.
89. Schmulson M, Chang L, Naliboff B, et al. Correlation of symptom criteria with perception thresholds during rectosigmoid distension in irritable bowel syndrome patients. Am J Gastroenterol 2000;95(1):152–6.
90. Drewes AM, Petersen P, Rossel P, et al. Sensitivity and distensibility of the rectum and sigmoid colon in patients with irritable bowel syndrome. Scand J Gastroenterol 2001;36(8):827–32.
91. Bouin M, Plourde V, Boivin M, et al. Rectal distention testing in patients with irritable bowel syndrome: sensitivity, specificity, and predictive values of pain sensory thresholds. Gastroenterology 2002;122(7):1771–7.
92. Bouin M, Lupien F, Riberdy M, et al. Intolerance to visceral distension in functional dyspepsia or irritable bowel syndrome: an organ specific defect or a pan intestinal dysregulation? Neurogastroenterol Motil 2004;16(3):311–4.
93. Rossel P, Pedersen P, Niddam D, et al. Cerebral response to electric stimulation of the colon and abdominal skin in healthy subjects and patients with irritable bowel syndrome. Scand J Gastroenterol 2001;36(12):1259–66.
94. Rossel P, Drewes AM, Petersen P, et al. Pain produced by electric stimulation of the rectum in patients with irritable bowel syndrome: further evidence of visceral hyperalgesia. Scand J Gastroenterol 1999;34(10):1001–6.
95. Costantini M, Sturniolo GC, Zaninotto G, et al. Altered esophageal pain threshold in irritable bowel syndrome. Dig Dis Sci 1993;38(2):206–12.
96. Rodrigues AC, Nicholas VG, Schmidt S, et al. Hypersensitivity to cutaneous thermal nociceptive stimuli in irritable bowel syndrome. Pain 2005;115(1–2):5–11.
97. Bouin M, Meunier P, Riberdy-Poitras M, et al. Pain hypersensitivity in patients with functional gastrointestinal disorders: a gastrointestinal-specific defect or a general systemic condition? Dig Dis Sci 2001;46(11):2542–8.
98. Gracely RH, Petzke F, Wolf JM, et al. Functional magnetic resonance imaging evidence of augmented pain processing in fibromyalgia. Arthritis Rheum 2002;46(5):1333–43.
99. Drossman DA. Brain imaging and its implications for studying centrally targeted treatments in irritable bowel syndrome: a primer for gastroenterologists. Gut 2005;54(5):569–73.
100. Rapps N, van Oudenhove L, Enck P, et al. Brain imaging of visceral functions in healthy volunteers and irritable bowel syndrome patients. J Psychosom Res 2008;64(6):599–604.
101. Giesecke T, Gracely RH, Grant MA, et al. Evidence of augmented central pain processing in idiopathic chronic low back pain. Arthritis Rheum 2004;50(2):613–23.
102. Langemark M, Jensen K, Jensen TS, et al. Pressure pain thresholds and thermal nociceptive thresholds in chronic tension-type headache. Pain 1989;38(2):203–10.
103. Gobel H, Weigle L, Kropp P, et al. Pain sensitivity and pain reactivity of pericranial muscles in migraine and tension-type headache. Cephalalgia 1992;12(3):142–51.

104. Flor H, Diers M, Birbaumer N. Peripheral and electrocortical responses to painful and non-painful stimulation in chronic pain patients, tension headache patients and healthy controls. Neurosci Lett 2004;361(1–3):147–50.
105. Jensen R, Rasmussen BK, Pedersen B, et al. Muscle tenderness and pressure pain thresholds in headache: a population study. Pain 1993;52(2):193–9.
106. Clauw DJ, Schmidt M, Radulovic D, et al. The relationship between fibromyalgia and interstitial cystitis. J Psychiatr Res 1997;31(1):125–31.
107. Ness TJ, Powell-Boone T, Cannon R, et al. Psychophysical evidence of hypersensitivity in subjects with interstitial cystitis. J Urol 2005;173(6):1983–7.
108. Giesecke J, Reed BD, Haefner HK, et al. Quantitative sensory testing in vulvodynia patients and increased peripheral pressure pain sensitivity. Obstet Gynecol 2004;104(1):126–33.
109. Danziger N, Gautron M, Le Bars D, et al. Activation of diffuse noxious inhibitory controls (DNIC) in rats with an experimental peripheral mononeuropathy. Pain 2001;91(3):287–96.
110. Edwards RR, Ness TJ, Weigent DA, et al. Individual differences in diffuse noxious inhibitory controls (DNIC): association with clinical variables. Pain 2003;106(3):427–37.
111. Le Bars D, Villanueva L, Bouhassira D, et al. Diffuse noxious inhibitory controls (DNIC) in animals and in man. Patol Fiziol Eksp Ter 1992;4:55–65.
112. King CD, Wong F, Currie T, et al. Deficiency in endogenous modulation of prolonged heat pain in patients with irritable bowel syndrome and temporomandibular disorder. Pain 2009;143(3):172–8.
113. de Souza JB, Potvin S, Goffaux P, et al. The deficit of pain inhibition in fibromyalgia is more pronounced in patients with comorbid depressive symptoms. Clin J Pain 2009;25(2):123–7.
114. Zubieta JK, Smith YR, Bueller JA, et al. Regional mu opioid receptor regulation of sensory and affective dimensions of pain. Science 2001;293(5528):311–5.
115. Diatchenko L, Nackley AG, Slade GD, et al. Catechol-O-methyltransferase gene polymorphisms are associated with multiple pain-evoking stimuli. Pain 2006;125(3):216–24.
116. Diatchenko L, Slade GD, Nackley AG, et al. Genetic basis for individual variations in pain perception and the development of a chronic pain condition. Hum Mol Genet 2005;14(1):135–43.
117. Nackley AG, Tan KS, Fecho K, et al. Catechol-O-methyltransferase inhibition increases pain sensitivity through activation of both beta2- and beta3-adrenergic receptors. Pain 2007;128(3):199–208.
118. Millan MJ. Descending control of pain. Prog Neurobiol 2002;66(6):355–474.
119. Yaksh TL. Pharmacology of spinal adrenergic systems which modulate spinal nociceptive processing. Pharmacol Biochem Behav 1985;22(5):845–58.
120. Bajic D, Proudfit HK, Van Bockstaele EJ. Periaqueductal gray neurons monosynaptically innervate extranuclear noradrenergic dendrites in the rat pericoerulear region. J Comp Neurol 2000;427(4):649–62.
121. Chang PF, Arendt-Nielsen L, Graven-Nielsen T, et al. Psychophysical and EEG responses to repeated experimental muscle pain in humans: pain intensity encodes EEG activity. Brain Res Bull 2003;59(6):533–43.
122. Giovengo SL, Russell IJ, Larson AA. Increased concentrations of nerve growth factor in cerebrospinal fluid of patients with fibromyalgia. J Rheumatol 1999;26(7):1564–9.

123. Sarchielli P, Mancini ML, Floridi A, et al. Increased levels of neurotrophins are not specific for chronic migraine: evidence from primary fibromyalgia syndrome. J Pain 2007;8(9):737–45.
124. Russell IJ, Orr MD, Littman B, et al. Elevated cerebrospinal fluid levels of substance P in patients with the fibromyalgia syndrome. Arthritis Rheum 1994; 37(11):1593–601.
125. Russell IJ. Neurochemical pathogenesis of fibromyalgia. Z Rheumatol 1998; 57(Suppl 2):63–6.
126. Harris RE, Clauw DJ, Scott DJ, et al. Decreased central mu-opioid receptor availability in fibromyalgia. J Neurosci 2007;27(37):10000–6.
127. Baraniuk JN, Whalen G, Cunningham J, et al. Cerebrospinal fluid levels of opioid peptides in fibromyalgia and chronic low back pain. BMC Musculoskelet Disord 2004;5:48.
128. Russell IJ. Neurotransmitters, cytokines, hormones and the immune system in chronic neuropathic pain. In: Wallace DJ, editor. Fibromyalgia and other central syndromes. Philadelphia: Lippincott Williams & Wilkins; 2005. p. 63–79.
129. Bryson HM, Wilde MI. Amitriptyline: a review of its pharmacological properties and therapeutic use in chronic pain states. Drugs Aging 1996;8(6):459–76.
130. van Ophoven A, Hertle L. Long-term results of amitriptyline treatment for interstitial cystitis. J Urol 2005;174(5):1837–40.
131. Lynch ME. Antidepressants as analgesics: a review of randomized controlled trials. J Psychiatry Neurosci 2001;26(1):30–6.
132. Arnold LM. Duloxetine and other antidepressants in the treatment of patients with fibromyalgia. Pain Med 2007;8(Suppl 2):S63–74.
133. Arnold LM, Goldenberg DL, Stanford SB, et al. Gabapentin in the treatment of fibromyalgia: a randomized, double-blind, placebo-controlled, multicenter trial. Arthritis Rheum 2007;56(4):1336–44.
134. Bergman S. Management of musculoskeletal pain. Best Pract Res Clin Rheumatol 2007;21(1):153–66.
135. Deuster PA. Exercise in the prevention and treatment of chronic disorders. Womens Health Issues 1996;6(6):320–31.
136. Williams DA. Cognitive and behavioral approaches to chronic pain. In: Wallace DJ, Clauw DJ, editors. Fibromyalgia and other central pain syndromes. Philadelphia: Lippincott Williams & Wilkins; 2005. p. 343–52.

Pediatric Fibromyalgia

Dan Buskila, MD

KEYWORDS

- Pediatric • Children • Adolescents
- Fibromyalgia • Tenderness

Fibromyalgia (FM) is an idiopathic chronic pain syndrome defined by widespread nonarticular musculoskeletal pain and generalized tender points. The syndrome is associated with a constellation of symptoms, including fatigue, nonrefreshing sleep, irritable bowel, and more.[1] Central nervous system sensitization is a major pathophysiologic aspect of FM; in addition, various external stimuli such as trauma and stress may contribute to development of the syndrome.

FM is most common in midlife, but may be seen at any age. Relative to the volume of literature on FM in adults, less work has been published concerning children. Diffuse musculoskeletal pains in children and adolescents are common. Girls are affected relatively more often. Whereas growing pains and joint hypermobility as possible causes tend to occur in younger children, FM seems to be more frequent in adolescents.[2]

This article reviews the epidemiology, clinical characteristics, etiology, management, and outcome of pediatric FM.

EPIDEMIOLOGY

The prevalence of FM was assessed in 338 subjects between the ages of 9 and 15 years (179 boys and 159 girls) in Israel.[3] Twenty-one of 338 (6.2%) were found to have FM. Using dolorimetry at specific tender point sites, boys exhibited less tenderness than girls; subjects who had FM had a lower tenderness threshold compared with the subjects who did not have FM. These data demonstrating effects on tenderness associated with gender in children confirm our experience in adults.[4] Another study of 2408 Italian subjects aged 8 to 21 years found an incidence of FM in 1.2%.[5] Clark and colleagues[6] reported that the prevalence of FM in schoolchildren in Mexico reached 1.2%, which is fivefold lower than the previous report from Israel.[3] This variance may result from racial and sociocultural differences between populations and from differences in methodological approach. Indeed, the author and associates have found that tenderness thresholds varied across three ethnic groups in Israel. Israeli-born Jewish children exhibited less tenderness than Bedouin Arab children, who in turn had less tenderness than Ethiopian Jewish children.[7] Among 1756 third

Division of Internal Medicine, Department of Medicine H, Soroka Medical Center, Ben Gurion University, P.O. Box 151, 84101 Beer Sheva, Israel
E-mail address: dbuskila@bgu.ac.il

Rheum Dis Clin N Am 35 (2009) 253–261
doi:10.1016/j.rdc.2009.06.001
0889-857X/09/$ – see front matter © 2009 Elsevier Inc. All rights reserved.

rheumatic.theclinics.com

and fifth graders in Finland, the prevalence of FM was 1.3%.[8] FM is more prevalent in children attending pediatric rheumatologic clinics. Malleson and colleagues[9] reported on 81 children at a pediatric rheumatology clinic who had localized or diffuse musculoskeletal pain for which no cause could be found. Forty-one children had localized idiopathic pain and 40 had diffuse idiopathic pain. Twenty-four of the subjects who had localized idiopathic pain fulfilled criteria for definite reflex neurovascular dystrophy. Thirty-five patients who had diffuse idiopathic pain fulfilled criteria for FM.

Two sets of classification criteria have been used in studies assessing the prevalence of FM in children. The older set of criteria, proposed in 1985 by Yunus,[10] was used in earlier studies, and the 1990 American College of Rheumatology (ACR) criteria for classification of FM were used in most new studies.[11] However, the 1990 ACR criteria have never been validated in children. The authors compared two methods for assessing tenderness in children: an 18-site points count by manual palpation and dolorimetry in nine tender point sites and four control sites.[12]

The sensitivity and specificity of the dolorimetry methods was 100% and 58.7%, respectively, when the dolorimetry thresholds for defining tenderness was 4 kg, as suggested by the ACR criteria for adults. However, when a 3 kg threshold was used, the sensitivity and specificity were 89.3% and 93.5%, respectively. It was therefore suggested that in children the dolorimetry threshold for defining tenderness should be 3 kg and not 4 kg as in adults.[12] There is a need for establishing newer classification criteria for the diagnoses of pediatric FM. Such criteria will enhance research in the field of juvenile FM, including epidemiologic studies and drug trials.

CLINICAL CHARACTERISTICS

Yunus & Masi[10] found that, as in adult patients who have FM, associated nonmusculoskeletal symptoms were common in pediatric FM, including fatigue, poor sleep, anxiety, stress, headaches, and paresthesias. Physical examination revealed multiple tender points at characteristic soft tissue sites and no objective evidence of arthritis. Mikkelsson and colleagues[8] reported that children who had widespread pain had significantly higher total emotional and behavioral scores than controls, according to child and parent evaluation. Children who had FM had significantly higher scores on the Children's Depression Inventory than the children who had widespread pain but no FM.

In patients referred to a pediatric rheumatology clinic, FM was characterized by diffuse pain and sleep disturbance, the latter being more common than in adults.[13] The mean number of tender points summed over all visits was fewer than the criterion of 11 established for adults at a single visit.[13] Gedalia and colleagues[14] reported on their experience with pediatric FM. Diffuse aching was reported in 97%, headaches in 76%, and sleep disturbances in 69%. Less common were stiffness in 29%, subjective joint swelling in 24%, fatigue in 20%, abdominal pain in 17%, joint hypermobility in 14%, and depression in 7% of children.[14]

FM is part of a spectrum of syndromes termed functional somatic syndromes, which include conditions such as chronic fatigue syndrome, irritable bowel syndrome, and posttraumatic stress disorder. Around 30% of children for whom chronic fatigue syndrome was diagnosed were found to have concomitant FM.[15] Those children who met FM criteria had a statistically greater degree of subjective muscle pain, sleep disturbance, and neurologic symptoms than did those who did not meet the FM criteria. There was no statistical difference between groups in degree of fatigue, headache, sore throat, abdominal pain, concentration difficulty, eye pain, and joint pain.[15]

ETIOLOGY

The etiology and pathogenesis of FM is not entirely understood, although much progress has been achieved in its understanding. The current concept views FM as the result of central nervous system malfunction, resulting in amplification of pain transmission and interpretation.[16,17] Several factors have been suggested to predispose the development of FM in children, including psychologic factors, sleep disturbance, sexual abuse, familial, and genetic factors.

Intrinsic factors potentially contributing to chronic pain in children include low pain thresholds, female gender, joint hypermobility, poor perceived control over pain, maladaptive pain-coping strategies, and difficult temperament.[18] A number of possible extrinsic factors predisposing to the development of chronic pain include previous pain experiences, physical or sexual abuse, sleep disturbance, decreased fitness, and more.[18]

Few studies have assessed sleep disturbances in pediatric FM. Yunus and Masi[10] reported poor sleep in 67% of 33 subjects younger than 17 years of age who have FM. Siegel and colleagues[13] found that, of a possible 15 symptoms associated with FM in 33 pediatric subjects who have FM, a mean of eight symptoms were reported, with more than 90% experiencing diffuse pain and sleep disturbance. Roizenblatt and colleagues[19] observed a significant concordance regarding FM diagnosis in children and their mothers. Sleep complaints and polysomnography findings were less prominent in affected children compared with mothers who had FM. In addition, they observed a significant correlation between polysomnographic indexes, sleep anomalies, and pain manifestations in children and their mothers.[19]

Abnormalities in sleep architecture have been demonstrated in children, including prolonged sleep latency, shortened total sleep, decreased sleep efficiency, and increased wakefulness during sleep.[20] Periodic limb movements in sleep were also noted in a significant number of subjects.[20]

Some studies have documented an association between chronic pain in adults and physical or sexual abuse, including sexual abuse in childhood. However the data regarding the role of sexual abuse in the development of juvenile FM are conflicting. Many children who have idiopathic musculoskeletal pain syndromes, including FM, had potentially important stressors, including single-parent families, histories of sexual abuse, and learning difficulties.[9] In another study,[21] subjects who have FM showed the highest score of childhood adversities. In addition to sexual and physical maltreatment, the subjects who have FM more frequently reported a poor emotional relationship with both parents, a lack of physical affection, experiences of the parent's physical quarrels, alcoholism or other problems of addiction in the mother, separation, and a poor financial situation before 7 years of age. These experiences were found to a similar extent in subjects who have somatoform pain disorders, but distinctly less frequently in the control group.[21]

Raphael and colleagues[22] concluded that any overall relationship between childhood abuse and pain in adulthood probably is modest in magnitude, if it exists at all.[22] A report by Ciccone and colleagues[23] examined lifetime sexual and physical abuse histories in a community sample of women who met ACR criteria for FM. When compared with the women who did not have FM, self reported sexual and physical abuse histories were not elevated among women who had FM. Thus, prior studies reporting elevated rates of abuse in patients who have FM have likely overestimated the relationship by focusing on care-seeking samples of individuals.[24]

Current evidence points toward the existence of a genetic basis for FM, and information has been accumulated regarding the role of a number of candidate genes in

FM pathogenesis.[25–27] It is currently well established that familial aggregation is characteristic of FM. Fifty-eight offspring aged 5 to 46 years from 20 complete nuclear families ascertained through mothers affected with FM were clinically evaluated by the authors for FM.[28] Sixteen offspring (28%) were found to have FM. We further expanded our observations on the prevalence of FM in relatives of patients who have FM, and studied 30 female subjects who have FM and 117 of their close relatives.[29]

The prevalence of FM among blood relatives of subjects FM was 26%. FM prevalence in male relatives was 14% and in female relatives 41%. Arnold and colleagues[30] studied 533 relatives of 78 probands with FM as well as 272 relatives of 40 probands with rheumatoid arthritis. FM aggregated strongly in families: the odds ratio for FM in a relative of a FM proband versus FM in a relative of a rheumatoid arthritis proband was 8.5. Recent evidence suggests a role for polymorphisms of genes in the serotoninergic, dopaminergic, and catecholaminergic systems in the pathogenesis of FM.[31–33] Environmental factors, including distress and trauma, may trigger the development of FM in genetically predisposed individuals.

The authors tested the hypothesis that joint hypermobility may play a part in the pathogenesis of pain in FM in children.[34] We studied 338 subjects (179 boys, 159 girls) with a mean age of 11.5 years. Forty-three subjects (13%) were found to have joint hypermobility and 21 subjects (6%) had FM. Eighty-one percent (17/21) of the subjects who had FM had joint hypermobility, and 40% (17) of the 43 subjects who had joint hypermobility had FM. This study indicated a strong association between joint hypermobility and FM in children.

Peripheral trauma factors in joint hypermobility may initially cause localized joint pain, which would then cause neuroendocrine dysfunction through central nervous system plasticity, leading to widespread pain and tenderness.[34] Hudson and colleagues[35] confirmed the association between hypermobility and soft tissue rheumatic complaints. Hakim and Grahame[36] concluded that nonmusculoskeletal symptoms are common in patients who have joint hypermobility syndrome and that individuals who have these symptoms may express more fatigue, anxiety, migraine, flushing, night sweats, and poor sleep than their peers. It was suggested that the pathophysiologic basis for these symptoms needs to be explored further but may be a complication of autonomic dysfunction.[36]

Growing pains exemplify a type of noninflammatory pain syndrome typically affecting the extremities. Growing pains are the most common form of recurrent musculoskeletal pains in children and are present in 10%–20% of children, mainly between 3 and 12 years.[37] Interestingly, children who have growing pains were found to have more tender points and lower pain thresholds than children who did not have growing pains, indicating that growing pains may represent a variant of a noninflammatory pain syndrome in younger children.[38]

There are some data suggesting that early experiences that include unusual and frequent exposure to pain are risk factors for pain vulnerability years later.[18] Circumcised infants showed a stronger pain response to subsequent routine vaccination than uncircumcised infants.[39] Among the circumcised group, preoperative treatment with EMLA (lidocaine–prilocaine cream) attenuated the pain response to vaccination.[39] The authors assessed the tenderness threshold in adolescents born prematurely in a case-control study.[40] The preterm-born children had significantly more tender points and lower tenderness thresholds, as measured by a dolorimeter, than children born at full term. In both groups, girls had significantly more tender points and lower tenderness thresholds. Despite their increased tenderness, most of the children born prematurely did not report pain or other related symptoms. It was suggested that it is important to follow-up on these preterm-born children, since one would predict that they would be more likely to develop pain syndromes in future years than the pain-free full-term–born subjects.[40] An adverse early environment as evidenced by reduced birth- or infant weight is associated with enhanced autonomic and hypothalamic pituitary adrenal axis responses to experimental psychologic stress.[41,42]

Children and adolescents who have juvenile primary FM syndrome demonstrate more temperamental instability, increased levels of depression and anxiety, less family cohesion, and higher pain sensitivity compared with children who have arthritis and with healthy controls.[43] Parents of children who have FM, in rating themselves, also reported higher levels of anxiety and depression and lower overall psychologic adjustment compared with parents of children in the other groups. Kashikar-Zuck and colleagues[44] reported that children and adolescents who have FM were highly vulnerable to emotional difficulties, with the majority of patients who have FM meeting criteria for at least one current (67.1%) or lifetime (71.2%) psychiatric diagnosis. It was suggested that future research should explore whether early anxiety symptoms are predictive of long-term functioning. Adolescents who have FM who were seen in a pediatric rheumatology clinic setting were more likely to be having significant difficulties with peer relationships, including social rejection and isolation, unlike patients who have other rheumatic conditions such as juvenile idiopathic arthritis.[45] Increased distress and chronic pain were evident in families of adolescents who have FM, and there was an impact on family relationships.[43]

MANAGEMENT

Because FM is a complex syndrome associated with a wide range of symptoms, treatment should be tailored to the particular needs of the individual child, targeting their most distressing symptoms. A multidisciplinary approach to treatment should be used, using pharmacologic and nonpharmacologic interventions.

Nonpharmacologic Treatment/Education

Education about the illness, its outcome, and treatment modalities are very important. Parents should be encouraged by their pediatrician to participate in educational sessions to better understand their child's symptoms and difficulties. Realistic goals for treatment should be established by health care providers. It has been shown that a 1.5-day multidisciplinary FM treatment program has a significant positive effect on the impact of illness among patients who have FM with or without concomitant depression and may be a cost-effective model for the treatment of these patients.[46]

Aerobic Exercise Training

Exercise interventions in adults who have FM have been successful in improving physical fitness, reducing pain and fatigue, and improving overall quality of life.[47] Stephens and colleagues[48] reported that it is feasible to conduct an exercise intervention trial in children who have FM. In their study, significant improvements in physical function, FM symptoms, quality of life, and pain were demonstrated in two exercise groups; the aerobic group tolerated moderate-intensity exercise without exacerbating their disease and performed better in several measures compared with the qigong group.

Complementary and Alternative Medicine

Recent work suggests that the use of complementary and alternative medicine (CAM) in pediatric populations is increasing substantially.[49] Tsao and colleagues[50] examined treatment preferences in pediatric subjects who were offered a choice of CAM therapies for chronic pain. Over 60% of subjects elected to try at least one CAM approach for pain. The most preferred CAM therapies were biofeedback, yoga, and hypnosis, with moderate preference for acupuncture, massage, and craniofacial therapy; the least preferred were art therapy and energy healing.

Patients with a diagnosis of FM were the most likely to try CAM versus those with other pain diagnoses. In multivariate analyses, pain duration emerged as a significant predictor of CAM preferences.

Cognitive Behavioral Therapy

Cognitive behavioral therapy (CBT) is a psychotherapeutic approach that aims to influence problematic and dysfunctional emotions, behaviors, and cognitions through a goal-oriented systematic procedure. Both operant behavioral and cognitive behavioral treatments may be effective in treating adult patients with FM.[51] Sixty-seven children who have FM and their parents were recruited to participate in an 8-week intervention that included modules of pain management psychoeducation, sleep hygiene, and activities of daily living. Children were taught techniques of cognitive restructuring, thought stopping, distraction, relaxation, and self-reward.[52] Following CBT, children reported significant reductions in pain, somatic symptoms, anxiety, and fatigue, as well as improvement in sleep quality. Additionally, children reported improved functional ability and had fewer school absences.[52]

Pharmacologic Treatment

Clinical studies demonstrated the effectiveness of the alpha-2-delta ligands (gabapentin and pregabalin) and the norepinephrine serotonin reuptake inhibitors (duloxetine and milnacipran) in FM in adults.[53] In children who have FM, however, there have been no well-controlled, systematic studies of drugs. Analgesics and nonsteroidal antiinflammatory drugs are not very effective. There are only limited data for the efficacy of cyclobenzaprine and amitriptyline.[54] No data are available on the effect of SSRIs and SNRIs in pediatric FM.

Treatment of pediatric FM should begin with nonpharmacologic modalities, including education and reassurance, exercise treatment, and CBT.

Outcome

There are limited data on the outcome and prognosis of juvenile FM. Although a few studies have suggested a poor prognosis,[9,55] our and others' experience does not corroborate those results.[13,14,56] The authors assessed the outcome of FM in a 30-month follow-up study of children who have FM.[56] After 30 months, 73% of the children who had FM were no longer fibromyalgic. The mean point count significantly decreased from 12.5 to 4.6 ($P<.001$) and the mean tenderness threshold of nine tender sites increased from 2.4 to 3.4 kg ($P<.01$). We have concluded that the outcome of FM in children is more favorable than in adults. Siegel and colleagues[13] found that the majority of pediatric patients who have FM improved over 2 to 3 years of follow-up. Gedalia and colleagues[14] reported that 60% of children who have FM who were available for follow-up at 18 months had improved.

More follow-up studies of children who have FM are needed to clarify long-term outcomes of this syndrome.

SUMMARY

Pediatric FM has been less studied than FM in adults, although the clinical features of FM in children are similar to those in adults. The outcome of pediatric FM, however, is more favorable than in adults. Management of pediatric FM should begin with non-pharmacologic modalities, including education and reassurance, exercise treatment, and psychologic interventions. No systematic studies assessing the efficacy of drugs in pediatric FM are available; therefore, controlled, well-designed studies are needed to assess the prevalence, outcome, and efficacy of drugs in pediatric FM.

REFERENCES

1. Ablin J, Neumann L, Buskila D. Pathogenesis of fibromyalgia—a review. Joint Bone Spine 2008;75(3):273–9.
2. Gedalia A, Press J, Buskila D. Diffuse musculoskeletal pain syndromes in pediatric practice. J Clin Rheumatol 1996;2(6):325–30.
3. Buskila D, Press J, Gedalia A, et al. Assessment of nonartricular tenderness and prevalence of fibromyalgia in children. J Rheumatol 1993;20(2):368–70.
4. Smythe HA, Lee D, Rush P, et al. Tender shins and steroid therapy. J Rheumatol 1991;18(10):1568–72.
5. Sardini S, Ghirardini M, Betelemme L, et al. Epidemiological study of a primary fibromyalgia in pediatric age (article in Italian). Minerva Pediatr 1996;48(2): 543–50.
6. Clark P, Burgos-Vargas R, Medina-Palma C, et al. Prevalence of fibromyalgia in children: a clinical study of Mexican children. J Rheumatol 1998;25(10):2009–14.
7. Buskila D, Neumann L, Press J, et al. Assessment of nonarticular tenderness of children in different ethnic groups. J Musculoskeletal Pain 1995;3(2):83–90.
8. Mikkelsson M, Sourander A, Piha J, et al. Psychiatric symptoms in preadolescents with musculoskeletal pain and fibromyalgia. Pediatrics 1997;100(2 Pt 1):220–7.
9. Malleson PN, al-Matar M, Petty RE. Idiopathic musculoskeletal syndromes in children. J Rheumatol 1992;19(11):1786–9.
10. Yunus MB, Masi AT. Juvenile primary fibromyalgia syndrome. A clinical study of thirty-three patients and matched normal controls. Arthritis Rheum 1985;28(2): 138–45.
11. Wolfe F, Smythe HA, Yunus MB, et al. The American College of Rheumatology 1990 criteria for the classification of fibromyalgia. Report of the multicenter criteria committee. Arthritis Rheum 1990;33(2):160–72.
12. Neumann L, Smythe HA, Buskila D. Performance of point count and dolorimetry in assessing nonarticular tenderness in children. J Musculoskeletal Pain 1996; 4(2):29–35.
13. Siegel DM, Janeway D, Braun J. Fibromyalgia syndrome in children and adolescents: clinical features at presentation and status at follow up. Pediatrics 1998; 101(3pt1):377–82.
14. Gedalia A, Garcia CO, Molina JF, et al. Fibromyalgia syndrome: experience in a pediatric rheumatology clinic. Clin Exp Rheumatol 2000;18(3):415–9.
15. Bell DS, Bell KM, Cheney PR. Primary juvenile fibromyalgia syndrome and chronic fatigue syndrome in adolescents. Clin Infect Dis 1994;18(Suppl 1): S21–3.
16. Gracely RH, Petzke F, Wolf JM, et al. Functional magnetic resonance imaging evidence of augmented pain processing in fibromyalgia. Arthritis Rheum 2002; 46(5):1333–43.
17. Staud R, Vierck CJ, Cannon RL, et al. Abnormal sensitization and temporal summation of second pain (wind up) in patients with fibromyalgia syndrome. Pain 2001;91(1–2):165–75.

18. Malleson PN, Connell H, Bennett SM, et al. Chronic musculoskeletal and other idiopathic pain syndromes. Arch Dis Child 2001;84(3):189–92.
19. Roizenblatt S, Tufik S, Goldenberg J, et al. Juvenile fibromyalgia: clinical and polysomnographic aspects. J Rheumatol 1997;24(3):579–85.
20. Tayag-Kier CE, Keenan GF, Scalzi LV, et al. Sleep and periodic limb movement in sleep in juvenile fibromyalgia. Pediatrics 2000;106(5):E70.
21. Imbierowicz K, Egle UT. Childhood adversities in patients with fibromyalgia and somatoform pain disorder. Eur J Pain 2003;7(2):113–9.
22. Raphael KG, Chandler HK, Ciccone DS. Is childhood abuse a risk factor for chronic pain in adulthood? Curr Pain Headache Rep 2004;8(2):99–110.
23. Ciccone DS, Elliott DK, Chandler HK, et al. Sexual and physical abuse in women with fibromyalgia syndrome: a test of the trauma hypothesis. Clin J pain 2005; 21(5):378–86.
24. Russell IJ, Raphael KG. Fibromyalgia syndrome: presentation, diagnosis, differential diagnosis, and vulnerability. CNS Spectr 2008;13(3 Suppl 5):6–11.
25. Buskila D, Neumann L, Press J. Genetic factors in neuromuscular pain. CNS Spectr 2005;10(4):281–4.
26. Buskila D, Neumann L. Genetics of fibromyalgia. Curr Pain Headache Rep 2005; 9(3):313–5.
27. Buskila D. Genetics of chronic pain states. Best Pract Res Clin Rheumatol 2007; 21(3):535–47.
28. Buskila D, Neumann L, Hazanov I, et al. Familial aggregation in the fibromyalgia syndrome. Semin Arthritis Rheum 1996;26(3):605–11.
29. Buskila D, Neumann L. Fibromyalgia syndrome (FM) and nonarticular tenderness in relatives of patients with FM. J Rheumatol 1997;24(5):941–4.
30. Arnold LM, Hudson JI, Hess EV, et al. Family study of fibromyalgia. Arthritis Rheum 2004;50(3):944–52.
31. Cohen H, Buskila D, Neumann L, et al. Confirmation of an association between fibromyalgia and serotonin transporter promoter region (5HTTLPR) polymorphism, and relationship to anxiety related personality traits. Arthritis Rheum 2002;46(3):845–7.
32. Buskila D, Cohen H, Neumann L, et al. An association between fibromyalgia and the dopamine D4 receptor exon III repeat polymorphism and relationship to novelty seeking personality traits. Mol Psychiatry 2004;9(8):730–1.
33. Vargas-Alarcon G, Fragoso JM, Gruz Robles D, et al. Catechol-O-methyltransferanse gene haployotpes in Mexican and Spanish patients with fibromyalgia. Arthritis Res Ther 2007;9(5):R110.
34. Gedalia A, Press J, Klein M, et al. Joint hypermobility and fibromyalgia in schoolchildren. Ann Rheum Dis 1993;52(7):494–6.
35. Hudson N, Starr MR, Esdaile JM, et al. Diagnostic associations with hypermobility in rheumatology patients. Br J Rheumatol 1995;34(12):1157–61.
36. Hakim AJ, Grahame R. Non-musculoskeletal symptoms in joint hypermobility syndrome. Indirect evidence for autonomic dysfunction. Rheumatology 2004; 43(9):1194–5.
37. Uziel Y, Hashkes PJ. Growing pains in children. (Article in Hebrew). Harefuah 2008;147(10):809–11.
38. Hashkes PJ, Friedland O, Jaber L, et al. Decreased pain threshold in children with growing pains. J Rheumatol 2004;31(3):610–3.
39. Taddio A, Katz J, Ilersich AL, et al. Effect of neonatal circumcision on pain response during subsequent routine vaccination. Lancet 1997;349(9052): 599–603.

40. Buskila D, Neumann L, Zmora E, et al. Pain sensitivity in prematurely born adolescents. Arch Pediatr Adolesc Med 2003;157(11):1079–82.
41. Phillips DIW, Jones A. Fetal programming of autonomic and HPA function: do people who were small babies have enhanced stress response? J Physiol 2006;572(Pt 1):45–50.
42. Conte PM, Walco GA, Kimura Y. Temperament and stress response in children with juvenile primary fibromyalgia syndrome. Arthritis Rheum 2003;48(10): 2923–30.
43. Kashikar-Zuck S, Lynch AM, Slater S, et al. Family factors, emotional functioning, and functional impairment in juvenile fibromyalgia syndrome. Arthritis Rheum 2008;59(10):1392–8.
44. Kashikar-Zuck S, Parkins IS, Graham TP, et al. Anxiety, mood, and behavioral disorders among pediatric patients with juvenile fibromyalgia syndrome. Clin J Pain 2008;24(7):620–6.
45. Kashikar-Zuck S, Lynch AM, Graham TB, et al. Social functioning and peer relationships of adolescents with juvenile fibromyalgia syndrome. Arthritis Rheum 2007;57(3):474–80.
46. Pfeiffer A, Thompson JM, Nelson A, et al. Effects of a 1.5 day multidisciplinary out patient treatment program for fibromyalgia: a pilot study. Am J Phys Med Rehabil 2003;82(3):186–91.
47. Jones KD, Adams D, Winters-Stone K, et al. A comprehensive review of 46 exercise treatment studies in fibromyalgia (1988–2005). Health Qual Life Outcomes 2006;4:67.
48. Stephens S, Feldman BM, Bradley N, et al. Feasibility and effectiveness of aerobic exercise program in children with fibromyalgia: results of a randomized controlled pilot trial. Arthritis Rheum 2008;59(10):1399–406.
49. Ottolini MC, Hamburger EK, Loprieato Jo, et al. Complementary and alternative medicine use among children in the Washington, DC, area. Ambul Pediatr 2001;1(2):122–5.
50. Tsao JC, Meldrum M, Kim SC, et al. Treatment preferences for CAM in children with chronic pain. Evid Based Complement Alternat Med 2007;4(3):367–74.
51. Thieme K, Flor H, Turk DC. Psychological pain treatment in fibromyalgia syndromes: efficacy of operant behavioral and cognitive behavioral treatment. Arthritis Res Ther 2006;8(4):R121.
52. Degotardi PJ, Klass ES, Rosenberg BS, et al. Development and evaluation of a cognitive behavioral intervention for juvenile fibromyalgia. J Pediatr Psychol 2006;31(7):714–23.
53. Crofford LJ. Pain management in fibromyalgia. Curr Opin Rheumatol 2008;20(3): 246–50.
54. Romano TJ. Fibromyalgia in children, diagnosis and treatment. W V Med J 1991; 87(3):112–4.
55. Rabinovich CE. A follow-up study of pediatric fibromyalgia patients. Arthritis Rheum 1990;33:S146.
56. Buskila D, Neumann L, Hershman E, et al. Fibromyalgia syndrome in children—an outcome study. J Rheumatol 1995;22(3):525–8.

Abnormal Pain Modulation in Patients with Spatially Distributed Chronic Pain: Fibromyalgia

Roland Staud, MD

KEYWORDS

- Modulation • Fibromyalgia • Chronic pain
- Diffuse noxious inhibitory control • Analgesia

Population surveys estimate the prevalence of chronic pain in the United States at more than 45% of the general population,[1] with minimal recovery rates over 4-year follow-up periods.[2] Furthermore, the total cost of chronic pain is estimated at more than 100 billion dollars annually.[3] Rheumatologists are frequently involved in the treatment of chronic pain syndromes, including various neuropathic and musculoskeletal pain syndromes, such as complex regional pain syndrome, postherpetic neuralgia (PHN), headache, facial pain, back pain, chronic fatigue syndrome, and fibromyalgia (FM), in addition to the painful aspects of such conditions as rheumatoid arthritis and osteoarthritis.

Although many chronic pain syndromes are defined by their anatomic location, they often share similar pathophysiologic mechanisms.[4,5] Many patients who have chronic pain syndromes (eg, FM, chronic headache, low back pain [LBP], temporomandibular disorder [TMD]) report insidious onsets, and their physical findings are often poor predictors of their symptoms, specifically pain. Similarly, easily apparent tissue damage (eg, in patients who have osteoarthritis, PHN, chronic postsurgical pain) often bears only a modest relation to reported symptoms, including pain. Thus, interindividual differences in pain sensitivity seem to play an important role for clinical pain, which is best illustrated by many patients who have PHN, postsurgical pain, or severe osteoarthritis and present with a similar extent of tissue damage but may have no pain at all or severe disabling pain. Such discrepancies in pain sensitivity suggest profound differences in pain processing of noxious stimulation.

Continuing nociceptive input can have many biologic, psychologic, and functional consequences, ranging from receptor modification and central sensitization to

Department of Medicine, University of Florida College of Medicine, PO Box 100221, Gainesville, FL 32610–0221, USA
E-mail address: staudr@ufl.edu

Rheum Dis Clin N Am 35 (2009) 263–274
doi:10.1016/j.rdc.2009.05.006
0889-857X/09/$ – see front matter © 2009 Elsevier Inc. All rights reserved.

depressed affect, inappropriate cognition, and social disruption. Thus, a persistent pain state may represent a disease entity in its own right.[6] Like any disease, the extent of experienced symptoms is greatly influenced by internal and external factors, particularly the environment; in other words, genetic, psychologic, and social factors strongly contribute to the perception and severity of persistent pain. Therefore persistent pain states cannot be defined solely by their associated tissue damage but are influenced by many other relevant contributors. Several characteristic features of many patients who have chronic pain are of special importance. First, there is substantial overlap among many pain conditions,[7] suggesting common pathophysiologic mechanisms. Second, many chronic pain syndromes are characterized by hyperalgesia and abnormal endogenous pain inhibition.[8] These pain conditions are often associated with secondary hyperalgesia at sites distant from the affected area, suggesting sensitization of the central nervous system (CNS) (eg, diabetic neuropathy, PHN).[9]

Individual differences in endogenous pain modulation may place people at increased or reduced risk for the development of chronic pain (eg, FM pain, headache, visceral pain); specifically, individuals who are highly sensitive to pain and who show the lowest degree of endogenous pain inhibition may be at greater risk for the onset and persistence of chronic pain.

INTERINDIVIDUAL DIFFERENCES OF PAIN IN ANIMALS AND HUMANS

Individual differences in the perception and modulation of pain have been reported in animals[10] and humans.[11,12] Most commonly, pain sensitivity is evaluated by psychophysical testing, including mechanical, thermal, and electrical threshold and suprathreshold stimuli.[13] Subjects usually rate the pain intensity of the stimulus using a validated pain rating scale, such as the visual analog scale[14] or the numeric pain scale.[14] Endogenous pain modulation can be assessed with phasic or tonic heat stimuli, by spatial summation,[15] or by simultaneous administering two noxious stimuli (counterirritation or diffuse noxious inhibitory controls [DNICs]) and measuring the resultant pain inhibition ("pain inhibits pain").[16,17] Importantly, high pain sensitivity and low endogenous pain inhibition have been observed in many patients who have chronic pain syndromes like FM.[18] Whereas pain thresholds and endogenous analgesia show only minor correlations,[19] the combination of high pain sensitivity with low endogenous pain inhibition seems to confer cumulative risk. Overall, individual differences in endogenous pain inhibition are better predictors of future chronic pain than increased pain sensitivity.[20]

WHAT ARE THE MECHANISMS FOR INDIVIDUAL DIFFERENCES IN PAIN SENSITIVITY?

The measures described previously are important indexes of CNS pain processing. Because pain is actively modulated by the nervous system at multiple levels of the pain pathways, testing individual differences in the endogenous modulation of pain is crucial for understanding the variability of pain responses.[21] Well-defined psychophysical methods, including heat and pressure stimuli, have been increasingly used to characterize interindividual differences in pain sensitivity.[12]

Individual differences in pain responses are normally distributed in the general population[22,23] and reflect a combination of genetic and environmental factors related to CNS pain processing. Human twin studies found heritability estimates for pain sensitivity ranging from 22% to 55% for several different pain stimuli.[24] Of specific interest were genetic effects on pain sensitivity, which explained 60% of the variance in cold-pressor pain and 26% of the variance in contact-heat pain. Importantly, there were distinct genetic and environmental factors influencing these two pain modalities. Only 6% of the variance in cold-pressor pain and 3% of the variance in heat pain were attributable to genetic factors that were common to both pain modalities. Similarly, only 5% of the variance in cold-pressor pain and 8% of the variance in heat pain were attributable to environmental factors that were common to both pain modalities.

Furthermore, genetic studies in human subjects show that single-nucleotide polymorphisms of several pain-related genes significantly contribute to basal pain sensitivity, including polymorphisms of the μ- and δ-opioid receptor genes,[25,26] the catechol-O-methyltransferase (COMT) gene,[27] and the guanosine triphosphatase (GTP) cyclohydrolase-1 gene.[28] These findings are supported by rodent studies,[29] which also emphasize the important effects of pain genes on sensitivity to noxious stimuli[29] and on analgesia.[30] Environmental influences can strongly influence pain sensitivity in animals and humans.[31] In particular, exposure to strong and prolonged pain[32] seems to alter individuals' subsequent pain sensitivity and increases their risk for more severe acute pain[33] and chronic pain.[34–37]

In addition to genetic and environmental factors, pain sensitivity is influenced by cognitive factors, such as catastrophizing. Specifically, high levels of catastrophizing seem to be associated with lower pain thresholds[38] and enhanced pain-related brain activation.[39] Therefore, individual differences in pain responsiveness may not only reflect the influence of genetic and environmental factors but may have an impact on an individual's risk for developing a variety of persistent pain conditions, including FM.

ACUTE PAIN INTENSITY AS A PREDICTOR OF CHRONIC PAIN

Several studies provide evidence that high preoperative pain sensitivity can be used to predict postoperative pain, particularly pain related to cesarean section,[20] hysterectomy,[40] limb amputation,[41] and cholecystectomy.[42] Experimental pain responses before surgery significantly predicted the magnitude of postoperative pain for several weeks after surgery. Specifically, patients who were highly sensitive to noxious heat or cold stimuli reported more severe pain after cesarean section.[20] These patients' preoperative ratings of noxious heat stimuli predicted more than 50% of the variance in their postoperative pain. This study also showed that suprathreshold heat stimuli seem to have clinical relevance as predictors of postsurgical pain.[13] Severe acute pain has been consistently demonstrated as a risk factor for the development of chronic pain after injury. For example, more than 50% of patients develop chronic pain syndromes after spinal cord injury or herpes zoster infection.[43,44] High pain ratings after surgery, such as mastectomy, cholecystectomy, amputation, thoracotomy, herniorrhaphy, prostatectomy, and total knee arthroplasty, also seem to increase the risk for developing persistent pain syndromes.[43,45–47] Some of the possible mechanisms contributing to future chronic pain may involve sensitization of the CNS[43] and inadequate pain modulation. Specifically, high pain sensitivity seems to predispose individuals to higher levels of acute pain after tissue trauma, resulting in sensitization of the CNS and subsequent chronic pain.

Several studies of healthy adults who were free of chronic pain demonstrated a significant relation between increased pain sensitivity and frequent pain complaints, such as headaches, backaches, and muscle aches, and impaired functional status.[48–50] These highly sensitive individuals not only rated noxious thermal stimuli as more painful[48] but showed the lowest levels of pain tolerance,[50] the greatest temporal summation of pain (central sensitization),[49] and the lowest levels of endogenous pain inhibition.[19] Similarly, high sensitivity to experimental pain also predicted more clinical pain and lower levels of physical functioning in patients who had chronic pain.[51,52]

VARIABILITY OF ANALGESIC RESPONSES

In animals and humans, the effect of genetic factors on pain sensitivity and analgesia seems to be moderate.[10,12,53,54] There seems to be a strong relation between high pain sensitivity and low analgesic responsiveness to opioid analgesics in animals[29,55,56] and humans, however, particularly in men.[57] These findings suggest concordance between high pain sensitivity and reduced analgesic responsiveness, both of which may predispose individuals to chronic pain while making them insensitive to opioid therapy.

PREDICTOR FOR NEW-ONSET CHRONIC MUSCULOSKELETAL PAIN

Most research on risk factors for new-onset chronic musculoskeletal pain has been done in patients with LBP[58] or knee pain.[59] Mechanical factors, including lifting and pulling heavy weights, seem to be important predictors of new-onset LBP and knee pain. Psychosocial and physical environment factors also seem to predict future pain significantly in both conditions, including monotonous work and poor working conditions. Work-related psychosocial and environmental factors seem to be most relevant in predicting new symptom onset, however.

Few studies have addressed the interaction of genetic or environmental factors with future FM pain.[60,61] One case-controlled study of previously healthy individuals found that 22% of patients with neck injury and 2% of patients with leg injury developed FM 1 year after a motor vehicle accident,[62] suggesting that neck trauma increases the risk for FM more than 10-fold in predisposed patients. Using individual differences in pain sensitivity as a predictor of new-onset TMD, a recent prospective study followed a large number of pain-free female participants over 3 years,[27] detecting new-onset TMD in 7.43% of study participants who were not only highly pain sensitive at study entry but shared mutations of the COMT gene (high or average pain sensitivity haplotype). Because of considerable overlap between TMD and FM, the results of this study suggest that similar genetic mutations may also contribute to the risk for future FM in predisposed individuals. Thus, multiple lines of evidence indicate that increased pain sensitivity may increase individuals' risk for the development of future chronic pain, including FM.

ABNORMAL PAIN MODULATION OF PATIENTS WHO HAVE FIBROMYALGIA

Several studies have provided psychophysical evidence that pain processing is abnormal in patients who have FM,[63–68] showing that perceived pain from experimental stimuli (mechanical, heat, cold, or electricity) was greater for patients who had FM compared with normal controls, as was the amount of temporal summation of pain or wind-up (WU) within a series of heat stimuli (**Fig. 1**). WU was used as a noninvasive method of assessing C-fiber–dependent central sensitization in human subjects. After multiple stimuli, WU aftersensations were greater in magnitude, lasted longer, and were more frequently painful in subjects who had FM. These results indicate augmentation and prolonged decay of nociceptive input in patients who have FM and provide convincing evidence for central sensitization in this syndrome. A couple of points related to central sensitization seem relevant for understanding FM pain. First, when central sensitization has occurred in patients who have chronic pain, including patients who have FM, little additional nociceptive input is required to maintain the

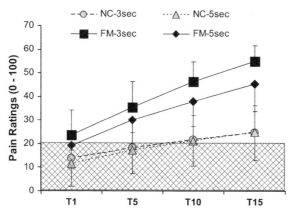

Fig. 1. WU pain ratings of normal controls (NC) and patients who have FM. All subjects received 15 mechanical stimuli to the adductor pollicis muscles of the hands at interstimulatory intervals (ISIs) of 3 and 5 seconds. The patients who have FM showed mechanical hyperalgesia during the first tap and greater temporal summation than the NC at both ISIs. A numeric pain scale was used (range: 0–100). The shaded area represents the pain threshold. T, mechanical tap.

sensitized state. Thus, seemingly innocuous daily activities may contribute to the maintenance of the chronic pain state. Second, the decay of painful sensations is prolonged in FM; therefore, patients may not experience robust changes in their pain levels during brief therapeutic interventions. Many frequently used analgesic medications do not improve central sensitization, and some medications, including opioids, have been shown to maintain or even worsen this CNS phenomenon.[69,70] Nevertheless, there is evidence that the antiepileptic drug pregabalin, which was recently approved for the treatment of FM, can reduce central sensitization.[71]

WIND-UP MEASURES AS PREDICTORS OF FIBROMYALGIA PAIN INTENSITY

The important role of central pain mechanisms for clinical pain is also supported by their usefulness as predictors of clinical pain intensity of patients who have FM. Heat WU ratings correlate well with clinical pain intensity (Peason's $r = 0.53$), thus emphasizing the important role of this pain mechanism for FM. In addition, hierarchic regression models that include tender point count, pain-related negative affect, and WU ratings have been shown to account for 50% of the variance in FM clinical pain intensity.[72]

MECHANISMS UNDERLYING ABNORMAL PAIN SENSITIVITY IN FIBROMYALGIA

The mechanisms underlying the central sensitization that occurs in patients who have FM relies on hyperexcitability of the spinal dorsal horn neurons that transmit nociceptive input to the brain. As a consequence, low-intensity stimuli delivered to the skin or deep muscle tissue generate high levels of nociceptive input to the brain in addition to the perception of pain. Specifically, intense or prolonged impulse input from A-δ and C afferents sufficiently depolarizes the dorsal horn neurons and results in the removal of the Mg^{2+} block of N-methyl-D-aspartate (NMDA)–gated ion channels. This is followed by the influx of extracellular Ca^{2+} and production of nitric oxide, which diffuses out of the dorsal horn neurons.[73] Nitric oxide, in turn, promotes the exaggerated release of excitatory amino acids and substance P from presynaptic afferent terminals and causes the dorsal horn neurons to become hyperexcitable.[74] Subsequently, low-intensity stimuli evoked by minor physical activity may be amplified in the spinal cord, resulting in painful sensations.[75]

ROLE OF GLIA IN CENTRAL SENSITIZATION

Accumulating evidence suggests that dorsal horn glia cells might have an important role in producing and maintaining abnormal pain sensitivity.[76,77] Synapses within the CNS are encapsulated by glia that do not normally respond to nociceptive input from local sites. After the initiation of central sensitization, however, spinal glia cells are activated by a wide array of factors that contribute to hyperalgesia, such as immune activation within the spinal cord, substance P, excitatory amino acids, nitric oxide, and prostaglandins. Precipitating events known to induce glial activation include viral infections, such as HIV, hepatitis C, and influenza.[78] Once activated, glia cells release proinflammatory cytokines, including tumor necrosis factor (TNF), interleukin (IL)-6 and IL-1, substance P, nitric oxide, prostaglandins, excitatory amino acids, ATP, and fractalkine,[79] which, in turn, further increase the discharge of excitatory amino acids and substance P from the A-δ and C afferents that synapse in the dorsal horn and also enhance the hyperexcitability of the dorsal horn neurons.[76,80] Recent evidence also points toward a possible role of NMDA receptors in glial activation and pain.[81]

POSSIBLE CAUSES OF CENTRAL SENSITIZATION IN FIBROMYALGIA

As a normal response to tissue trauma, injury is followed by repair and healing. Inflammation occurs, which results in a cascade of electrophysiologic and chemical events that resolve over time, and the patient becomes pain-free. In persistent pain, however, the local, spinal, and even supraspinal responses are considerably different from those that occur during acute pain. Although defining the relation between tissue events and pain is necessary for understanding the clinical context of these pathologic conditions, defining the relation between injury and specific and relevant nociceptive responses is crucial for understanding the central mechanisms of persistent pain in FM. It must be emphasized, however, that specific abnormalities have not been identified in persons who have FM that might produce the prolonged impulse input necessary to initiate the events underlying the development of central sensitization or spinal glia cell activation. After central sensitization has occurred, low-threshold A-β afferents, which normally do not serve to transmit a pain response, are recruited to transmit spontaneous and movement-induced pain. This central hyperexcitability is characterized by a WU response of repetitive C-fiber stimulation, expanding receptive field areas, and spinal neurons taking on properties of wide dynamic range neurons.[82] Ultimately, A-β fibers stimulate postsynaptic neurons to transmit pain, whereas these A-β fibers previously had no role in pain transmission, all leading to central sensitization. Nociceptive information is transmitted from the spinal cord to supraspinal sites, such as the thalamus and cerebral cortex, by ascending pathways.

MUSCLE TISSUE AS A SOURCE OF NOCICEPTIVE INPUT

A potential source of nociceptive input that might account for FM pain is muscle tissue.[83] Several types of muscle abnormalities have been reported in patients who have FM, including the appearance of ragged-red fibers, inflammatory infiltrates, and moth-eaten fibers.[84–86] Possible mechanisms for such muscle changes might include repetitive muscle microtrauma, which could contribute to the postexertional pain and other painful symptoms experienced by these patients. In addition, prolonged muscle tension and ischemia were found in muscles of patients who had FM.[87–89] Changes in muscle pH related to ischemia[90] might provide a powerful mechanisms for the sensitization of spinal and supraspinal pain pathways.[91] Investigations using ^{31}P nuclear magnetic resonance (NMR) spectroscopy have shown that patients who have FM display significantly lower phosphorylation potential and total oxidative capacity in the quadriceps muscle during rest and exercise.[92] Patients who have FM also exhibit significantly lower levels of muscle phosphocreatine and ATP, in addition to a lower phosphocreatine/inorganic phosphate ratio.[84,85] Furthermore, NMR testing of muscles in patients who had FM showed an increased prevalence of phosphodiester peaks, which have been associated with sarcolemmal membrane damage.[92,93]

Focal muscle abnormalities, including trigger points (TrPs), are frequently detectable in patients who have FM and may play an important role as pain generators. Using sensitive microdialysis techniques, concentrations of protons, bradykinin, calcitonin gene-related peptide, substance P, TNFα, IL-1b, serotonin, and norepinephrine have been found to be significantly higher in TrPs of patients who have myofascial pain than in normal muscle tissue.[94,95] Recent studies have shown that advanced glycation end products (AGEs) may also be relevant for FM pain. AGEs can trigger the synthesis of cytokines, particularly IL-1b and TNFα, and elevated AGE levels have been detected in interstitial connective tissue of muscles and in serum of patients who have FM.[96] All these biochemical mediators can sensitize muscle nociceptors, and thus indirectly contribute to central sensitization and chronic pain. Because nociceptive input from muscles is powerful in inducing and maintaining central sensitization,[97] FM muscle abnormalities may strongly contribute to pain through the important mechanism of pain amplification.

SUMMARY

Many different factors seem to contribute to current pain in patients who have chronic pain and may affect previously healthy individuals' risk for future musculoskeletal pain. These factors include individual variability of pain-facilitatory and analgesic mechanisms, such as temporal summation and analgesia from counterirritation (DNICs). Such individual differences in pain sensitivity or modulation can be readily assessed in the laboratory and could be used as sensitive biomarkers of current pain sensitivity and risk factors for future chronic pain. Which specific abnormalities, however, are critical for maintenance of the chronic pain state is unclear at this time. They most likely include a host of psychologic and physical stressors. There is accumulating evidence for genetic risk factors for chronic pain, specifically COMT and GTP cyclohydrolase-1 polymorphisms, which may interfere with pain modulation in patients who have chronic pain, including those who have FM. Because the effectiveness of treatments for chronic musculoskeletal pain is limited at this time, emphasis should be placed on prevention or modification of risk factors that may result in worsening of current pain and the occurrence of future chronic pain disorders. Specifically, highly pain-sensitive individuals should be identified, evaluated, and counseled about risk modifications for future chronic pain. Psychophysical test methods, including WU and DNICs, play an increasingly important role in the assessment of patients who have chronic pain and may become useful biomarkers for individual pain sensitivity and the ability to modulate pain.

REFERENCES

1. Elliott AM, Smith BH, Penny KI, et al. The epidemiology of chronic pain in the community. Lancet 1999;354(9186):1248–52.
2. Elliott AM, Smith BH, Hannaford PC, et al. The course of chronic pain in the community: results of a 4-year follow-up study. Pain 2002;99(1–2):299–307.
3. Turk DC. Clinical effectiveness and cost-effectiveness of treatments for patients with chronic pain. Clin J Pain 2002;18(6):355–65.
4. Max MB. Is mechanism-based pain treatment attainable? Clinical trial issues. J Pain 2000;1(Suppl 3):2–9.
5. Woolf CJ, Max MB. Mechanism-based pain diagnosis: issues for analgesic drug development. Anesthesiology 2001;95(1):241–9.
6. Siddall PJ, Cousins MJ. Persistent pain as a disease entity: implications for clinical management. Anesth Analg 2004;99(2):510–20.
7. Aaron LA, Burke MM, Buchwald D. Overlapping conditions among patients with chronic fatigue syndrome, fibromyalgia, and temporomandibular disorder. Arch Intern Med 2000;160(2):221–7.
8. Peters ML, Schmidt AJ, van den Hout MA. Chronic low back pain and the reaction to repeated acute pain stimulation. Pain 1989;39(1):69–76.
9. Sommer C. Painful neuropathies. Curr Opin Neurol 2003;16(5):623–8.
10. Mogil JS. The genetic mediation of individual differences in sensitivity to pain and its inhibition. Proc Natl Acad Sci U S A 1999;96(14):7744–51.
11. MacGregor AJ. The heritability of pain in humans. In: Mogil JS, editor. The genetics of pain. Progress in pain research and management, vol. 28. Seattle: IASP Press; 2004. p. 154–70.
12. Nielsen CS, Staud R, Price DD. Individual differences in pain sensitivity: measurement, causation, and consequences. J Pain 2009;10(3):231–7.
13. Edwards RR, Sarlani E, Wesselmann U, et al. Quantitative assessment of experimental pain perception: multiple domains of clinical relevance. Pain 2005;114(3):315–9.
14. Price DD, Patel R, Robinson ME, et al. Characteristics of electronic visual analogue and numeric scales for ratings of experimental pain in healthy subjects and fibromyalgia patients. Pain 2008;140:158–66.
15. Staud R, Vierck CJ, Robinson ME, et al. Spatial summation of heat pain within and across dermatomes in fibromyalgia patients and pain-free subjects. Pain 2004;111(3):342–50.
16. Edwards RR, Fillingim RB, Ness TJ. Age-related differences in endogenous pain modulation: a comparison of diffuse noxious inhibitory controls in healthy older and younger adults. Pain 2003;101(1–2):155–65.
17. Staud R, Robinson ME, Vierck CJ, et al. Diffuse noxious inhibitory controls (DNIC) attenuate temporal summation of second pain in normal males but not in normal females or fibromyalgia patients. Pain 2003;101:167–74.
18. Lautenbacher S, Rollman GB. Possible deficiencies of pain modulation in fibromyalgia. Clin J Pain 1997;13(3):189–96.
19. Edwards RR, Ness TJ, Weigent DA, et al. Individual differences in diffuse noxious inhibitory controls (DNIC): association with clinical variables. Pain 2003;106(3):427–37.
20. Granot M, Lowenstein L, Yarnitsky D, et al. Postcesarean section pain prediction by preoperative experimental pain assessment. Anesthesiology 2003;98(6):1422–6.
21. Edwards RR. Individual differences in endogenous pain modulation as a risk factor for chronic pain. Neurology 2005;65(3):437–43.

22. Gracely RH, Grant MAB, Giesecke T. Evoked pain measures in fibromyalgia. Best Pract Res Clin Rheumatol 2003;17(4):593–609.
23. Yarnitsky D, Sprecher E, Zaslansky R, et al. Heat pain thresholds: normative data and repeatability. Pain 1995;60(3):329–32.
24. Nielsen CS, Stubhaug A, Price DD, et al. Individual differences in pain sensitivity: genetic and environmental contributions. Pain 2008;136(1–2):21–9.
25. Fillingim RB, Kaplan L, Staud R, et al. The A118G single nucleotide polymorphism of the mu-opioid receptor gene (OPRM1) is associated with pressure pain sensitivity in humans. J Pain 2005;6(3):159–67.
26. Kim HS, Neubert JK, Miguel AS, et al. Genetic influence on variability in human acute experimental pain sensitivity associated with gender, ethnicity and psychological temperament. Pain 2004;109(3):488–96.
27. Diatchenko L, Slade GD, Nackley AG, et al. Genetic basis for individual variations in pain perception and the development of a chronic pain condition. Hum Mol Genet 2005;14(1):135–43.
28. Tegeder I, Costigan M, Griffin RS, et al. GTP cyclohydrolase and tetrahydrobiopterin regulate pain sensitivity and persistence. Nat Med 2006;12(11):1269–77.
29. Mogil JS, Wilson SG, Bon K, et al. Heritability of nociception I: responses of 11 inbred mouse strains on 12 measures of nociception. Pain 1999;80(1–2):67–82.
30. Mogil JS, Sternberg WF, Marek P, et al. The genetics of pain and pain inhibition. Proc Natl Acad Sci U S A 1996;93(7):3048–55.
31. MacGregor AJ, Griffiths GO, Baker J, et al. Determinants of pressure pain threshold in adult twins: evidence that shared environmental influences predominate. Pain 1997;73(2):253–7.
32. Taddio A, Katz J. The effects of early pain experience in neonates on pain responses in infancy and childhood. Paediatr Drugs 2005;7(4):245–57.
33. Fillingim RB, Wilkinson CS, Powell T. Self-reported abuse history and pain complaints among young adults. Clin J Pain 1999;15(2):85–91.
34. Aaron LA, Bradley LA, Alarcon GS, et al. Perceived physical and emotional trauma as precipitating events in fibromyalgia. Associations with health care seeking and disability status but not pain severity. Arthritis Rheum 1997;40(3):453–60.
35. Goldberg RT, Goldstein R. A comparison of chronic pain patients and controls on traumatic events in childhood. Disabil Rehabil 2000;22(17):756–63.
36. Lampe A, Doering S, Rumpold G, et al. Chronic pain syndromes and their relation to childhood abuse and stressful life events. J Psychosom Res 2003;54(4):361–7.
37. Ren TH, Wu J, Yew D, et al. Effects of neonatal maternal separation on neurochemical and sensory response to colonic distension in a rat model of irritable bowel syndrome. Am J Physiol Gastrointest Liver Physiol 2007;292(3):G849–56.
38. Sullivan MJL, Thorn B, Haythornthwaite JA, et al. Theoretical perspectives on the relation between catastrophizing and pain. Clin J Pain 2001;17(1):52–64.
39. Gracely RH, Geisser ME, Giesecke T, et al. Pain catastrophizing and neural responses to pain among persons with fibromyalgia. Brain 2004;127:835–43.
40. Brandsborg B, Nikolajsen L, Hansen CT, et al. Risk factors for chronic pain after hysterectomy: a nationwide questionnaire and database study. Anesthesiology 2007;106(5):1003–12.
41. Nikolajsen L, Ilkjaer S, Jensen TS. Relationship between mechanical sensitivity and postamputation pain: a prospective study. Eur J Pain 2000;4(4):327–34.
42. Bisgaard T, Kehlet H, Rosenberg J. Pain and convalescence after laparoscopic cholecystectomy. Eur J Surg 2001;167(2):84–96.
43. Perkins FM, Kehlet H. Chronic pain as an outcome of surgery. A review of predictive factors. Anesthesiology 2000;93(4):1123–33.

44. Putzke JD, Richards JS, Hicken BL, et al. Interference due to pain following spinal cord injury: important predictors and impact on quality of life. Pain 2002;100(3): 231–42.
45. Harden RN, Bruehl S, Stanos S, et al. Prospective examination of pain-related and psychological predictors of CRPS-like phenomena following total knee arthroplasty: a preliminary study. Pain 2003;106(3):393–400.
46. Stammberger U, Steinacher C, Hillinger S, et al. Early and long-term complaints following video-assisted thoracoscopic surgery: evaluation in 173 patients. Eur J Cardiothorac Surg 2000;18(1):7–11.
47. Widerstrom-Noga EG, Felipe-Cuervo E, Yezierski RP. Relationships among clinical characteristics of chronic pain after spinal cord injury. Arch Phys Med Rehabil 2001;82(9):1191–7.
48. Edwards RR, Fillingim RB. Ethnic differences in thermal pain responses. Psychosom Med 1999;61(3):346–54.
49. Edwards RR, Fillingim RB. Effects of age on temporal summation and habituation of thermal pain: clinical relevance in healthy older and younger adults. J Pain 2001;2(6):307–17.
50. Fillingim RB, Edwards RR, Powell T. The relationship of sex and clinical pain to experimental pain responses. Pain 1999;83(3):419–25.
51. Clauw DJ, Williams D, Lauerman W, et al. Pain sensitivity as a correlate of clinical status in individuals with chronic low back pain. Spine 1999;24(19):2035–41.
52. Edwards RR, Doleys DM, Fillingim RB, et al. Ethnic differences in pain tolerance: clinical implications in a chronic pain population. Psychosom Med 2001;63(2): 316–23.
53. Lariviere WR, Chesler EJ, Mogil JS. Transgenic studies of pain and analgesia: mutation or background genotype? J Pharmacol Exp Ther 2001;297(2): 467–73.
54. Lariviere WR, Wilson SG, Laughlin TM, et al. Heritability of nociception. III. Genetic relationships among commonly used assays of nociception and hypersensitivity. Pain 2002;97(1–2):75–86.
55. Elmer GI, Pieper JO, Negus SS, et al. Genetic variance in nociception and its relationship to the potency of morphine-induced analgesia in thermal and chemical tests. Pain 1998;75(1):129–40.
56. Mogil JS, Wilson SG, Bon K, et al. Heritability of nociception II. 'Types' of nociception revealed by genetic correlation analysis. Pain 1999;80(1–2):83–93.
57. Fillingim RB, Hastie BA, Ness TJ, et al. Sex-related psychological predictors of baseline pain perception and analgesic responses to pentazocine. Biol Psychol 2005;69(1):97–112.
58. Harkness EF, Macfarlane GJ, Nahit ES, et al. Risk factors for new-onset low back pain amongst cohorts of newly employed workers. Rheumatology (Oxford) 2003; 42(8):959–68.
59. Jones GT, Harkness EF, Nahit ES, et al. Predicting the onset of knee pain: results from a two year prospective study of new workers. Ann Rheum Dis 2006;doi: 10.1136/ard.2006.057570.
60. Al Allaf AW, Sanders PA, Ogston SA, et al. A case-control study examining the role of physical trauma in the onset of rheumatoid arthritis. Rheumatology 2001;40(3):262–6.
61. McLean SA, Clauw DJ, Abelson JL, et al. The development of persistent pain and psychological morbidity after motor vehicle collision: integrating the potential role of stress response systems into a biopsychosocial model. Psychosom Med 2005; 67(5):783–90.

62. Buskila D, Neumann L, Vaisberg G, et al. Increased rates of fibromyalgia following cervical spine injury. A controlled study of 161 cases of traumatic injury. Arthritis Rheum 1997;40(3):446–52.

63. Price DD, Staud R, Robinson ME, et al. Enhanced temporal summation of second pain and its central modulation in fibromyalgia patients. Pain 2002; 99:49–59.

64. Staud R. Evidence of involvement of central neural mechanisms in generating fibromyalgia pain. Curr Rheumatol Rep 2002;4(4):299–305.

65. Staud R, Domingo M. Evidence for abnormal pain processing in fibromyalgia syndrome. Pain Med 2001;2(3):208–15.

66. Staud R, Domingo M. New insights into the pathogenesis of fibromyalgia syndrome. Med Aspects Hum Sex 2001;1:51–7.

67. Staud R, Vierck CJ, Cannon RL, et al. Abnormal sensitization and temporal summation of second pain (wind-up) in patients with fibromyalgia syndrome. Pain 2001;91(1–2):165–75.

68. Vierck CJ, Staud R, Price DD, et al. The effect of maximal exercise on temporal summation of second pain (wind-up) in patients with fibromyalgia syndrome. J Pain 2001;2(6):334–44.

69. Celerier E, Rivat C, Jun Y, et al. Long-lasting hyperalgesia induced by fentanyl in rats: preventive effect of ketamine. Anesthesiology 2000;92(2):465–72.

70. Dunbar SA, Pulai IJ. Repetitive opioid abstinence causes progressive hyperalgesia sensitive to N-methyl-D-aspartate receptor blockade in the rat. J Pharmacol Exp Ther 1998;284(2):678–86.

71. Iannetti GD, Zambreanu L, Wise RG, et al. Pharmacological modulation of pain-related brain activity during normal and central sensitization states in humans. Proc Natl Acad Sci U S A 2005;102(50):18195–200.

72. Staud R, Robinson ME, Vierck CJ, et al. Ratings of experimental pain and pain-related negative affect predict clinical pain in patients with fibromyalgia syndrome. Pain 2003;105(1–2):215–22.

73. Coderre TJ, Melzack R. The role of NMDA receptor-operated calcium channels in persistent nociception after formalin-induced tissue injury. J Neurosci 1992;12(9): 3671–5.

74. Neugebauer V, Schaible HG, Weiretter F, et al. The involvement of substance P and neurokinin-1 receptors in the responses of rat dorsal horn neurons to noxious but not to innocuous mechanical stimuli applied to the knee joint. Brain Res 1994; 666(2):207–15.

75. Gracely RH, Lynch SA, Bennett GJ. Painful neuropathy: altered central processing maintained dynamically by peripheral input. Pain 1992;51(2):175–94.

76. Watkins LR, Milligan ED, Maier SF. Glial activation: a driving force for pathological pain. Trends Neurosci 2001;24(8):450–5.

77. Wieseler-Frank J, Maier SF, Watkins LR. Glial activation and pathological pain. Neurochem Int 2004;45(2–3):389–95.

78. Holguin A, O'Connor KA, Biedenkapp J, et al. HIV-1 gp120 stimulates proinflammatory cytokine-mediated pain facilitation via activation of nitric oxide synthase-1 (nNOS). Pain 2004;110(3):517–30.

79. Wieseler-Frank J, Maier SF, Watkins LR. Central proinflammatory cytokines and pain enhancement. Neurosignals 2005;14(4):166–74.

80. Watkins LR, Maier SF. When good pain turns bad. Curr Dir Psychol Sci 2003; 12(6):232–6.

81. Salter MW. Cellular signalling pathways of spinal pain neuroplasticity as targets for analgesic development. Curr Top Med Chem 2005;5(6):557–67.

82. Cook AJ, Woolf CJ, Wall PD, et al. Dynamic receptive field plasticity in rat spinal cord dorsal horn following C-primary afferent input. Nature 1987;325(7000): 151–3.
83. Henriksson KG. Is fibromyalgia a distinct clinical entity? Pain mechanisms in fibromyalgia syndrome. A myologist's view. Best Pract Res Clin Rheumatol 1999;13(3):455–61.
84. Bengtsson A, Henriksson KG, Jorfeldt L, et al. Primary fibromyalgia. A clinical and laboratory study of 55 patients. Scand J Rheumatol 1986;15(3):340–7.
85. Bengtsson A, Henriksson KG, Larsson J. Muscle biopsy in primary fibromyalgia. Light-microscopical and histochemical findings. Scand J Rheumatol 1986;15(1): 1–6.
86. Pongratz DE, Spath M. Morphologic aspects of fibromyalgia. Z Rheumatol 1998; 57:47–51.
87. Bennett RM, Clark SR, Goldberg L, et al. Aerobic fitness in patients with fibrositis. A controlled study of respiratory gas exchange and 133xenon clearance from exercising muscle. Arthritis Rheum 1989;32(4):454–60.
88. Elvin A, Siosteen AK, Nilsson A, et al. Decreased muscle blood flow in fibromyalgia patients during standardised muscle exercise: a contrast media enhanced colour Doppler study. Eur J Pain 2006;10(2):137–44.
89. Lund N, Bengtsson A, Thorborg P. Muscle tissue oxygen pressure in primary fibromyalgia. Scand J Rheumatol 1986;15(2):165–73.
90. de Kerviler E, Leroy-Willig A, Jehenson P, et al. Exercise-induced muscle modifications: study of healthy subjects and patients with metabolic myopathies with MR imaging and P-31 spectroscopy. Radiology 1991;181(1):259–64.
91. Sluka KA, Kalra A, Moore SA. Unilateral intramuscular injections of acidic saline produce a bilateral, long-lasting hyperalgesia. Muscle Nerve 2001;24(1):37–46.
92. Park JH, Phothimat P, Oates CT, et al. Use of P-31 magnetic resonance spectroscopy to detect metabolic abnormalities in muscles of patients with fibromyalgia. Arthritis Rheum 1998;41(3):406–13.
93. Jubrias SA, Bennett RM, Klug GA. Increased incidence of a resonance in the phosphodiester region of 31P nuclear magnetic resonance spectra in the skeletal muscle of fibromyalgia patients. Arthritis Rheum 1994;37(6):801–7.
94. Rosendal L, Kristiansen J, Gerdle B, et al. Increased levels of interstitial potassium but normal levels of muscle IL-6 and LDH in patients with trapezius myalgia. Pain 2005;119(1–3):201–9.
95. Shah JP, Phillips TM, Danoff JV, et al. An in vivo microanalytical technique for measuring the local biochemical milieu of human skeletal muscle. J Appl Physiol 2005;99(5):1977–84.
96. Ruster M, Franke S, Spath M, et al. Detection of elevated N-epsilon-carboxymethyllysine levels in muscular tissue and in serum of patients with fibromyalgia. Scand J Rheumatol 2005;34(6):460–3.
97. Wall PD, Woolf CJ. Muscle but not cutaneous C-afferent input produces prolonged increases in the excitability of the flexion reflex in the rat. J Physiol 1984;356:443–58.

The Significance of Dysfunctions of the Sleeping / Waking Brain to the Pathogenesis and Treatment of Fibromyalgia Syndrome

Harvey Moldofsky, MD, FRCPC

KEYWORDS

- Nonrestorative sleep • Fibromyalgia syndrome • Pain
- Fatigue • Treatment

Since the publication of the American College of Rheumatology (ACR) criteria for fibromyalgia (FM) in 1990,[1] the essential clinical features of widespread musculoskeletal pain and multiple tender points in specific anatomic sites have taken root in the scientific literature and the clinic to characterize a population of patients having a specific pain diagnosis or disease. This FM descriptive diagnostic label substituted for an earlier nonspecific ailment termed "fibrositis." The fibrositis term fell into disrepute because of a lack of confirmed evidence for inflammatory disease involving fibrous tissue. Nevertheless, the FM diagnosis continues to suggest a rheumatologic pathogenesis where the source of the pain resides in the muscles and connective tissue. Both the ACR clinical criteria and the presumed rheumatic pathogenesis, however, have generated considerable controversy within the rheumatology community. Some rheumatologists argue that the current ACR diagnostic criteria for FM are useful in identifying patients of rheumatologic interest;[2] others use epidemiologic methodology to argue that FM is not a specific rheumatologic entity.[3,4] Once more, some authors continue to hypothesize that the source of the illness lay in muscles[5] even though the specific sites of tenderness, which are designated as a clinical feature of FM, are not specific for characterizing such patients with diffuse pain.[6] Other authors

The author has served as a consultant to Pfizer, Eli Lilly, Pierre Fabre, and Jazz Pharmaceuticals.
Sleep Disorders Clinics of the Centre for Sleep & Chronobiology, University of Toronto, 340 College Street, Suite 580, Toronto, Ontario M5T 3A9, Canada
E-mail address: h.moldofsky@utoronto.ca

Rheum Dis Clin N Am 35 (2009) 275–283
doi:10.1016/j.rdc.2009.05.008
0889-857X/09/$ – see front matter © 2009 Elsevier Inc. All rights reserved.

argue against the significance of histopathological claims for muscle and fibrous tissue abnormalities.[7,8]

Because of the lack of definitive evidence for peripheral indications of muscular or fibrous tissue structural pathology, attention has shifted away from the idea of a peripheral painful disease. Current interest resides in the role of the nervous system in the clinical features and pathogenesis of FM. This article reviews the evidence in favor of the diffuse muscular pain and body tenderness being aspects of a clinical syndrome that includes dysfunctions of the sleeping/waking brain and its contribution to unrefreshing sleep, fatigue, psychological disturbances, and impaired quality of life of patients who have FM. In particular, the author proposes that the pathogenesis of the widespread pain of patients who have FM involves disturbances of the functions of the sleeping/waking brain and coincident adverse effects on somatic and behavioral functions. As such, the author intends to summarize some recent evidence of therapeutic agents that improve sleep physiology, thus facilitating restorative sleep and ameliorating the pain and fatigue symptoms.

CLINICAL STUDIES ON THE CONTRIBUTION OF UNREFRESHING SLEEP TO WIDESPREAD PAIN AND FATIGUE IN FIBROMYALGIA SYNDROME

Common experience, confirmed by numerous clinical research studies, reveal that poor nighttime sleep interferes with our energy, alertness, mood, and ability to think. If FM is a syndrome involving malfunctions of the sleeping/waking brain, then there should be clinical evidence for such disturbances in patients with widespread pain and fatigue. From a purely descriptive perspective, patients diagnosed with FM commonly complain of poor sleep.[9,10] Indeed, among the many features of patients who have FM, unrefreshing or nonrestorative sleep ranks with pain and fatigue as the most common of all symptoms. Furthermore, problems with sleep, low energy, emotional distress, and poor health are independent predictors of chronic widespread pain.[11]

A series of prospective clinical studies support the notion of the interplay of poor sleep and widespread pain. A prospective study of a group of subjects who have FM who completed sleep/wake behavioral diaries showed that a night of poorer sleep results in complaints of more pain the following day. A more painful day is followed by a night of poorer sleep.[11] A 15-month population-based study of subjects who initially had no symptoms of chronic widespread pain showed that poor sleep increases the risk of such pain symptoms.[12] In another large-scale prospective study of FM subjects, increased disturbances in sleep result in increased pain, then disability, followed by depression.[13]

These clinical research studies highlight a broader conception of FM than originally proposed by the ACR criteria.[1] This broader conception of FM is embraced by the Outcome Measures in Rheumatology Clinical Trials (OMERACT) FM working group, which proposes an extension of the ACR criteria to include unrefreshing sleep as one of the key outcome domains for assessing the treatment of patients who have FM.[14] Recently, the author and colleagues have incorporated the proposal into a simple six-item screening instrument known as the Fibromyalgia Moldofsky Questionnaire. In an United Kingdom epidemiologic study, this instrument proved to be a valid tool for identifying subjects with widespread pain, hyperesthesia, unrefreshing sleep, fatigue, psychological distress, and impaired quality of life.[15] The identification of people with this constellation of symptoms in the general population allows for more detailed clinical study of the prevalence of such patients in clinical practice and with it improved understanding of the pathogenesis of the FM syndrome (FMS) and its management.

DISORDERED SLEEPING/WAKING BRAIN AND THE PATHOGENESIS OF FIBROMYALGIA SYNDROME

In the absence of a definitive etiology for FMS, various hypotheses are proposed that involve functional disturbances of the nervous system, including neurotransmitter, neuroendocrine, neuroimmune, and autonomic disturbances, and psychological stress factors. Whereas various stressful factors are suggested as likely etiologies, in some patients there is no evidence for a specific triggering distressful event. In patients who have chronic fatigue syndrome, which commonly overlaps with FMS, both genetic and environmental triggering agents are proposed to activate specific genes that affect sleep disturbances, which then become involved in the evolution of these syndromes.[16]

There is growing evidence that the sleeping/waking brain and its influence on peripheral functions promote hyperalgesia or bodily hypersensitivity and fatigue.[17] The author initially proposed this etiologic concept approximately 35 years ago, showing that the experimental disruption of slow wave sleep (SWS) in healthy sleeping subjects induced musculoskeletal pain and fatigue symptoms.[18] Since then, various experimental studies have confirmed these seminal clinical observations, although the differing methodologies may have resulted in some inconsistent results.[19–22] For example, one study that did not schedule an initial adaptation night to the sleep experimental procedures failed to show differences in tenderness after the subject's sleep was disrupted.[19] Another study that used an automated computerized system for analyzing sleep electroencephalography (EEG) failed to demonstrate the artificial production of the alpha frequency (7–11.5 Hz) EEG sleep arousal anomaly. Possibly, the computerized methodology was not able to differentiate between EEG awakenings and noise-induced sleep EEG arousals.[20] Other studies that employed total sleep deprivation or specific deprivation of SWS or of rapid eye movement (REM) sleep have demonstrated alteration in pain measures in normal subjects. For example, 40 hours of total sleep deprivation reduced pain thresholds, which returned to baseline values only after sleep was undisturbed, thus permitting restoration of SWS.[22] Studies of the effects of either REM or SWS deprivation followed by a night of undisturbed sleep show that both conditions reduce thresholds of pressure–pain tolerance. An increase in SWS on the recovery night is associated with an increase in pain-tolerance threshold.[23] This study also showed that sleep deprivation induces hyperalgesia without altering somatosensory functions.[23] REM sleep deprivation in animals and the loss of 4 hours of sleep, which interferes with occurrence of REM sleep in human subjects, induce a hyperalgesic state. Four hours of sleep versus 8 hours of sleep over 12 consecutive nights produce a 15% reduction in psychosocial behavior and a 3% increase in generalized body pain, back pain, and stomach pain.[24]

The results of these experimental sleep studies are consistent with neurophysiological studies, which demonstrate that patients with FMS are predisposed to central nervous system (CNS) hypersensitivity and not peripheral pain sensitization.[25] This CNS hypersensitivity may occur as the result of a loss of CNS sensory inhibitory functions. Indeed, the fragmentation of SWS in healthy subjects causes interference in the nervous system's inhibitory response to painful noxious stimuli and increases sensitivity to various nonpainful stimuli, eg, bright light, loud sounds, and strong odors.[26] These nonpainful, unpleasant sensory experiences are relevant to patients who have FMS who commonly report not only the widespread pain and tenderness, but also overall somatic hypersensitivity, or an inability to acclimatize readily to various noxious environmental stimuli (H. Moldofsky, unpublished data).

DISORDERED SLEEP PHYSIOLOGY IN FIBROMYALGIA SYNDROME

Patients who have FMS commonly have disturbances of their EEG sleep. The studies show a disorder in sleep architecture with a delayed onset to EEG sleep,[27,28] reduced sleep efficiency,[22,29] and reduced SWS and REM sleep.[27–30] There may be increased motor activity during sleep and generalized restlessness.[27–29,31–35] Commonly, there is an increase in alpha-EEG activity during non-REM sleep.[22,28,30,36–41] This sleep anomaly is commonly associated with unrefreshing sleep, which may be associated with various health problems and is not specific to FMS.[17]

Patients who have FMS often have fragmented sleep as the result of periodic arousal disturbances of their nocturnal polysomnography. These intrinsic or primary periodic sleep disturbances include periodic involuntary limb movements (PLMs)/restless legs, obstructive sleep apnea, and a high frequency of the cyclic alternating pattern (CAP) in the sleep EEG.[42] The frequent occurrence of CAP in patients who have FMS may account for the finding of the low frequency of sleep EEG spindles in stage 2 or intermediate sleep.[43] This high index of periodic arousal disturbances in the sleep EEG, which is an indicator of sleep instability, is accompanied by less efficient and unrefreshing sleep and is correlated to the severity of clinical symptoms in FMS patients.[42]

Since the sleeping/waking brain is intimately involved in circadian changes in metabolic functions of the body, we would expect that such abnormalities in neuroendocrine metabolic functions to be found in FMS. For example, much of the growth hormone production by the body occurs soon after falling asleep and is associated with the emergence of SWS or deep sleep. Patients who have FMS have decreased growth hormone,[44–46] its metabolites,[47] and disturbances in the hypothalamic–cortical adrenal axis.[48–50] Furthermore, various neurotransmitters govern the sleeping/waking brain. Specific dysfunctions in neurotransmitter functions contribute to bodily hypersensitivity and disordered sleep. For example, inhibition of serotonin (5HT) synthesis by p-chlorophenylalanine induces insomnia and a hyperalgesic state in animals and humans.[51] The increased levels of substance P (SP), which are found in the cerebrospinal fluid of FM patients,[52] led to experimental studies that demonstrated that SP operates through a neurokinin (NK) pathway to influence nociception and sleep. Intracerebral ventricular administration of SP in mice in sufficient quantities that did not induce nociceptive response delayed their ability to fall asleep and provoked awakenings from their sleep. An NK-1 receptor antagonist reversed the interfering effect upon sleep by SP.[53] This research, demonstrating the blocking of the SP-induced insomnia by prior treatment of the mice with NK-1 receptor antagonist, provides support to the notion of the arousing effect of SP on the sleeping/waking brain. Moreover, these experimental findings suggest an experimental animal model for studying sleep disturbances and musculoskeletal pain in FMS.

Increased overnight sympathetic activity using electrocardiographic methodology is consistent with the notion of circadian autonomic metabolic dysfunction associated with an arousal disturbance during the sleep of patients who have FM.[54] In addition to the chronobiological physiologic abnormalities, there are diurnal changes in behavior. FMS subjects who have light unrefreshing sleep commonly report daytime sleepiness, fatigue, negative mood, and show diurnal impairment in speed of performance with complex cognitive tasks.[55] Such behavioral difficulties may account for the functional disabilities that occur in the workplace or in social situations.

THERAPIES FOR NONRESTORATIVE SLEEP BENEFIT FIBROMYALGIA SYNDROME

If nonrestorative sleep is involved in the pathogenesis of widespread pain, then the corollary would be that restorative sleep should result in improvement in pain. Indeed, in the 15-month prospective study of subjects in the United Kingdom with chronic widespread pain symptoms, those who reported improvement in sleep quality, that is, restorative sleep, were likely to report the resolution of chronic widespread pain and return to musculoskeletal health.[56] These observations suggest that therapeutic agents that improve sleep physiology and sleep quality should benefit the pain and fatigue of patients who have FMS. Early on, the assessment of this hypothesis with a double-blind, parallel 1-week study demonstrated that 100 mg chlorpromazine, but not 5 Gm L-tryptophan, increased SWS and reduced alpha-EEG sleep physiology and symptoms of FM.[57] The nonspecific and potential adverse effects of chlorpromazine did not make this a desirable drug for the long-term management of the disorder. 5-hydroxytryptophan, a direct precursor of brain serotonin, tends to improve pain and sleep quality,[58] but its effect on the sleep physiology of patients who have FMS has not been studied. Whereas cyclobenzaprine 10–30 mg decreases evening fatigue and increases total sleep time, a small-scale study did not show a beneficial effect on pain measures, mood ratings, and alpha-EEG sleep disorder.[59] A similar tricyclic drug, amitriptyline, provides short term remedial effects on symptoms, but more than two months of treatment does not result in improvement in the arousal disturbances in sleep physiology or pain symptoms.[40]

Recently approved serotonin–adrenaline reuptake inhibitors for the treatment of FM, duloxetine and milnacipran, which are also used for treating depression, are helpful in improving pain symptoms of FM.[60] Similar to other agents that are also known to have antidepressant effect, duloxetine and milnacipran induce a delay in onset to REM sleep and a reduction of REM sleep. However, unlike SSRI antidepressant drugs that are disruptive to non-REM sleep, duloxetine 80 mg and milnacipran 50 mg twice a day improve sleep continuity and quality.[61] Duloxetine increases in stage 3 SWS[62] and milnacipran facilitates non-REM stage 2 sleep[63] in depressed patients. As yet there are no published sleep physiological studies on either of these two drugs in patients who have FMS.

A dopamine agonist, pramipexole, is reported to improve pain, fatigue, and overall function in a subset of FMS patients, but half of them were also taking narcotics.[64,65] Properly controlled studies of dopamine agonists should determine whether those who benefit have a remedial effect on RLS/PLMs, which occur in a subset of patients with FMS.

Traditional sedatives and hypnotic benzodiazepines alone do not provide any specific benefit. Nonbenzodiazepine hypnotic drugs (such as zopiclone and zolpidem) improve subjective sleep and daytime tiredness but do not modify alpha-EEG sleep or benefit pain symptoms. Recently assessed novel sleep promoting agents, however, demonstrate beneficial effects in sleep physiology, restorative sleep, pain, and fatigue. For example, the nocturnal administration of sodium oxybate, which improves SWS and reduces arousal disturbances in sleep physiology, tends to induce restorative sleep, and reduce pain and fatigue symptoms.[66,67] Pregabalin, which reduces stage 1 (light) sleep, wakefulness after sleep onset and increases SWS,[68] has shown improvement in the pain, quality of sleep, and fatigue in FMS.[69]

Furthermore, such nondrug physical methods as ultrasound and interferential current treatments decrease unrefreshing sleep, fatigue, pain, and tender points while increasing SWS and decreasing the percentage of stage 1 (light) sleep.[70] Transcranial direct current stimulation of the primary motor cortex benefits pain and sleep quality with improvement in sleep efficiency and decrease in arousals from sleep.[71]

ACKNOWLEDGMENTS

Acknowledgments of funding sources supporting research that is the primary subject of discussion in the article include the following pharmaceutical companies: Pfizer, Eli Lilly, Jazz Pharmaceuticals.

REFERENCES

1. Wolfe F, Smythe HA, Yunus MB, et al. The American College of Rheumatology 1990 criteria for the classification of fibromyalgia. Report of the Multicenter Criteria Committee. Arthritis Rheum 1990;33:160–72.
2. Crofford LJ, Clauw DJ. Fibromyalgia: where are we a decade after the American College of Rheumatology classification criteria were developed? Arthritis Rheum 2002;46:1136–8.
3. Wolfe F. The relation between tender points and fibromyalgia symptom variables: evidence that fibromyalgia is not a discrete disorder in the clinic. Ann Rheum Dis 1997;56:268–71.
4. Wessely S, Hotopf M. Is fibromyalgia a distinct clinical entity? Historical and epidemiological evidence. Best Pract Res Clin Rheumatol 1999;13:427–36.
5. Katz DL, Greene L, Ali A, et al. The pain of fibromyalgia syndrome is due to muscle hypoperfusion induced by regional vasomotor dysregulation. Med Hypotheses 2007;69(3):517–25.
6. Gupta A, McBeth J, Macfarlane GJ, et al. Pressure pain thresholds and tender point counts as predictors of new chronic widespread pain in somatising subjects. Ann Rheum Dis 2007;66:517–21.
7. Simms RW. Is there muscle pathology in fibromyalgia syndrome? Rheum Dis Clin North Am 1996;22:245–66.
8. Le Goff P. Is fibromyalgia a muscle disorder? Joint Bone Spine 2006;73:239–42.
9. Hauser W, Zimmer C, Felde E, et al. [What are the key symptoms of fibromyalgia? Results of a survey of the German Fibromyalgia Association]. Schmerz 2008; 22(2):176–83 [in German].
10. Bennett RM, Jones J, Turk DC, et al. An internet survey of 2,596 people with fibromyalgia. BMC Musculoskelet Disord 2007;8:27.
11. Affleck G. Sequential daily relations of sleep, pain intensity, and attention to pain among women with fibromyalgia. Pain 1996;68:363–8.
12. Gupta A, Silman AJ, Ray D, et al. The role of psychosocial factors in predicting the onset of chronic widespread pain: results from a prospective population-based study. Rheumatology 2007;46:666–71.
13. Bigatti SM, Hernandez AM, Cronan TA, et al. Sleep disturbances in fibromyalgia syndrome: relationship to pain and depression. Arthritis Rheum 2008;59:961–7.
14. Mease PJ, Arnold LM, Crofford LJ, et al. Identifying the clinical domains of fibromyalgia: contributions from clinician and patient Delphi exercises. Arthritis Rheum 2008;59:952–60.
15. Moldofsky H, Le Lay K, Bousetta S, et al. Fibromyalgia Moldofsky Questionnaire (FMQ): validation of a tool to aid diagnosis. Poster at annual meeting of the American College of Rheumatology meeting San Francisco, October 24–29, 2008.
16. Gurbaxani BM, Jones JF, Goertzel BN, et al. Linear data mining the Wichita clinical matrix suggests sleep and allostatic load involvement in chronic fatigue syndrome. Pharmacogenomics 2006;7(3):455–65.
17. Moldofsky H. The significance of the sleeping-waking brain for the understanding of widespread musculoskeletal pain and fatigue in fibromyalgia syndrome and allied syndromes. Joint Bone Spine 2008;75(4):397–402.

18. Moldofsky H, Scarisbrick P, England R, et al. Musculoskeletal symptoms and non-REM sleep disturbance in patients with "fibrositis syndrome" and healthy subjects. Psychosom Med 1975;37:341–51.

19. Older SA, Battafarano DF, Danning CL, et al. The effects of delta wave sleep interruption on pain thresholds and fibromyalgia-like symptoms in healthy subjects: correlations with insulin-like growth factor I. J Rheumatol 1998;25:1180–6.

20. Lentz MJ, Landis CA, Rothermel J, et al. Effects of selective slow wave sleep disruption on musculoskeletal pain and fatigue in middle aged women. J Rheumatol 1999;26:1586–92.

21. Drewes AM, Nielson KD, Arendt-Nielson L, et al. The effect of cutaneous and deep pain on the electroencephalogram during sleep: an experimental study. Sleep 1997;20:632–40.

22. Onen SH, Alloui A, Gross A, et al. The effects of total sleep deprivation, selective sleep interruption and sleep recovery on pain tolerance thresholds in healthy subjects. J Sleep Res 2001;10:35–42.

23. Kundermann B, Spernal J, Huber MT, et al. Sleep deprivation affects thermal pain thresholds but not somatosensory thresholds in healthy volunteers. Psychosom Med 2004;66:932–7.

24. Roehrs T, Hyde M, Blaisdell B, et al. Sleep loss and REM sleep loss are hyperalgesic. Sleep 2006;29(2):145–51.

25. Staud R, Bovee CE, Robinson ME, et al. Cutaneous C-fiber pain abnormalities of fibromyalgia patients are specifically related to temporal summation. Pain 2008; 139:315–23.

26. Smith MT, Edwards RR, McCann UD, et al. The effects of sleep deprivation on pain inhibition and spontaneous pain in women. Sleep 2007;30:494–505.

27. Horne JA, Shackell BS. Alpha-like EEG activity in non-REM sleep and the fibromyalgia (fibrositis) syndrome. Electroencephalogr Clin Neurophysiol 1991;79: 271–6.

28. Branco J, Atalaia A, Paiva T. Sleep cycles and alpha-delta sleep in fibromyalgia syndrome. J Rheumatol 1994;21:1113–7.

29. Touchon J, Besset A, Billiard M, et al. Fibrositis syndrome: polysomnographic and psychological aspects. In: Koella WP, Obál F, Schulz H, editors. Sleep' 86. New York: Gustav Fischer, Verlag; 1988. p. 445–7.

30. Drewes AM, Nielsen KD, Taagholt SJ, et al. Sleep intensity in fibromyalgia: focus on the microstructure of the sleep process. Br J Rheumatol 1995;34: 629–35.

31. Shaver JL, Lentz M, Landis CA, et al. Sleep, psychological distress, and stress arousal in women with fibromyalgia. Res Nurs Health 1997;20:247–57.

32. Wittig RM, Zorick FJ, Blumer D, et al. Disturbed sleep in patients complaining of chronic pain. J Nerv Ment Dis 1982;70:429–31.

33. Molony RR, MacPeek DM, Schiffman PL, et al. Sleep, sleep apnea, and fibromyalgia syndrome. J Rheumatol 1986;13:797–800.

34. Clauw D, Blank C, Hiltz R, et al. Polysomnography in fibromyalgia patients. [abstract]. Arthritis Rheum 1994;37(Suppl 9):S348.

35. Staedt J, Windt H, Hajaki G, et al. Cluster arousal analysis in chronic pain-disturbed sleep. J Sleep Res 1993;2:134–7.

36. Roizenblatt S, Tufik S, Goldenberg J, et al. Juvenile fibromyalgia: clinical and polysomnographic aspects. J Rheumatol 1977;24:579–85.

37. Drewes AM, Gade J, Nielsen KD, et al. Clustering of sleep electroencephalopathic patterns in patients with the fibromyalgia syndrome. Br J Rheumatol 1995;34:1151–6.

38. Perlis ML, Giles DE, Bootzin RR, et al. Alpha sleep and information processing, perception of sleep, pain and arousability in fibromyalgia. Int J Neurosci 1997; 89:265–80.
39. Ware JC, Russell IJ, Campos E. Alpha intrusions into the sleep of depression and fibromyalgia syndrome (fibrositis) patients [abstract]. Sleep Res 1986;15:210.
40. Carette S, Oakson G, Guimont C, et al. Sleep electroencephalography and the clinical response to amitriptyline in patients with fibromyalgia. Arthritis Rheum 1995;38:1211–7.
41. Roizenblatt S, Moldofsky H, Benedito AA, et al. Alpha sleep characteristics in fibromyalgia. Arthritis Rheum 2001;44:222–30.
42. Rizzi M, Sarzi-Puttini P, Atzeni F, et al. Cyclic alternating pattern: a new marker of sleep alteration in patients with fibromyalgia? J Rheumatol 2004;31:1193–9.
43. Landis CA, Lentz MJ, Rothermel J, et al. Decreased sleep spindles and spindle activity in midlife women with fibromyalgia and pain. Sleep 2004;27:741–50.
44. Landis CA, Lentz MJ, Rothermel J, et al. Decreased nocturnal levels of prolactin and growth hormone in women with fibromyalgia. J Clin Endocrinol Metab 2001; 86:1672–8.
45. Paiva ES, Deodhar A, Jones KD, et al. Impaired growth hormone secretion in fibromyalgia patients: evidence for augmented hypothalamic somatostatin. Arthritis Rheum 2002;46:440–50.
46. Bennett RM. Adult growth hormone deficiency in patients with fibromyalgia. Curr Rheumatol Rep 2002;4:306–12.
47. Bennett RM, Clark SC, Campbell SM, et al. Low levels of somatomedin C in patients with the fibromyalgia syndrome: a possible link between sleep and muscle pain. Arthritis Rheum 1992;35:1113–6.
48. Demitrack MA, Crofford LJ. Evidence for and pathophysiologic implications of the hypothalamic-pituitary-adrenal axis dysregulation in fibromyalgia and chronic fatigue syndrome. Ann N Y Acad Sci 1998;840:684–97.
49. Adler GK, Kinsley BT, Hurwitz S, et al. Reduced hypothalamic-pituitary-adrenal and sympathoadrenal responses to hypoglycemia in women with fibromyalgia syndrome. Am J Med 1999;106:534–43.
50. Klerman EB, Goldenberg DL, Brown EN, et al. Circadian rhythms of women with fibromyalgia. J Clin Endocrinol Metab 2001;86:1034–9.
51. Moldofsky H. Rheumatic pain modulation syndrome: the inter-relationships between sleep, central nervous system serotonin, and pain. In: Critchley M, Freedman AP, Sicuteri F, editors, Advances in neurology, vol. 33. New York: Raven Press; 1982. p. 51–7.
52. Russell IJ. The promise of substance P inhibitors in fibromyalgia. Rheum Dis Clin North Am 2002;28(2):329–42.
53. Andersen ML, Nascimento DL, Machado RB, et al. Sleep disturbance induced by substance P in mice. Behav Brain Res 2006;167:212–8.
54. Martinez-Lavin M, Hermosillo AG, Rosas M, et al. Circadian studies of autonomic nervous balance in patients with fibromyalgia: a heart rate variability analysis. Arthritis Rheum 1998;41:1966–71.
55. Coté KA, Moldofsky H. Sleep, daytime symptoms, and cognitive performance in patients with fibromyalgia. J Rheumatol 1997;24:2014–23.
56. Davies KA, Macfarlane GJ, Nicholl BI, et al. Restorative sleep predicts the resolution of chronic widespread pain: results from the EPIFUND study. Rheumatology (Oxford) 2008;47:1809–13.

57. Moldofsky H, Lue FA. The relationship of alpha and delta EEG frequencies to pain and mood in 'fibrositis' patients treated with chlorpromazine and L-tryptophan. Electroencephalogr Clin Neurophysiol 1980;50:71–80.
58. Caruso I, Sarzi Puttini P, Cazzola M, et al. Double-blind study of 5-hydroxytryptophan versus placebo in the treatment of primary fibromyalgia syndrome. J Int Med Res 1990;18(3):201–9.
59. Reynolds WJ, Moldofsky H, Saskin P, et al. The effects of cyclobenzaprine on sleep physiology and symptoms in patients with fibromyalgia. J Rheumatol 1991;18:452–4.
60. Arnold LM. Duloxetine and other antidepressants in the treatment of patients with fibromyalgia. Panminerva Med 2007;8(Suppl 2):S63–74.
61. Chalon S, Pereira A, Lainey E, et al. Comparative effects of duloxetine and desipramine on sleep EEG in healthy subjects. Psychopharmacologia 2005;177(4): 357–65.
62. Kluge M, Schüssler P, Steiger A. Duloxetine increases stage 3 sleep and suppresses rapid eye movement (REM) sleep in patients with major depression. Eur Neuropsychopharmacol 2007;17:527–31.
63. Lemoine P, Faivre T. Subjective and polysomnographic effects of milnacipran on sleep in depressed patients. Hum Psychopharmacol 2004;19(5):299–303.
64. Holman AJ, Myers RR. A randomized, double blind, placebo controlled trial of pramipexole, a dopamine agonist, in patients with fibromyalgia receiving concomitant medications. Arthritis Rheum 2005;52:2495–505.
65. Moldofsky H, Lue FA, Mously C, et al. The effect of zolpidem in patients with fibromyalgia: a dose ranging, double blind, placebo controlled, modified crossover study. J Rheumatol 1996;23(3):529–33.
66. Scharf MB, Baumann M, Berkowitz DV. The effect of sodium oxybate on clinical symptoms and sleep patterns in patients with fibromyalgia. J Rheumatol 2003; 30:1070–4.
67. Russell IJ, Bennett RM, Michalek JE, Oxybate for FMS Study Group. Sodium oxybate relieves pain and improves function in fibromyalgia syndrome: a randomized, double-blind, placebo-controlled, multicenter clinical trial. Arthritis Rheum 2009;60:299–309.
68. Hindmarch I, Dawson J, Stanley N. A double-blind study in healthy volunteers to assess the effects on sleep of pregabalin compared with alprazolam and placebo. Sleep 2005;28(2):187–93.
69. Crofford LJ, Rowbotham MC, Mease PJ, et al. Pregabalin for the treatment of fibromyalgia syndrome: results of a randomized, double-blind, placebo-controlled trial. Arthritis Rheum 2005;52:1264–73.
70. Almeida TF, Roizenblatt S, Benedito-Silva AA, et al. The effect of combined therapy (ultrasound and interferential current) on pain and sleep in fibromyalgia. Pain 2003;104(3):665–72.
71. Roizenblatt S, Fregni F, Gimenez R, et al. Site-specific effects of transcranial direct current stimulation on sleep and pain in fibromyalgia: a randomized, sham-controlled study. Pain Pract 2007;7(4):297–306.

Complex Adaptive Systems Allostasis in Fibromyalgia

Manuel Martinez-Lavin, MD*, Angelica Vargas, MD

KEYWORDS

- Fibromyalgia • Autonomic nervous system
- Complex adaptive systems • Allostasis
- Neuropathic pain • Dorsal root ganglia
- Complexity science • Holism

Prevailing linear-reductionist medical models seem unable to explain complex diseases like fibromyalgia (FM) and similar maladies fully. In contrast, paradigms derived from the new complexity theory seem to provide a more coherent explanation for the pathogenesis of these intangible illnesses. Different lines of investigation have shown that patients who have FM experience degradation of their main complex adaptive system, namely, the autonomic nervous system (ANS). It has been proposed that such autonomic dysfunction may cause the multiple symptoms of FM, including chronic widespread pain.[1]

This article is divided into two parts. The first part intends to be evidence based and reviews basic concepts of the ANS related to pain generation. This first part also reviews all controlled studies listed in PubMed looking at ANS performance in FM. The second part of the article contains a holistic pathogenetic proposal for FM based on the new complexity science paradigms. In this second section, "allostasis" and "allostatic load" are proposed as pertinent concepts for FM. This holistic model intends to be hypothesis generating; therefore, it needs to be tested with appropriate scientific studies.

PART ONE
Autonomic Nervous System: Basic Concepts Related to Pain Generation

The ANS is the portion of the nervous system that controls the function of the different organs and systems of the body. One striking characteristic of this system is the rapidity and intensity of the onset of its action and its dissipation. This unpredictable performance has chaotic features. The ANS is activated by centers located in the

Rheumatology Department, National Cardiology Institute, Juan Badiano 1, 14080 Mexico City, Mexico
* Corresponding author.
E-mail address: mmlavin@terra.com.mx (M. Martinez-Lavin).

Rheum Dis Clin N Am 35 (2009) 285–298
doi:10.1016/j.rdc.2009.05.005

spinal cord, brain stem hypothalamus, and thalamus. These centers also receive input from the limbic system and other higher brain areas. These connections enable the ANS to serve as the principal part of the stress response system in charge of fight or flight reactions.

The peripheral autonomic system is divided into two branches: sympathetic and parasympathetic. These two branches have harmonious antagonistic actions on most bodily functions; thus, their proper balance preserves homeostasis. The action of these two branches is mediated by neurotransmitters. Catecholamines are the sympathetic neurotransmitters, whereas acetylcholine acts in the parasympathetic periphery.

The naturally occurring sympathetic catecholamines that act as neurotransmitters within the central nervous system are norepinephrine, epinephrine, and dopamine. Norepinephrine also acts in peripheral postganglionic nerve endings and exerts its effects locally in the immediate vicinity of its release, whereas epinephrine is the circulating hormone of the adrenal medulla and influences processes throughout the body. The major metabolic transformation of catecholamines involves methylation and oxidative deamination. Methylation is catalyzed by the enzyme catechol-O-methyltransferase (COMT), whereas oxidative deamination is promoted by monoamine oxidase.[2] The COMT enzyme has been a focus of interest because of its relation to pain susceptibility in healthy women. There are several polymorphisms in the COMT gene that are associated with a defective catecholamine-clearing enzyme. Women who possess these polymorphisms are more susceptible to experiencing pain.[3]

Catecholamines act by binding to adrenergic receptors (ARs). ARs are fundamental parts of the sympathetic nervous system for maintenance of homeostasis. ARs are G-related proteins expressed on virtually every cell type in the body, including lymphocytes and platelets. As result of this receptor ubiquity, sympathetic activation may influence other major networks of the body, such as the immune system or the coagulation system. ARs are subject to many regulatory factors, including desensitization, down-regulation, and internalization. This dynamic plasticity may serve as a buffer against excessive agonist stimulation.[4] ARs are key players in cardiovascular homeostasis, such as blood pressure regulation during orthostatic challenges. ARs are also involved in pain sensitivity. Healthy women with a particular type of β-AR haplotype termed *haplotype 2* are prone to have low blood pressure and to develop chronic painful conditions.[5]

Clinical Assessment of Autonomic Nervous System Function

The complex function of the ANS cannot be properly appreciated with linear methods, such as static blood or urine levels of catecholamines. Changes in breathing pattern, mental stress, or even posture alter the sympathetic/parasympathetic balance immediately and completely. Opportunely, two nonlinear research instruments have been introduced to aid in clinical research of cardiovascular autonomic function: heart rate variability (HRV) analysis and head-up tilt-table test (HUT).[6–8] These two measuring tools have provided important clues to the pathogenesis of FM.

Heart rate variability analysis

This method is based on the well-known fact that the heart rate is not fixed; rather, it varies from beat to beat in a seemingly random way. Computers are able to discern and measure the influence of the sympathetic or parasympathetic branch of the ANS on this constant variability. HRV can be studied in the time domain in which the basic units are milliseconds. Time domain mathematic calculations include, among others, the standard deviation of the duration of all R-R intervals and the percentage of adjacent pairs of R-R intervals that differ by more than 50 milliseconds from each other in a given time period. The higher time domain variability indexes signify the more parasympathetic influx on the sinus node.

HRV can be also studied in the frequency domain using spectral analysis, in which the basic units are hertz (cycles per second). Pharmacologic and clinical studies have established that the high-frequency band spectral power reflects parasympathetic activity on the heart, whereas the low-frequency band power is modulated mostly by sympathetic impulses. Because the two branches of the ANS have harmonious antagonistic effects on the sinus node, the low-frequency band/high-frequency band ratio is regarded as a reflection of sympathetic activity.[7]

This new method has several advantages. Because it is noninvasive, patients are subjected to no discomfort. The equipment is portable; thus, recording can be accomplished while subjects perform their routine activities. Finally, the method is based on computerized calculations; therefore, it has boundless development potentials.

It should be noted, however, that HRV is a measuring tool that provides indirect information on the function of the ANS because it is a proxy; it measures ANS influence on heart rate, and is therefore an indirect measure of ANS reactivity.

Tilt-table test

This is another useful procedure for studying orthostatic intolerance and syncope. It is based on the physiologic changes that occur after adopting an upright posture with pooling of approximately 700 mL of blood in the lower parts of the body. In normal circumstances, the ANS quickly compensates for this relative volume loss by increasing vascular tone and cardiac output. This mechanism avoids hypotension and inadequate cerebral perfusion. Tilt-table testing examines this response in a controlled environment. With passive orthostasis, additional stress is exerted on the sympathetic nervous system by blocking the influence of muscle contraction that could increase venous return. In the first step, subjects are positioned supine for 30 minutes. The subject is then tilted upright for 30 to 45 minutes at an angle of 60° to 80°. Pharmacologic stimulation with isoproterenol is sometimes used as an additional step.

The normal response to tilting consists of an increased heart rate by 10 to 15 beats per minute, elevation of diastolic blood pressure by approximately 10 mm Hg, and little change in systolic pressure. There are two types of abnormal responses. The first is orthostatic hypotension, defined as a reduction of systolic blood pressure of at least 20 mm Hg or a reduction of diastolic blood pressure of at least 10 mm Hg. This hypotension may induce syncope. Another type of abnormal response is postural orthostatic tachycardia, which consists of a sustained heart rate increase of at least 30 beats per minute or a sustained pulse rate of 120 beats per minute. The HUT has been used mostly to study syncope in patients with no evidence of structural heart disease.[6–8]

Sympathetic Nervous System and Pain

The recognition of the sympathetic nervous system dates back to the early times of medicine. The greatest anatomist and physiologist of antiquity, Galen, discovered the sympathetic ganglia. Etymologically, the term *sympathetic* means "sharing emotions." Galen described sympathetic nerves as hollow connecting wires that allowed concerted performance of internal organs.[9]

For more than a century, it has been assumed that abnormal activity of the sympathetic nervous system may be involved in the pathogenesis of protracted pain syndromes. This assumption was based mainly on the observations that the pain is spatially correlated with signs of autonomic dysfunction and that blocking the efferent sympathetic supply to the affected region relieves the pain. This latter premise led to the clinical concept of sympathetically maintained pain, which is applied to those neuropathic pain cases that respond to sympatholytic maneuvers.[10] The nociceptive and autonomic systems interact at the level of the periphery, spinal cord, brain stem, and forebrain. Spinal and visceral afferents provide converging information to spino-thalamic neurons in the dorsal horn and to neurons of the nucleus tractus solitarius and parabrachial nuclei. These structures project to areas involved in reflex, homeostatic, and behavioral control of autonomic outflow; endocrine function; and nociception.[11] Dorsal root ganglia (DRG) are also important autonomic-nociceptive short-circuit sites.[12] Recent genetic studies have implicated key sympathetic system elements, such as the COMT enzyme or AR, in amplified pain sensitivity.[13,14]

The concept of sympathetically maintained pain has strong and ample foundations in the animal model.[10,15,16] Under normal circumstances, primary afferent nociceptors do not have catecholamine sensitivity; however, under pathologic conditions, partic-ularly after trauma, a sympathetic-afferent interaction can be established at the peripheral and central levels.

In a rabbit model, after peripheral nerve injury, sympathetic stimulation and norepi-nephrine are excitatory for a subset of skin C-fiber nociceptors that express α_2- adren-ergic–like receptors.[15] Perhaps more germane to the pathogenesis of sympathetically maintained pain are the experimental models that have been extensively reproduced in which sympathetic sprouting at the DRG becomes apparent after nerve injury and forms basket-like structures around large-diameter axotomized sensory neurons; sympathetic stimulation can activate such neurons repetitively.[16] Another site of abnormal posttraumatic connections occurs in the dorsal horn of the spinal cord, where there are A-fibers sprouting into the superficial layers, thus provoking tactile stimuli that may be painful. This mechanism may explain allodynia.

Dorsal Root Ganglia, Sodium Channels, and Sympathetic Pain

DRG are nodules that lie along the spinal column. They house the cell bodies of sensory neurons, the dendrites of which are located in the skin, muscles, tendons, joints, and internal organs. These dendrites monitor touch, stretching, temperature, and pain. Sodium channels located in DRG (particularly Nav1.7) act as molecular gate-keepers of pain detection at peripheral nociceptors. Different infecting agents may lie dormant for years in DRG. Trauma or infection reactivation can induce neuroplasticity with overexpression of sympathetic fibers and sodium channels in DRG. Nerve growth factor mediates these phenotypic changes. Such neuroplasticity enables catechol-amines or sympathetic impulses to activate nociceptors. Several DRG sodium "chan-nelopathies" have recently been associated with rare painful dysautonomic syndromes, such as primary erythermalgia and paroxysmal extreme pain disorder (formerly called familial rectal pain syndrome).[12]

Autonomic Nervous System Dysfunction in Fibromyalgia

Different groups of investigators using diverse methods have shown ANS dysfunction in patients who have FM. **Table 1** contains all controlled studies assessing ANS func-tion in FM published in the PubMed database up to April 2009.[13,17–45] To obtain this information, the authors accessed the PubMed database, with the key words "fibro-myalgia" and "autonomic" or "sympathetic." All abstracts were reviewed searching for controlled studies; there were 31 controlled studies using different methods to test dysautonomia, including muscle sympathetic nerve activity, electrodermal studies, HRV analyses, and sympathetic response to orthostatic or mental stressors. Essentially all the reported studies found evidence of autonomic dysfunction in FM.

Most published studies found basal sympathetic hyperactivity accompanied by an attenuated sympathetic response to different types of stressors. This seemingly paradoxical behavior of the ANS (hyperactivity with hyporeactivity to stress) nevertheless agrees with a basic physiologic principle: excessive AR stimulation leads to receptor desensitization and down-regulation.[4]

Mechanisms whereby such autonomic dysfunction may lead to FM have already been discussed and are summarized in **Fig. 1**. Briefly, the authors have proposed that persistent sympathetic hyperactivity induces insomnia, irritable bowel, anxiety, and dryness in the eyes and mouth. Sympathetic hyporeactivity may cause fatigue. The key FM domain of widespread pain could be sympathetically maintained.[46] The following two arguments favor the notion that sympathetic hyperactivity is the cause and not the effect of FM chronic pain: (1) patients who have FM have norepinephrine-evoked pain,[31] and (2) genetic variations linked to sluggish catecholamine-degrading enzymes are also associated with increased pain sensitivity in healthy persons and in patients who have FM.[13]

Genetic Studies of Key Sympathetic Elements in Patients Who Have Fibromyalgia

Genetic studies of the COMT enzyme and AR support the dysautonomic nature of FM. In Turkish[47] and Spanish populations, a single-nucleotide polymorphism (SNP) of the COMT gene associated with sluggish COMT enzyme occurs significantly more frequently in patients who have FM than in healthy controls.[13] In Mexican patients, such SNPs are related to several FM syndrome domains.[13] Defective COMT enzyme may induce pain sensitivity by means of AR activation.[48] Patients who have FM have an increased frequency of AR SNPs associated with pain sensitivity.[14]

PART TWO
Holistic Approach to Fibromyalgia Based on the New Complexity Sciences

The prevailing medical paradigm is supported in a linear-reductionist algorithm: the clinical-pathologic correlation. In this construct, a group of symptoms and signs (the effect) is linearly explained by a discrete anatomic lesion or an abnormal laboratory test result (the cause). Reductionism proposes that the whole can be understood by analyzing each of its parts. Accordingly, at present, MRI scans, biopsies, or blood tests are able to explain the cause of many clinical syndromes. The existence of medical specialties is another reductionist scheme. Ophthalmologists, cardiologists, urologists, and other specialists have a deep but fractioned view of patients and their suffering.

There is no doubt that this linear-reductionist approach helped enormously in the understanding of many linear diseases (those with clinical-pathologic correlation). In contrast, this approach is less helpful in understanding such complex diseases as FM and similar maladies.[49]

Complexity theory and holism

There is a new scientific perspective that may have a profound impact on the practice of medicine: complexity theory. This paradigm derives from cybernetics and computer modeling of natural phenomena, such as weather changes. Basically, this new theory proposes that the universe is full of complex systems composed of many agents interacting in parallel at different levels. Such systems are open, elastic, and constantly adapting to the environment through positive and negative feedback loops (complex adaptive systems). The systems have nonlinear behavior; as such, the intensity of the stimulus is dissimilar to the magnitude of the response. These systems cannot be understood by analyzing each of their elements individually because complex

Table 1
Controlled studies of autonomic nervous system function in fibromyalgia published in PubMed up to April 2009

No.	Authors (Reference)	Publication Year	No. Patients who had FM	No. Controls	Method	Main Finding
1	Bengtsson and Bengtsson[17]	1988	28	20	Stellate ganglion blockade	Regional reduction of pain and tender points
2	Vaerøy et al[18]	1989	27	29	Auditive stimulation, cold pressor test	Fewer vasoconstrictive responses
3	Qiao et al[19]	1991	27	29	Electrodermal studies	Less vasoconstriction during acoustic stimulation and cold pressor tests
4	van Denderen et al[20]	1992	10	10	Bicycle and step ergometer until exhaustion	Decreased cortisol, epinephrine, and norepinephrine after exercise
5	Elam et al[21]	1992	8	8	Muscle sympathetic nerve activity	Normal basal sympathetic activity, attenuated response to handgrip
6	Visuri et al[22]	1992	17	20	Orthostatic, deep breathing, Valsalva maneuver, and handgrip tests	Altered orthostatic response
7	Martínez-Lavín et al[23]	1997	19	19	HRV response to orthostatic test	Orthostatic sympathetic derangement
8	Bou-Holaigah et al[24]	1997	20	20	HUT	Abnormal drop in blood pressure, provocation of FM symptoms during tilting
9	Martínez-Lavín et al[25]	1998	30	30	24-hour HRV analysis	Changes consistent with sympathetic hyperactivity

#	Study	Year			Method	Changes consistent with
10	Cohen et al[26]	2000	22	22	HRV analysis	Changes consistent with sympathetic hyperactivity
11	Torpy et al[27]	2000	13	8	Corticotropin cortisol and catecholamine plasma levels after administration of interleukin-6	Exaggerated norepinephrine responses to interleukin-6
12	Raj et al[28]	2000	17	14	HRV, HUT	Sympathetic hyperactivity, with hyporeactivity to tilt
13	Cohen et al[29]	2001	19	19	HRV, HUT	Sympathetic hyperactivity with hyporeactivity to stress
14	Naschitz et al[30]	2001	38	30 who had CFS, 37 controls	HRV, HUT	HRV score values differed significantly between patients who had FM and patients who had CFS, suggesting that homeostatic responses are dissimilar in both diseases
15	Martínez-Lavin et al[31]	2002	20	20 who had RA, 20 controls	Norepinephrine injections	Patients who had FM had norepinephrine-evoked pain
16	Martínez-Lavin et al[32]	2003	20	20 who had RA, 20 controls	Leeds Assessment of Neuropathic Symptoms and Signs pain scale questionnaire	Patients who had FM had neuropathic pain features
17	Kooh et al[33]	2003	11	10	HRV, polysomnography	More arousal/awakening episodes, increased nocturnal sympathovagal balance

(continued on next page)

Table 1
(continued)

No.	Authors (Reference)	Publication Year	No. Patients who had FM	No. Controls	Method	Main Finding
18	Tang[34]	2004	18 (23.7%) who had SLE and FM	76 who had SLE	HUT	No increased hypotension in patients who had concurrent SLE and FM
19	Friederich et al[35]	2005	28	15	HRV baroreflex sensitivity under mental stress and passive orthostatism	Hyporeactivity to stress
20	Furlan et al[36]	2005	16	16	HRV, HUT, muscle sympathetic activity, catecholamines	Basal sympathetic hyperactivity with hyporeactivity to HUT
21	Thieme and Turk[37]	2006	90	30	EMG, heart rate, skin conductance levels at rest and during stress	Lower basal EMG levels, elevated heart rate and skin conductance levels
22	Unlü et al[38]	2006	28	18	Sympathetic skin response	Abnormal sympathetic skin response
23	Ulas et al[39]	2006	34	22	SSR and HRV analysis.	Abnormal sympathetic skin response, decreased HRV
24	Ozgocmen et al[40]	2006	29	22	Sympathetic skin response and HRV	Decreased HRV and abnormal sympathetic skin response
25	Nilsen et al[41]	2007	23	29 who had shoulder-neck pain, 35 controls	Blood pressure, heart rate, finger skin blood flow, and respiration before, during, and after stressful task	Abnormal cardiovascular responses to a 60-minute stressful task in patients who had FM

26	Giske et al[42]	2008	19	19	Maximal voluntary contraction and repetitive isometric contractions, EMG, catecholamines	Attenuated adrenergic response to repetitive isometric exercise
27	Vargas-Alarcon et al[13]	2007	57 Mexican, 78 Spanish	33 Mexican, 80 Spanish	COMT SNPs	In Spanish patients, association of FM with COMT SNPs, in Mexican patients with FIQ scores
28	Figueroa et al[43]	2008	10	9	Resistance exercise training, HRV, BRS	Resistance exercise training improves HRV
29	Jones et al[44]	2008	106	101	Intervention with pyridostigmine and exercise	Pyridostigmine improved anxiety and sleep, exercise improved fatigue
30	Solano et al[45]	2009	30	30	Composite Autonomic Symptom Scale	Patients who had FM had symptoms related to different expressions of dysautonomia
31	Doğru et al[46]	2009	50	30	HRV, orthostatic tests	HRV changes consistent with basal sympathetic hyperactivity that persisted during stress test

Abbreviations: BRS, baroreflex sensitivity; CFS, chronic fatigue syndrome; EMG, electromyography; FIQ, Fibromyalgia Impact Questionnaire; RA, rheumatoid arthritis; SLE, systemic lupus erythematosus; SNP, single-nucleotide polymorphism; SSR, skin sympathetic reactivity.

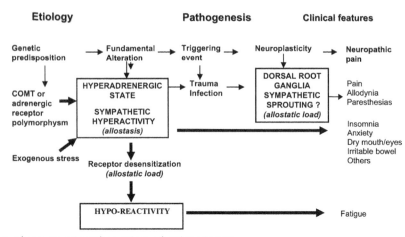

Fig. 1. Theoretic etiopathogenic mechanisms in FM.

adaptive systems have emergent properties that are not found in their components. Therefore, for them, the whole is different than the sum of its parts. Examples of complex adaptive systems include the following: democratic societies, stock markets, ant colonies, and the major homeostatic systems of the human body. Healthy complex systems have seemingly disorderly (chaotic) behaviors. If a system becomes rigid, it loses complexity, experiences degradation, and ultimately dies.[50]

The best way to understand complex systems is with a holistic approach: viewing the system dynamics in their entirety and observing their interactions with the environment. Complexity theory provides a scientific foundation for holism. Rather than opponents, holism and reductionism should be regarded as complementary medical paradigms; both perspectives are needed for a proper account of reality.

Autonomic nervous system as a complex adaptive system
The ANS is a good example of a complex adaptive system. It is a hierarchic and decentralized self-regulatory system, from cells to neurons and from neurons to nerve system. Each level upholds a measure of independence while contributing to a higher level of organization. The ANS maintains the critical physiologic parameter autonomously and contributes to adjust to the external changing environment without additional interventions. The ANS is able to learn, to measure, and to adapt. On the face of external perturbations (physical or mental stressors), it immediately recomposes its performance to maintain homeostasis.[51]

Complexity theory may have important clinical implications. Diseases like FM may result from excessive allostasis of our complex systems in an effort to adapt to a hostile environment.

Allostasis and allostatic load: two concepts relevant to fibromyalgia
The concept of allostasis was proposed by Sterling and Eyre[53] in 1988 to describe the additional effort needed to re-establish homeostasis. Literally, the term *allostasis* means maintaining stability through change.[52] *Allostatic load*, a term introduced by McEwen,[54] refers to the price the body pays for being forced to adapt to adverse psychosocial or physical situations, and it represents the presence of too much stress or the inefficient operation of the stress response system.

These two concepts seem relevant to FM pathogenesis. Modern environment has become inhospitable in different ways. As an example, we have lost the night. Nowadays, there is still light, noise, and activity after sunset. In addition, exercise is lacking, diets are aberrant, and working conditions are often tedious and monotonous. The authors propose that in many individuals, allostasis to a hostile environment is achieved through persistent sympathetic hyperactivity. This persistent allostasis may eventually lead to a dysfunctional system. In cases of FM, the allostatic load is manifested by the inability of the sympathetic nervous system to respond to further stress and by abnormal sympathetic-nociceptive short circuits leading to a chronic sympathetically maintained pain syndrome (see **Fig. 1**).[54]

Holistic treatment in fibromyalgia

Conventional (linear) medical visit, in which the patient acts as a passive consumer of medications and advice is likely to be less effective. For patients who have FM, a biopsychosocial approach is recommended instead. The following list outlines those procedures having scientific or expert group support.[55,56] Most of the discussed methods have been shown to improve resting autonomic tone.[1]

- Information: Explain the complex characteristics of FM. A well-written and well-annotated book is useful in achieving this task. In the authors' experience, most patients can appreciate the dysautonomia model. Points to highlight to patients are as follows: validation of symptoms, role of genetics and external stressors on the hyperadrenergic state, and the neuropathic nature of pain.
- Self-help groups: Such groups operate precisely as a complex adaptive system, in which the agents (patients) engage in an active change to a healthy lifestyle. Well-coordinated assertive group therapies are effective and less expensive, and they free physician time.
- Diet: Many patients who have FM have irritable bowel. Their diet should be predominantly vegetarian. Search for lactose or gluten intolerance.
- Avoidance of sympathomimetic substances: Avoid caffeine and nicotine.
- Exercise: pool-based, dance, light aerobics, diaphragmatic, T'ai Chi.
- Biofeedback techniques: Use methods based on electromyography or HRV.
- Sleep hygiene.
- Cognitive-behavioral therapy: Use cognitive behavioral therapy and other self-efficacy techniques.
- Psychologic or psychiatry counseling.
- Pharmacologic therapy: Several drugs that target excessive nociceptive signaling in the central nervous system, such as pregabalin, or augment pain inhibitory pathways in the central nervous system, such as duloxetine and milnacipran, have been approved for the treatment of FM based on controlled studies. Some analgesic medications, such as tramadol, have shown efficacy in FM, as have older neuromodulatory drugs, such as the tricyclics. Other types of drugs may be helpful in alleviating associated symptoms, such as sleep dysfunction, irritable bowel, and depression or anxiety. A rational combination of targeted therapies may be warranted but needs to be tested with appropriate controlled studies. Excessive polypharmacy should be avoided.

REFERENCES

1. Martinez-Lavin M. Fibromyalgia conundrum. Is scientific holism the answer? The Rheumatologist 2008;2(7):26–7.

2. Westfall TC, Westfall DP. Neurotransmission. The autonomic and somatic motor nervous systems. In: Brunton, editor. Goodman and Gilman's the pharmacological basis of therapeutics. 11th edition. New York: McGraw-Hill; 2006. p. 137–82.

3. Diatchenko L, Slade GD, Nackley AG, et al. Genetic basis for individual variation of pain perception and the development of a chronic pain condition. Hum Mol Genet 2005;14(1):135–43.

4. Small KM, McGraw DW, Liggett SB. Pharmacology and physiology of human adrenergic receptor polymorphisms. Annu Rev Pharmacol Toxicol 2003;43: 381–411.

5. Diatchenko L, Anderson AD, Slade GD, et al. Three major haplotypes of the beta2 adrenergic receptor define psychological profile, blood pressure, and the risk for development of a common musculoskeletal pain disorder. Am J Med Genet B Neuropsychiatr Genet 2006;141:449–62.

6. Hermosillo AG, Marquez MF, Jauregui-Renau K, et al. Orthostatic hypotension 2001. Cardiol Rev 2001;9:339–41.

7. Task Force of the European Society of Cardiology and the North American Society of Pacing and Electrophysiology. Heart rate variability standards of measurement, physiological interpretation, and clinical use. Circulation 1996;93:1043–65.

8. Lamarre-Cliche M, Cusson J. The fainting patients: value of the head-upright tilt-table test in adult patients with orthostatic intolerance. CMAJ 2001;164:372–6.

9. Ackerknecht EH. The history of the discovery of the vegetative (autonomic) nervous system. Med Hist 1974;18(1):1–8.

10. Baron R, Levina JD, Fields HL. Causalgia and reflex sympathetic dystrophy: does the sympathetic nervous system contribute to the generation of pain? Muscle Nerve 1999;22:678–95.

11. Benarroch EE. Pain-autonomic interactions: a selective review. Clin Auton Res 2001;11:343–9.

12. Martinez-Lavin M, Solano C. Dorsal root ganglia, sodium channels, and fibromyalgia sympathetic pain. Med Hypotheses 2009;72(1):64–6.

13. Vargas-Alarcón G, Fragoso JM, Cruz-Robles D, et al. Catechol-O-methyltransferase gene haplotypes in Mexican and Spanish patients with fibromyalgia. Arthritis Res Ther 2007;9(5):R110. Available at: http://arthritis-research.com/content/9/5/R110.

14. Vargas-Alarcón G, Fragoso JM, Cruz-Robles D, et al. Association of adrenergic receptor gene polymorphisms with different fibromyalgia syndrome domains. Arthritis Rheum, in press.

15. Sato J, Perl ER. Adrenergic excitation of cutaneous pain receptors induced by peripheral nerve injury. Science 1991;251:1608–10.

16. McLachlan EM, Jäning W, Devor M, et al. Peripheral nerve injury triggers noradrenergic sprouting within dorsal root ganglia. Nature 1993;363:543–6.

17. Bengtsson A, Bengtsson M. Regional sympathetic blockade in primary fibromyalgia. Pain 1988;33(2):161–7.

18. Vaerøy H, Qiao ZG, Mørkrid L, et al. Altered sympathetic nervous system response in patients with fibromyalgia (fibrositis syndrome). J Rheumatol 1989; 16(11):1460–5.

19. Qiao ZG, Vaerøy H, Mørkrid L. Electrodermal and microcirculatory activity in patients with fibromyalgia during baseline, acoustic stimulation and cold pressor tests. J Rheumatol 1991;18(9):1383–9.

20. van Denderen JC, Boersma JW, Zeinstra P, et al. Physiological effects of exhaustive physical exercise in primary fibromyalgia syndrome (PFS): is PFS a disorder of neuroendocrine reactivity? Scand J Rheumatol 1992;21(1):35–7.

21. Elam M, Johansson G, Wallin BG. Do patients with primary fibromyalgia have an altered muscle sympathetic nerve activity? Pain 1992;48(3):371–5.
22. Visuri T, Lindholm H, Lindqvist A, et al. Cardiovascular functional disorder in primary fibromyalgia: a noninvasive study in 17 young men. Arthritis Care Res 1992;5(4):210–5.
23. Martínez-Lavín M, Hermosillo AG, Mendoza C, et al. Orthostatic sympathetic derangement in subjects with fibromyalgia. J Rheumatol 1997;24(4):714–8.
24. Bou-Holaigah I, Calkins H, Flynn JA, et al. Provocation of hypotension and pain during upright tilt table testing in adults with fibromyalgia. Clin Exp Rheumatol 1997;15(3):239–46.
25. Martínez-Lavín M, Hermosillo AG, Rosas M, et al. Circadian studies of autonomic nervous balance in patients with fibromyalgia: a heart rate variability analysis. Arthritis Rheum 1998;41(11):1966–71.
26. Cohen H, Neumann L, Shore M, et al. Autonomic dysfunction in patients with fibromyalgia: application of power spectral analysis of heart rate variability. Semin Arthritis Rheum 2000;29(4):217–27.
27. Torpy DJ, Papanicolaou DA, Lotsikas AJ, et al. Responses of the sympathetic nervous system and the hypothalamic-pituitary-adrenal axis to interleukin-6: a pilot study in fibromyalgia. Arthritis Rheum 2000;43(4):872–80.
28. Raj SR, Brouillard D, Simpson CS, et al. Dysautonomia among patients with fibromyalgia: a noninvasive assessment. J Rheumatol 2000;27(11):2660–5.
29. Cohen H, Neumann L, Alhosshle A, et al. Abnormal sympathovagal balance in men with fibromyalgia. J Rheumatol 2001;28(3):581–9.
30. Naschitz JE, Rozenbaum M, Rosner I, et al. Cardiovascular response to upright tilt in fibromyalgia differs from that in chronic fatigue syndrome. J Rheumatol 2001;28(6):1356–60.
31. Martínez-Lavín M, Vidal M, Barbosa RE, et al. Norepinephrine-evoked pain in fibromyalgia. A randomized pilot study [ISRCTN70707830]. BMC Musculoskelet Disord 2002;3:2. Available at: http://www.biomedcentral.com/1471-2474/3/2.
32. Martínez-Lavín M, López S, Medina M, et al. Use of the Leeds assessment of neuropathic symptoms and signs questionnaire in patients with fibromyalgia. Semin Arthritis Rheum 2003;32(6):407–11.
33. Kooh M, Martínez-Lavín M, Meza S, et al. Simultaneous heart rate variability and polysomnographic analyses in fibromyalgia. Clin Exp Rheumatol 2003;21(4):529–30.
34. Tang S, Calkins H, Petri M. Neurally mediated hypotension in systemic lupus erythematosus patients with fibromyalgia. Rheumatology 2004;43(5):609–14.
35. Friederich HC, Schellberg D, Mueller K, et al. Stress and autonomic dysregulation in patients with fibromyalgia syndrome. Schmerz 2005;19(3):185–8.
36. Furlan R, Colombo S, Perego F, et al. Abnormalities of cardiovascular neural control and reduced orthostatic tolerance in patients with primary fibromyalgia. J Rheumatol 2005;32(9):1787–93.
37. Thieme K, Turk DC. Heterogeneity of psychophysiological stress responses in fibromyalgia syndrome patients. Arthritis Res Ther 2006;8(1):R9. Available at: http://arthritis-research.com/content/8/1/R9.
38. Unlü E, Ulaş UH, Gürçay E, et al. Genital sympathetic skin responses in fibromyalgia syndrome. Rheumatol Int 2006;26(11):1025–30.
39. Ulas UH, Unlu E, Hamamcioglu K, et al. Dysautonomia in fibromyalgia syndrome: sympathetic skin response and RR interval analysis. Rheumatol Int 2006;26:383–7.
40. Ozgocmen S, Yoldas T, Yigiter R, et al. R-R interval variation and sympathetic skin response in fibromyalgia. Arch Med Res 2006;37(5):630–4.

41. Nilsen KB, Sand T, Westgaard RH, et al. Autonomic activation and pain in response to low-grade mental stress in fibromyalgia and shoulder/neck pain patients. Eur J Pain 2007;11(7):743–55.
42. Giske L, Vøllestad NK, Mengshoel AM, et al. Attenuated adrenergic responses to exercise in women with fibromyalgia—a controlled study. Eur J Pain 2008;12(3): 351–60.
43. Figueroa A, Kingsley JD, McMillan V, et al. Resistance exercise training improves heart rate variability in women with fibromyalgia. Clin Physiol Funct Imaging 2008; 28(1):49–54.
44. Jones KD, Burckhardt CS, Deodhar AA, et al. A six-month randomized controlled trial of exercise and pyridostigmine in the treatment of fibromyalgia. Arthritis Rheum 2008;58(2):612–22.
45. Solano C, Martinez A, Becerril L, et al. Autonomic dysfunction in fibromyalgia assessed by the Composite Autonomic Symptoms Scale (COMPASS). J Clin Rheumatol 2009; [Epub ahead of print].
46. Doğru MT, Aydin G, Tosun A, et al. Correlations between autonomic dysfunction and circadian changes and arrhythmia prevalence in women with fibromyalgia syndrome. Anadolu Kardiyol Derg 2009;9:110–7.
47. Martínez-Lavín M, Hermosillo AG. Autonomic nervous system dysfunction may explain the multisystem features of fibromyalgia. Semin Arthritis Rheum 2000; 29(4):197–9.
48. Gursoy S, Erdal E, Herken H, et al. Significance of catechol-O-methyltransferase gene polymorphism in fibromyalgia syndrome. Rheumatol Int 2003;23(3):104–7.
49. Nackley AG, Tan KS, Fecho K, et al. Catechol-O-methyltransferase inhibition increases pain sensitivity through activation of both beta2- and beta3-adrenergic receptors. Pain 2007;128(3):199–208.
50. Martínez-Lavín M, Infante O, Lerma C. Hypothesis: the chaos and complexity theory may help our understanding of fibromyalgia and similar maladies. Semin Arthritis Rheum 2008;37(4):260–4.
51. Goldberger AL. Non-linear dynamics for clinicians: chaos theory, fractals, and complexity at the bedside. Lancet 1996;347(9011):1312–4.
52. Long B. Autonomic computing. Available at: http://kbs.cs.tuberlin.de/teaching/ sose2006/oc/folien/AutonomicComputingPaper.pdf. Accessed April 13, 2009.
53. Sterling P, Eyer J. Allostasis: a new paradigm to explain arousal pathology. In: Fischer S, Reason J, editors. Handbook of life stress, cognition and health. New York: John Wiley & Sons; 1988. p. 629–49.
54. McEwen BS. Protective and damaging effects of stress mediators. N Engl J Med 1998;338(3):171–9.
55. Martínez-Lavín M. Biology and therapy of fibromyalgia. Stress, the stress response system and fibromyalgia. Arthritis Res Ther 2007;9(4):216. Available at: http://arthritis-research.com/content/9/4/216.
56. Carville SF, Arendt-Nielsen S, Bliddal H, et al. EULAR evidence based recommendations for the management of fibromyalgia syndrome. Ann Rheum Dis 2008;67:536–41.

Review of Cognitive Dysfunction in Fibromyalgia: A Convergence on Working Memory and Attentional Control Impairments

Jennifer M. Glass, PhD[a,b],*

KEYWORDS

- Fibromyalgia • Cognitive function • Neuropsychologic function
- Dyscognition • Working memory

Widespread musculoskeletal pain is the hallmark of fibromyalgia (FM), but patients frequently experience several other symptoms as well, including memory and concentration problems. In a 2001 article, Glass and Park[1] summarized the small extant body of research on cognitive dysfunction in FM. The evidence at that time supported the existence of cognitive deficits relative to healthy control participants, with indications of particular problems in working memory, episodic memory, and semantic memory access. Briefly, working memory is a system of short-term storage (on the order of seconds) combined with other mental processes, as would be used to briefly remember two numbers and add them together mentally.[2] Episodic memory refers specifically to storage of particular episodes or events, and semantic memory refers to stored knowledge and facts. Remembering a list of items to buy at the grocery store is an example of episodic memory; knowing that eggs and milk are sources of protein is an example of semantic memory.[3] In the 2001 review, it was noted that psychologic factors such as depression or anxiety were sometimes related to cognitive function in FM, but these factors did not seem to explain the observed cognitive dysfunction. In

[a] Department of Psychiatry, University of Michigan, 4250 Plymouth Road, Ann Arbor, MI 48109-2700, USA
[b] Institute for Social Research, University of Michigan, 426 Thompson Street, Ann Arbor, MI 48104, USA
* Department of Psychiatry, University of Michigan, 4250 Plymouth Road, Ann Arbor, MI 48109-2700.
E-mail address: jglass@umich.edu

Rheum Dis Clin N Am 35 (2009) 299–311
doi:10.1016/j.rdc.2009.06.002
0889-857X/09/$ – see front matter © 2009 Elsevier Inc. All rights reserved.

rheumatic.theclinics.com

the studies where such data were presented, pain was significantly correlated with cognitive performance, as was fatigue. In 2001, the conclusion was that demonstrable cognitive dysfunction exists in FM that cannot be attributed solely to concomitant psychiatric conditions such as depression, but does seem to be related to the level of pain. Questions remained regarding the exact nature of the cognitive dysfunction and its impact on patients. Which cognitive abilities were most affected? What was the cause of cognitive dysfunction in FM? What can be done to ameliorate the dysfunction? More recent contributions to this field of research are added to the earlier review in the discussion below.

IMPORTANCE AND IMPACT OF DYSCOGNITION FOR FIBROMYALGIA PATIENTS

Since 2001, several new reports of dyscognition in FM have been published that verify the importance of these symptoms to patients who have FM. The term dyscognition is used here to refer to the patient-experienced impact of both the self-reported cognitive problems and the dysfunction observed in performance-based measures of cognition and neuropsychologic function. For example, Zachrisson and colleagues[4] reported a 95% incidence rate for "Concentration Difficulties" and a 93% incidence rate for "Failing Memory" on their FibroFatigue scale. Additionally, patients who have FM report more cognitive problems and dissociative states than other rheumatology patients.[5,6] In a large Internet survey of individuals who have FM, forgetfulness and problems with concentration were the fifth and sixth most prevalent symptoms, with stiffness, fatigue, nonrestorative sleep, and pain at the top of the list.[7] Arnold and colleagues[8] reported the results of patient focus groups that assessed important symptoms and the impact of these symptoms from a patient perspective. Patients reported that memory and concentration problems were very disruptive—affecting their ability to express themselves due to word-finding difficulties, their ability to organize and plan ahead, their ability to respond quickly to questions, and their ability to drive. Mease and colleagues[9] reported the results of Delphi exercises with patients and with clinicians, who confirmed patient perceptions that memory and concentration problems are very common symptoms in FM and are quite disruptive for patients. Given the frequency with which patients cite dyscognition as a troubling symptom, it is curious that only one study has used a well-validated questionnaire of self-report cognitive function in subjects who have FM. In a study of beliefs about memory, Glass and colleagues[10] found that subjects who have FM reported lower memory capacity, more negative change in memory, and more anxiety about memory performance than controls. Interestingly, subjects who have FM also reported more use of strategies to support memory while at the same time reporting lower self-efficacy over memory performance. Altogether, these reports demonstrate quite conclusively the salience of dyscognition and its impact on daily life for patients who have FM.

WHICH COGNITIVE MECHANISMS ARE MOST AFFECTED BY FIBROMYALGIA?

Along with the growing awareness of the salience of dyscognition symptoms described above, there have been some new studies of cognitive performance in FM. Remarkably, these studies have been quite consistent with our observation in 2001 that the most marked impairment was seen on measures of working memory, followed by episodic memory, and access to semantic memory. In addition, a new focus has emerged that points to a particular difficulty in dealing with distracting information. The studies of cognitive performance in FM are described below.

Working Memory

Working memory is critical to accurate performance in demanding cognitive situations.[2] A busy work environment requires an employee to hold some information in mind while using that information for further processing. In the laboratory, working memory is measured by determining how well people can both store and process information. A quick laboratory index of working memory function is how many digits an individual can listen to and then repeat in backward order. There are now several studies that have reported impairment in this important cognitive function in subjects who have FM, using a variety of different tests of working memory. For example, there are at least five reports using the paced auditory serial attention test (PASAT)[11] in FM compared with controls. Commonly called a test of attention, the PASAT is also a challenging working memory test. Participants listen to a series of digits, mentally add together the most recent two digits and state the answer out loud. Thus, if the auditory digits were 2, 7, 3, 4….the correct answers would be "nine," "ten," "seven," and so on. Most studies using the PASAT found lower performance in subjects who have FM compared with controls,[12–15] although Suhr[16] did not find differences.

Another commonly used test is the auditory consonant trigram (ACT) test.[17] A list of three consonants is presented for a short period and then the consonants are replaced by a delay period (9, 18, or 36 seconds), during which the participant counts backward by threes from a randomly chosen number to prevent rehearsal of the to-be-remembered consonant trigram. After the delay period, the participant recalls the trigram. Both Leavitt and Katz[15] and Dick and colleagues[18] found that subjects who have FM recalled fewer of the trigrams correctly, and many performed in the impaired range compared with the control participants.

Two separate studies have reported lower performance on the reading span task,[19] a working memory test used extensively to study age-related decline in working memory. During the reading span task, participants hear factual sentences and are asked multiple choice questions about the sentences immediately after hearing the sentence. At the same time, they also tried to remember the last word in each sentence. After a certain number of sentences (between one and six), participants recall the words from the sentences in the same order in which they were presented. Park and colleagues[20] and Dick and colleagues[18] found that subjects who have FM perform more poorly than age-matched controls. Furthermore, Park and colleagues found that performance in the subjects who have FM was not different from control subjects who were 20 years older.

In addition to the neuropsychologic and laboratory tests described above, Dick and colleagues[18,21] have used the Test of Everyday Attention (TEA), a standardized test designed to have high ecological validity. All components of this test take place within the context of a sightseeing trip. The working memory tests involve keeping track of which floor an elevator occupied by counting the tones, with and without distraction. The results showed that subjects who have FM had lower scores on the working memory component of the TEA.[22]

The wide variety of working memory tests that demonstrate lower performance in FM is striking, suggesting that this deficit is quite robust. This is a crucial finding since working memory is a basic cognitive mechanism that underlies successful performance on many other cognitive tasks.[2] Because deficits in working memory ability have repercussive effects on other aspects of cognition, a small deficit in working memory may have a large impact on performance on complex tasks. Future research is necessary to understand in more detail the effects of FM on working memory. For example, is short-term storage deficit to blame or difficulty managing competing information (central executive), or both? To this end, it is interesting to note that Landro and colleagues[23] did not find performance differences between subjects who have FM and controls using simple short-term storage tests (digit span), which suggests that processes that control and manage the contents of working memory are more likely than storage mechanisms to be disrupted in FM.

Episodic Memory

Episodic memory is the ability to remember specific events or episodes (eg, the memory of your first car or, in a laboratory setting, your ability to remember a list of words). Several researchers have found deficits in episodic memory in subjects who have FM using a wide variety of standardized neuropsychologic tests and some laboratory tests. However, the results of episodic memory testing do not seem to be as robust as the working memory results. Among researchers using the Wechsler Memory Scale-Revised (WMS-R), Grace and colleagues[24] found significant differences on the general memory, verbal memory, and delayed recall components of the WMS-R, but not on the visual memory or attention/concentration components. Leavitt and Katz[15] found that subjects who have FM performed slightly below the norm on logical memory and paired associates, but the effect was not nearly as large as seen with the working memory tests (PASAT, ACT). There are a few reports using the Rey Auditory Verbal Learning Test, again with mixed results. Munguia-Izquierdo and Legaz-Arrese[14] found significantly lower performance in subjects who have FM compared with controls, but neither Grace and colleagues[24] nor Suhr[16] found differences using this test. Landro and colleagues[23] reported significant differences using the Randt Memory Test and the Code Memory Test but not with the Kimura Recurring Recognition Figures Test. Park and colleagues[20] used two laboratory tests of episodic memory: a recall task and a recognition memory task. On both tests, subjects who have FM recalled significantly fewer items than matched controls. In another list learning task, Glass and colleagues[25] found that subjects who have FM recalled fewer words, and their memory was most impaired when combined with a distracting secondary task at both list learning and recall.

In the main, the findings concerning episodic memory do suggest a mild deficit for patients who have FM, but it does not seem to be as large nor as robust as the findings with working memory. Perhaps, as Leavitt and Katz[15] suggested, memory function in FM may be strong enough to perform well under the ideal conditions, but performance decrements are observed in the presence of distraction. Memory failures are a common complaint in FM, so further study is warranted.

Semantic Memory

Semantic memory is the knowledge of words and facts and can be measured in a number of ways. One method uses verbal fluency to measure how quickly and efficiently stored knowledge about words can be accessed. Typically, participants write down (or say out loud) as many words as they can that start with a given letter, as in the FAS verbal fluency tests. Several studies indicate impairment on verbal fluency tests in subjects who have FM. Park and colleagues[20] found that subjects who have FM produced fewer words during an FAS fluency test than age-matched controls, and Landro and colleagues[23] and Munguia-Izquierdo and Legaz-Arrese[14] reported similar findings. However, Suhr[16] did not find any difference between subjects who have FM and controls on a fluency test.

In addition to verbal fluency deficits, Park and colleagues[20] and Glass and colleagues[10] also found that subjects who have FM perform more poorly than education-matched controls on tests of vocabulary, another test of semantic memory.

Leavitt and Katz[26] reported a naming speed deficit in FM, consistent with the verbal fluency results. Thus, patients who have FM seem to have a deficit in accessing stored knowledge. This deficit can make it difficult for patients to think quickly and to come up with the right word for a given situation and indeed, several patients indicated this kind of word-finding difficulty in the patient focus groups.[8,9] Further research is necessary to confirm and fully understand semantic memory problems in FM.

Attention and Concentration

In the cognitive psychology literature, attention and working memory are very closely linked because attention mechanisms are used to control the items that are stored and processed in working memory.[2] In the section on working memory, it was suggested that patients who have FM have working memory problems that are due to the management of the contents of working memory rather than the loss of storage capacity in working memory. This view is consistent with patients' perspective of difficulty dealing with complex, rapidly changing environments, and it is also supported by several studies of attention and distraction. For example, Leavitt and Katz[15] suggest that the typical setting for testing neuropsychologic function where distractions are minimized may not be the most sensitive way to find cognitive problems in patients who have FM. They found the most impairment on tasks where distraction from a competing source of information was prominent (PASAT, ACT) in contrast to tasks without distraction (digit span, logical memory, paired associate). Other findings demonstrate that memory in subjects who have FM is more disrupted than healthy controls during conditions of maximal distraction, in which attention was divided while learning a word list and while recalling the word list.[10] Dick and colleagues[18,22] have reported that subjects who have FM perform at a lower level than healthy controls on the TEA, a test of attention with high ecological validity. Subjects who have FM score lower overall and have particular difficulty with the working memory components of the test. Taken together, these results strongly suggest that dealing with distraction, or controlling what is attended to, is a particular problem in FM. The ability to manage distraction is part of executive function. In a recent study, Verdejo-Garcia and colleagues[27] examined executive function and decision making in FM using the Wisconsin Card Sorting Task (WCST) and the Iowa Gambling Task (IGT). They found that subjects who have FM achieved a lower number of categories and made more nonperseverative errors on the WCST. On the IGT, subjects who have FM showed an altered learning curve that suggested a hypersensitivity to reward. These new data on executive function fit well with the attention control difficulties noted in this section and points to a need for more research on executive function in FM. Further speculation about a possible cause (ie, the disruptive nature of pain) for this problem are included in the section below.

WHY DO FIBROMYALGIA PATIENTS EXPERIENCE COGNITIVE PROBLEMS?

Many of the common comorbid symptoms in FM, such as depressed mood, anxiety, fatigue, poor sleep, and pain, have the potential to negatively impact cognitive function. Several studies have examined these variables and are discussed below.

Depression and Anxiety

Early studies of cognitive function in FM focused on psychologic comorbidities such as depression and anxiety as important factors that may explain dyscognition. Thus, Landro and colleagues[23] split their sample of subjects who have FM into those with and without a lifetime history of major depressive disorder. When subjects with a lifetime history were excluded, the investigators no longer found significant differences between subjects who have FM and controls. However, this may well have been due to a reduction in statistical power when the FM group was reduced, because the scores on memory tests for the subjects with and without a lifetime history of depression were very similar to one another. Grace and colleagues[24] reported that anxiety (but not depression) was correlated with measures of memory and concentration. Sephton and colleagues[28] found that depressive symptoms were negatively correlated with verbal recall. Suhr[16] also found that depressive symptoms were related to memory. Similarly, Dick and colleagues[18] found a relationship between depression and anxiety and cognitive function. However, they reported significant differences on cognitive function between FM and healthy controls even when controlling for depression and anxiety. In contrast to the above studies, Park and colleagues[20] screened subjects to rule out major depressive disorder; nonetheless, subjects who have FM still endorsed more symptoms of depression and anxiety than controls. However, neither depression nor anxiety was correlated with performance on any of the cognitive measures. Similarly, Verdejo-Garcia and colleagues[27] did not find a significant correlation between the affective distress scale (from the West Haven–Yale Multidimensional Pain Inventory) and any of their neuropsychologic measures. In summary, it does seem that psychologic variables such as depression and anxiety can contribute to cognitive dysfunction in FM, but do not entirely explain it. Whether a significant relationship is found between depressive symptoms and cognitive function most likely depends on sampling strategies. Samples rigorously screened for depressive symptoms may not show this relationship and may offer a more "pure" test of cognitive function in FM. However, the results will not be informative for the many patients who have FM who are experiencing symptoms of depression. This is an important point for both researchers and reviewers to bear in mind, and the field is still in need of research that can rule out the effects of depression on cognition as well as research that can provide information on the combined effect of depression and FM on cognitive function.

Sleep

Disturbed sleep is another common symptom in FM, and impaired sleep is known to have a negative impact on cognitive function.[29] Cote and Moldofsky[30] were the first to investigate this and reported a possible relationship between altered sleep architecture and cognitive function. Suhr[16] reported that fatigue was significantly related to measures of psychomotor speed, as well as self-reported cognitive complaints. However, Dick and colleagues[18] reported that significant differences remained between FM and healthy control groups even when controlling for self-reported sleep disruption (number of awakenings per night). Therefore, as with the psychologic variables discussed above, poor sleep probably contributes to cognitive dysfunction in FM, but does not entirely explain it, and further research is warranted to understand the impact of poor sleep on cognitive function in FM.

Pain

Chronic pain is a condition for FM diagnosis, and it is known that pain, both chronic and acute, can have a negative impact cognitive function. Neuropsychologic performance is lower in chronic pain states (see Hart[31] for a review). Indeed, there is a growing body of research about the effects of chronic pain (including many different pain conditions) on brain morphology, physiology, and function in both animal[32] and human models. In humans, subjects who have chronic pain (including a recent study of FM) show impaired learning on a decision-making task,[27,33] and an attentional bias to pain-related stimuli.[34] For example, a modified Stroop task has been used in several studies to investigate an attentional bias to pain-related words. In the original Stroop interference task, participants are shown words that spell color names (ie, blue, red, green) printed in colored ink. The interference task is to name the color of the ink, while ignoring the actual word. People in general are much slower at this than naming the color of the ink when it is presented as a nonword, showing that there is interference from the word itself. There is some evidence that chronic pain subjects are impaired (ie, have more interference) on the original Stroop task.[35] In the modified version of the Stroop test, pain-related words are used instead of color words. For example, the word "aching" is written in colored ink and the patient's task is to name the color of the ink. Slower responses for the pain words among chronic pain subjects compared with healthy controls is indication of greater interference because the pain word is presumed to be more salient to the subject who has pain and therefore harder to inhibit. In a meta-analysis of five modified Stroop tests with chronic pain subjects (including subjects who have FM), Roelofs and colleagues[34] reported that chronic pain subjects show evidence of greater interference from both sensory and affective pain words, indicating a tendency among subjects to selectively attend to pain words. Other cognitive methods have been tested in chronic pain syndromes with the overall conclusion that pain interferes with attention and that chronic pain subjects show an attentional bias to pain-related information.[36–40]

These studies frequently test a mix of chronic pain subjects (sometimes including subjects who have FM), so we cannot know how specific the findings would be for FM; nonetheless, the results are intriguing enough to warrant further study exclusively with subjects who have FM. There already exists a convincing collection of results showing that pain is related to cognitive function in FM. Self-reported level of pain is correlated with cognitive performance among subjects who have FM in a number of studies.[10,18,20,24,27,41] These results suggest that pain may disrupt the normal function of the attention system. Indeed, Dick and colleagues[18] reported that the significant differences observed between subjects who have FM and controls on the TEA were reduced to nonsignificant levels when self-reported pain was included as a covariant in the analyses. This is particularly interesting because this was not the case when they controlled for depression and anxiety, or sleep disturbance.

Of further interest is the mechanism through which pain interferes with cognitive function. A painful sensation automatically garners attention from many levels of the cognitive system, including attention networks that are not typically under conscious control.[39,42,43] Many have speculated that chronic pain states may therefore interfere with attention in everyday settings and the studies described above represent an effort to delineate the cognitive/attention mechanisms involved in pain-related disruption using experimental/cognitive science methods. This line of investigation has not been pursued specifically in FM, in spite of the strong suggestion from extant data that pain is related to cognitive dysfunction in these patients.

Effort

An important consideration when testing neuropsychologic function is whether performance is affected by poor effort. Fibromyalgia subjects might devote less effort to neuropsychologic and cognitive testing due to ongoing pain and fatigue or the belief that they will not perform well. To date, very little research has been done regarding formalized effort testing in subjects who have FM, although the findings of normal function on some tests (eg, pattern comparison)[20] contrasted with poor performance on other tests in the same sample of subjects does provide a suggestion that the results are not due to lower effort in the subjects who have FM. The one study using formal effort testing in subjects who have FM (Test of Memory Malingering or TOMM) found that among the 54 subjects tested, none failed the TOMM. This implies that poor effort is not a typical finding in FM. However, future studies need to address this issue, particularly in studies using standardized neuropsychologic tests in which subjects fall into the impaired range.

To summarize, the evidence suggests that many of the comorbid symptoms (depression, anxiety, fatigue, disturbed sleep) often present in FM can have a negative impact on cognitive function, but these do not seem to completely explain the phenomenon. Stronger evidence exists for the role of pain, both in its ability to disrupt attention and from central nervous system reorganization in the face of chronic pain. Patients who have FM seem to devote adequate effort to cognitive testing, although there is only one study that has reported findings using formal effort testing.

CAN COMPUTERIZED BATTERIES TEST COGNITIVE FUNCTION IN FIBROMYALGIA?

There are now several companies with computerized batteries of neuropsychologic tests. The advantage of these computer batteries is that they allow easy and identical administration and capture data electronically, eliminating the need for a separate data entry step. These batteries are ideal for large clinical trials whereby data are gathered in multiple sites. To date, only one study of FM using a computerized neuropsychologic battery has been published, with no significant effects between subjects who have FM and controls.[44] This null result may have been due to the types of tests included in the battery, because none of them involved significant distraction, nor was there a working memory test in this battery. However, given the advantages of computerized batteries, it is expected that new studies using these assessment tools will soon be available. Other batteries do contain some modules that overlap with the types of cognitive tests that have been shown to be sensitive to differences in subjects who have FM and could therefore be adapted for use in FM trials.

NEUROIMAGING IN FIBROMYALGIA

Several neuroimaging techniques are available that can be used to connect brain function to cognitive performance, including event-related potentials (ERP) whereby electrical activity in the brain is measured on the scalp and is time locked with events in a cognitive task. For example, Montoya and colleagues[45] used ERP to study attention and cognitive processing of pain-related words in subjects who have FM. Both subjects and controls showed enhanced p300 amplitudes to the pain-related words compared with neutral words. In contrast, controls but not subjects showed enhanced late potential complex (LPC) amplitudes in response to pain-related words. Increased LPC amplitudes are common in ERP studies of emotional stimuli, thought to reflect ongoing processing of emotionally arousing material. Thus, the finding that LPC was not influenced by the emotional content of the words in subjects who have FM is counterintuitive, but could reflect activity related to coping with the emotional material. Further research is necessary to understand the implication of these ERP findings, but they do illustrate differences between subjects who have FM and controls in the neurocognitive processing of pain-related information. In another study, Montoya and colleagues[46] measured ERPs while subjects who have FM and controls received nonpainful tactile stimulation. During the tactile stimulation, participants viewed pictures from the International Affective Picture System with either pleasant or unpleasant contents. For subjects who have FM, viewing unpleasant pictures significantly increased the early tactile ERP components, demonstrating increased sensitivity to the tactile stimuli. The authors hypothesized that subjects who have FM have an abnormal vulnerability to the negative emotional context in which pain occurs. Although further studies are necessary, these results demonstrate the complex inter- action between sensory processing, attention, cognition, and emotion that can occur in the face of chronic pain.

Other neuroimaging techniques such as positron emission tomography and MRI (both structural and functional) measure brain activity by way of changes in blood flow. In FM, some abnormalities of cerebral blood flow have been reported;[47,48] in contrast, one study found normal cerebral glucose metabolism.[49] Functional imaging during painful stimulation shows augmented activation in pain-processing areas of the brain in subjects who have FM,[50–53] a finding that may be informative for cognitive function because painful stimulation activates some areas of the brain that are also involved in attention-demanding cognitive tasks. More recently, proton magnetic resonance spectroscopy has been used to study regional brain metabolism in FM. Harris and colleagues[54] have found that improvements in pain are correlated with changes in glutamate in the insula, and that pain is related to choline variations in the dorsolateral prefrontal cortex.[55] Emad and colleagues[56] reported dysfunctional levels of N-acetylaspartate in the hippocampus in subjects who have FM. These results have implications for cognitive function, because the insula, hippocampus, and prefrontal cortex all are involved in many cognitive tasks. To date, no functional imaging studies have been published with subjects who have FM performing cognitive tasks, but there is preliminary evidence that subjects who have FM activate more cortical areas during a working memory task.[57]

CAN COGNITIVE FUNCTION BE IMPROVED IN FIBROMYALGIA?

The data presented in this review make it clear that dyscognition is a real and troubling symptom for FM sufferers. The obvious question is, what can be done about it? Unfor- tunately there are still very few data that address this question. In a study with chronic pain subjects, Dick and Rashiq[58] found no improvement in cognitive function with short-term local analgesia. On a more positive note, Munguia-Izquierdo and Lagaz- Arrese[13,14] found that aquatic therapy (exercise in warm water) improved many symp- toms in FM, including cognitive function. Their measures of cognition included working memory, episodic memory, and semantic memory tasks. At baseline, the subjects who have FM had significantly lower scores on all of these tests compared with healthy controls. After 16 weeks, the subjects who have FM in the exercise group had significant improvements in all cognitive measures, whereas the subjects who have FM in the control group did not show these improvements. In a recent study, Leavitt and Katz[59] found that rehearsal helped subjects who have FM overcome the effects of distraction in a memory test. These studies give hope that the cognitive effects can be ameliorated. It is not yet known if any of the pharmacologic therapies are helpful for the cognitive domain.

SUMMARY

The evidence continues to mount that dyscognition is a real and troubling symptom in FM, and further corroborates earlier speculation that the cognitive mechanisms most affected in FM are working memory, episodic memory, and semantic memory. A new focus that has emerged since our 2001 review is that patients who have FM seem especially sensitive to distraction. There may be a particular difficulty in managing the items that are held in working memory/conscious attention such that distracting or competing sensory stimuli are not filtered. The effects seen on working memory tests are consistent with this hypothesis, as is the finding that patients who have

FM are sensitive to other sensory modalities beside pain sensation. For example, Geisser and colleagues[60,61] found that subjects who have FM were more sensitive to unpleasant auditory stimulation as well as to painful pressure applied to the thumbnail.

Further work is needed to understand the causes and contributors to dyscognition in FM. In particular, a study with a large sample of subjects who have varied levels of depression, anxiety, pain, fatigue, and sleep disruption would allow the use of multivariate methods to assess the contributions of these comorbid symptoms to dyscognition. A large study like this should ideally make use of both self-report cognitive symptoms and performance-based measures of working memory, episodic memory, and semantic memory. The use of a computerized neuropsychologic battery would greatly help in this scenario, allowing for consistent testing across multiple sites.

There is also a need for smaller, more focused studies that would help to delineate the specific cognitive mechanisms that are disrupted. Results from studies such as these would inform the search for treatments, both pharmaceutic and nonpharmaceutic because they would highlight the brain systems involved. This initiative would go hand-in-hand with neuroimaging studies that take full advantage of the new and existing technologies for exploring the human brain. In order for these types of studies to have their full impact, there ought to be a greater use of and appreciation for the methods in cognitive science in the FM field. These methods use cognitive tasks where some part of the task is manipulated, and the effects of this manipulation on performance can be used to understand the cognitive mechanisms underlying the performance. For example, a memory test could be paired with different levels of distraction to assess the effects of distraction on either the learning of the to-be-remembered material, or on the recall of the material. Thus, the recall with distraction would be compared with the recall without distraction within the same individual as well as across groups (eg, subjects versus controls). An experiment like this could show whether memory is more vulnerable during learning or during recall in healthy controls and whether the pattern of vulnerability is different in a particular patient group. Cognitive science methods are crucial for functional neuroimaging of cognitive function, because the methods are used to design tests that will detect activity in brain areas associated with specific cognitive mechanisms. This kind of testing is differentiated from standardized neuropsychologic testing where the goal is to administer the tests in a highly consistent manner so that the results can be compared with published norms, or to a group of control participants. Both types of testing are useful, but yield answers to different kinds of questions, and these converging methods are necessary if we are to understand the nature of cognitive dysfunction in FM.

Dyscognition is a very real symptom for people who have FM. The evidence points to particular problems with working memory and attentional control. Further work is necessary to understand the precise cognitive mechanisms and brain systems that are involved. This work will help guide theoretic advances about the effects of chronic pain on brain/cognitive function and will inform efforts (both pharmaceutic and nonpharmeceutic) to find effective treatments for all of the symptoms experienced by people who have FM.

REFERENCES

1. Glass JM, Park DC. Cognitive dysfunction in fibromyalgia. Curr Rheumatol Rep 2001;3(2):123–7.
2. Jonides J, Smith EE, Osherson DN. Working memory and thinking. An invitation to cognitive science: thinking. Cambridge (MA): MIT Press; 1995. p. 215–65.

3. Squire LR, Zola SM. Structure and function of declarative and nondeclarative memory systems. Proc Natl Acad Sci U S A 1996;93(24):13515–22.
4. Zachrisson O, Regland B, Jahreskog M, et al. A rating scale for fibromyalgia and chronic fatigue syndrome (the FibroFatigue scale). J Psychosom Res 2002;52(6):501–9.
5. Katz RS, Heard AR, Mills M, et al. The prevalence and clinical impact of reported cognitive difficulties (fibrofog) in patients with rheumatic disease with and without fibromyalgia. J Clin Rheumatol 2004;10(2):53–8.
6. Leavitt F, Katz RS, Mills M, et al. Cognitive and dissociative manifestations in fibromyalgia. J Clin Rheumatol 2002;8(2):77–84.
7. Bennett RM, Jones J, Turk DC, et al. An internet survey of 2,596 people with fibromyalgia. BMC Musculoskelet Disord 2007;8:27.
8. Arnold LM, Crofford LJ, Mease PJ, et al. Patient perspectives on the impact of fibromyalgia. Patient Educ Couns 2008;73(1):114–20.
9. Mease PJ, Arnold LM, Crofford LJ, et al. Identifying the clinical domains of fibromyalgia: contributions from clinician and patient Delphi exercises. Arthritis Care Res 2008;59(7):952–60.
10. Glass JM, Park DC, Minear M, et al. Memory beliefs and function in fibromyalgia patients. J Psychosom Res 2005;58(3):263–9.
11. Gronwall DM. Paced auditory serial-addition task: a measure of recovery from concussion. Percept Mot Skills 1977;44(2):367–73.
12. Sletvold H, Stiles TC, Landro NI. Information processing in primary fibromyalgia, major depression and healthy controls. J Rheumatol 1995;22(1):137–42.
13. Munguia-Izquierdo D, Legaz-Arrese A. Assessment of the effects of aquatic therapy on global symptomatology in patients with fibromyalgia syndrome: a randomized controlled trial. Arch Phys Med Rehabil 2008;89(12):2250–7.
14. Munguia-Izquierdo D, Legaz-Arrese A. Exercise in warm water decreases pain and improves cognitive function in middle-aged women with fibromyalgia. Clin Exp Rheumatol 2007;25(6):823–30.
15. Leavitt F, Katz RS. Distraction as a key determinant of impaired memory in patients with fibromyalgia. J Rheumatol 2006;33(1):127–32.
16. Suhr JA. Neuropsychological impairment in fibromyalgia: relation to depression, fatigue, and pain. J Psychosom Res 2003;55:321–9.
17. Boone KB, Ponton MO, Gorsuch RL, et al. Factor analysis of four measures of prefrontal lobe functioning. Arch Clin Neuropsychol 1998;13(7):585–95.
18. Dick BD, Verrier MJ, Harker KT, et al. Disruption of cognitive function in fibromyalgia syndrome. Pain 2008;139:610–6.
19. Salthouse TA, Babcock RL. Decomposing adult age differences in working memory. Dev Psychol 1991;27(5):763–76.
20. Park DC, Glass JM, Minear M, et al. Cognitive function in fibromyalgia patients. Arthritis Rheum 2001;44(9):2125–33.
21. Dick B, Eccleston C, Crombez G. Attentional functioning in fibromyalgia, rheumatoid arthritis, and musculoskeletal pain patients. Arthritis Rheum 2002;47(6):639–44.
22. Robertson IH, Ward T, Ridgeway V, et al. The structure of normal human attention: the test of everyday attention. J Int Neuropsychol Soc 1996;2(6):525–34.
23. Landro NI, Stiles TC, Sletvold H. Memory functioning in patients with primary fibromyalgia and major depression and healthy controls. J Psychosom Res 1997;42(3):297–306.
24. Grace GM, Nielson WR, Hopkins M, et al. Concentration and memory deficits in patients with fibromyalgia syndrome. J Clin Exp Neuropsychol 1999;21(4):477–87.

25. Glass JM, Park DC, Crofford LJ. Memory performance with divided attention in fibromyalgia (FM) patients [abstract]. Arthritis Rheum 2004;50(Suppl Issue): S489.
26. Leavitt F, Katz RS. Speed of mental operations in fibromyalgia: a selective naming speed deficit. J Clin Rheumatol 2008;14(4):214–8.
27. Verdejo-Garcia A, Lopez-Torrecillas F, Calandre EP, et al. Executive function and decision-making in women with fibromyalgia. Arch Clin Neuropsychol 2009;24(1):113–22.
28. Sephton SE, Studts JL, Hoover K, et al. Biological and psychological factors associated with memory function in fibromyalgia syndrome. Health Psychol 2003;22(6):592–7.
29. Balkin TJ, Bliese PD, Belenky G, et al. Comparative utility of instruments for monitoring sleepiness-related performance decrements in the operational environment. J Sleep Res 2004;13(3):219–27.
30. Cote KA, Moldofsky H. Sleep, daytime symptoms, and cognitive performance in patients with fibromyalgia. J Rheumatol 1997;24(10):2014–23.
31. Hart RP, Martelli MF, Zasler ND. Chronic pain and neuropsychological functioning. Neuropsychol Rev 2000;10(3):131–49.
32. Metz AE, Yau HJ, Centeno MV, et al. Morphological and functional reorganization of rat medial prefrontal cortex in neuropathic pain. Proc Natl Acad Sci U S A 2009; 106(7):2423–8.
33. Apkarian AV, Sosa Y, Krauss BR, et al. Chronic pain patients are impaired on an emotional decision-making task. Pain 2004;108(1–2):129–36.
34. Roelofs J, Peters ML, Zeegers MP, et al. The modified Stroop paradigm as a measure of selective attention towards pain-related stimuli among chronic pain patients: a meta-analysis. Eur J Pain 2002;6(4):273–81.
35. Grisart JM, Plaghki LH. Impaired selective attention in chronic pain patients. Eur J Pain 1999;3(4):325–33.
36. Van Damme S, Crombez G, Lorenz J. Pain draws visual attention to its location: experimental evidence for a threat-related bias. J Pain 2007;8(12):976–82.
37. Van DS, Crombez G, Eccleston C, et al. Hypervigilance to learned pain signals: a componential analysis. J Pain 2006;7(5):346–57.
38. Van DS, Crombez G, Eccleston C, et al. Impaired disengagement from threatening cues of impending pain in a crossmodal cueing paradigm. Eur J Pain 2004;8:227–36.
39. Eccleston C, Crombez G. Pain demands attention: a cognitive-affective model of the interruptive function of pain. Psychol Bull 1999;125(3):356–66.
40. Crombez G, Van DS, Eccleston C. Hypervigilance to pain: an experimental and clinical analysis. Pain 2005;116(1–2):4–7.
41. Glass JM, Williams DA, Gracely RH, et al. Relationship of self-reported pain, tender-point count, and evoked pressure pain sensitivity to cognitive function in fibromyalgia. J Pain 2004;5(Suppl):S38.
42. McCabe C, Lewis J, Shenker N, et al. Don't look now! Pain and attention. Clin Med 2005;5(5):482–6.
43. Eccleston C, Crombez G. Attention and pain: merging behavioural and neuroscience investigations. Pain 2005;113(1–2):7–8.
44. Walitt B, Roebuck-Spencer T, Bleiberg J, et al. Automated neuropsychiatric measurements of information processing in fibromyalgia. Rheumatol Int 2008; 28(6):561–6.
45. Montoya P, Pauli P, Batra A, et al. Altered processing of pain-related information in patients with fibromyalgia. Eur J Pain 2005;9(3):293–303.

46. Montoya P, Sitges C, Garcia-Herrera M, et al. Abnormal affective modulation of somatosensory brain processing among patients with fibromyalgia. Psychosom Med 2005;67(6):957–63.
47. Bradley LA, McKendree-Smith NL, Alberts KR, et al. Use of neuroimaging to understand abnormal pain sensitivity in fibromyalgia. Curr Rheumatol Rep 2000;2(2):141–8.
48. Kwiatek R, Barnden L, Tedman R, et al. Regional cerebral blood flow in fibromyalgia: single-photon-emission computed tomography evidence of reduction in the pontine tegmentum and thalami. Arthritis Rheum 2000;43(12):2823–33.
49. Yunus MB, Young CS, Saeed SA, et al. Positron emission tomography in patients with fibromyalgia syndrome and healthy controls. Arthritis Rheum 2004;51(4): 513–8.
50. Gracely RH, Petzke F, Wolf JM, et al. Functional magnetic resonance imaging evidence of augmented pain processing in fibromyalgia. Arthritis Rheum 2002; 46(5):1333–43.
51. Cook DB, Lange G, Ciccone DS, et al. Functional imaging of pain in patients with primary fibromyalgia. J Rheumatol 2004;31(2):364–78.
52. Wik G, Fischer H, Finer B, et al. Retrospenial cortical deactivation during painful stimulation of fibromyalgic patients. Int J Neurosci 2006;116(1):1–8.
53. Gracely RH, Geisser ME, Giesecke T, et al. Pain catastrophizing and neural responses to pain among persons with fibromyalgia. Brain 2004;127(Pt 4): 835–43.
54. Harris RE, Sundgren PC, Pang Y, et al. Dynamic levels of glutamate within the insula are associated with improvements in multiple pain domains in fibromyalgia. Arthritis Rheum 2008;58(3):903–7.
55. Petrou M, Harris RE, Foerster BR, et al. Proton MR spectroscopy in the evaluation of cerebral metabolism in patients with fibromyalgia: comparison with healthy controls and correlation with symptom severity. AJNR Am J Neuroradiol 2008; 29(5):913–8.
56. Emad Y, Ragab Y, Zeinhom F, et al. Hippocampus dysfunction may explain symptoms of fibromyalgia syndrome. A study with single-voxel magnetic resonance spectroscopy. J Rheumatol 2008;35(7):1371–7.
57. Bangert A, Glass JM, Welsh RC, et al. Functional magnetic resonance imaging of working memory in fibromyalgia. Arthritis Rheum 2003;48(9):S90.
58. Dick BD, Rashiq S. Disruption of attention and working memory traces in individuals with chronic pain. Anesth Analg 2007;104(5):1223–9, tables.
59. Leavitt F, Katz RS. Normalizing memory recall in fibromyalgia with rehearsal: a distraction-counteracting effect. Arthritis Rheum 2009;61(6):740–4.
60. Geisser ME, Strader Donnell C, Petzke F, et al. Comorbid somatic symptoms and functional status in patients with fibromyalgia and chronic fatigue syndrome: sensory amplification as a common mechanism. Psychosomatics 2008;49(3): 235–42.
61. Geisser ME, Glass JM, Rajcevska LD, et al. A psychophysical study of auditory and pressure sensitivity in patients with fibromyalgia and healthy controls. J Pain 2008;9(5):417–22.

Neuroimaging of Fibromyalgia

Mary B. Nebel, BSE, Richard H. Gracely, PhD*

KEYWORDS

- Fibromyalgia • fMRI • Neuroimaging • Tenderness
- Cerebral activity • Widespread pain

Fibromyalgia is a significant medical problem characterized by chronic widespread pain. Although the diagnostic criteria for fibromyalgia are, in part, based on tenderness in more than 10 of 18 defined sites,[1] recent evidence suggests fibromyalgia tenderness is not confined to these classic sites or to muscle.[2] The general and widespread nature of pain in fibromyalgia implicates the involvement of generalized mechanisms that facilitate spontaneous pain and increase the body's sensitivity to painful blunt pressure.

INFERRING BRAIN ACTIVITY FROM REGIONAL CEREBRAL BLOOD FLOW

Functional neuroimaging of the brain has opened a window into supraspinal processes in health and disease. The majority of recent interest has been in methods that infer neural activity in the brain by evaluating the time course of highly localized changes in regional cerebral blood flow (rCBF) occurring in response to changes in neuronal metabolic demand. rCBF increases after a hemodynamic delay of a few seconds and is closely coupled to the magnitude and duration of the underlying neuronal activity.

FIRST IMAGING STUDIES OF BASELINE REGIONAL CEREBRAL BLOOD FLOW IN FIBROMYALGIA USING SINGLE-PHOTON EMISSION COMPUTED TOMOGRAPHY

The pioneering application of functional neuroimaging to the investigation of pain in fibromyalgia used single-photon emission computed tomography (SPECT), a method that involves detecting the distribution in the brain of a radioactive tracer injected into the vascular system before scanning. Using SPECT, Mountz and coworkers[3] compared baseline levels of rCBF in large predefined regions of interest (ROIs) in ten patients with fibromyalgia and seven control subjects. In this initial study, patients who had fibromyalgia demonstrated lower rCBF reflecting reduced neural activity

Center for Neurosensory Disorders, University of North Carolina School of Dentistry, 2110-A Old Dental Building, CB#7455, Chapel Hill, NC 27599, USA
* Corresponding author.
E-mail address: rgracely@med.umich.edu (R.H. Gracely).

Rheum Dis Clin N Am 35 (2009) 313–327
doi:10.1016/j.rdc.2009.06.004
0889-857X/09/$ – see front matter © 2009 Published by Elsevier Inc.

rheumatic.theclinics.com

bilaterally in the thalamus and in the caudate nucleus relative to controls. Kwiatek and colleagues[4] subsequently performed a similar SPECT study with a larger sample of fibromyalgia patients and healthy controls and observed decreased rCBF in the right thalamus, in the inferior pontine tegmentum, and near the right lentiform nucleus. The consistent finding of reduced resting rCBF in the right thalamus was replicated by Bradley and coworkers,[5] and reduced perfusion of the thalamus has also been observed in patients with other chronically painful conditions such as traumatic peripheral neuropathy[6] and metastatic breast cancer.[7] Although the cause of thalamic decreases in rCBF is unknown, inhibition of activity in this region is associated with prolonged excitatory nociceptive input.[6] The persistent excitatory input associated with ongoing and spontaneous pain in fibromyalgia may be sufficient to activate pain inhibitory mechanisms. One consequence of this inhibition appears to be reduced resting and evoked activity in the thalamus.

FUNCTIONAL MAGNETIC RESONANCE IMAGING STUDIES OF FIBROMYALGIA

While these initial SPECT studies of fibromyalgia were occurring, functional MRI (fMRI) methods were being developed that could assess brain activity with greater temporal and spatial resolution than either SPECT or positron emission tomography (PET). Unlike SPECT and PET, fMRI relies on an intrinsic tracer, the oxygenation state of hemoglobin, to track changes in rCBF. Whether or not oxygen is attached to hemoglobin alters the magnetic properties of the transporter protein and its effect on the local magnetic field. The higher the regional concentration of deoxygenated hemoglobin, the faster the MR signal emitted from brain tissue will deteriorate. Because oxygen supply increases more than oxygen consumption during neuronal firing, the regional concentration of deoxygenated hemoglobin decreases, and the fMRI signal is observed to increase or light up in active brain regions. This is referred to as the blood oxygenation level dependent (BOLD) signal.

TASK ACTIVATION STUDIES: BRAIN ACTIVITY EVOKED BY A PAINFUL STIMULUS
Pain Augmentation

The first fMRI study of fibromyalgia investigated cortical responses to painful blunt pressure applied to the thumb.[8] The thumb was chosen for its dense innervation, for its large representation in the primary somatosensory cortex (SI), and to test implicitly the hypothesis that tenderness in fibromyalgia is not due to muscle sensitivity or confined to muscles but is a property of deep tissue, with fibromyalgia tenderness being generally expressed over the entire body. To account for the increased sensitivity that characterizes the fibromyalgia participants' perception of evoked pain stimuli, cortical responses to pressure stimuli were evaluated in the context of equal stimulus intensities for patients and controls and under conditions of equal perceptual intensities. For each of the 32 participants (16 fibromyalgia), pressures that evoked pain described as near "slightly intense" on a calibrated pain scale[2,9] were determined using a 1-cm diameter hard rubber probe attached to a hydraulic cylinder. During a 10-minute fMRI scan, subjects experienced 30-second blocks of slightly intense painful pressure interleaved with 30-second blocks of nonpainful pressure. The comparison of the effects of these subjectively equal evoked pain sensations on the BOLD response (produced by pressure amplitudes approximately half as small for fibromyalgia patients as for controls) defined the equal pain contrast. The healthy control subjects underwent an additional fMRI scan in which stimuli delivered during the 30-second blocks of painful pressure were reduced to the amplitudes of pressure delivered to the patients (equal pressure contrast); however, these pressures were consistently reported as "not painful" or only "faintly painful" by the control subjects.

Group results demonstrated that stimuli that evoked similar levels of perceived pain intensity in fibromyalgia and control subjects evoked significant changes in neural activity in a similar network of brain regions implicated in pain processing. These increases were observed in structures involved in sensory discriminative processing (contralateral primary [SI] and secondary somatosensory cortices [SII]), sensory association (contralateral superior temporal gyrus, inferior parietal lobule), motor responses (contralateral putamen and ipsilateral cerebellum), and affective processing (contralateral insula). Fibromyalgia and control subjects also shared a similar region of decreased neural activation in ipsilateral SI.

In contrast to the numerous common activations observed between fibromyalgia subjects and controls when subjective pain perception was equated, no common activations were observed between the two groups when pressure stimulus intensities were equated. The relatively low pressure stimuli evoked significantly greater activity in most of the previously mentioned regions for fibromyalgia subjects; in contrast, controls only demonstrated greater evoked activity in the ipsilateral medial frontal gyrus. These findings suggest that the greater perceived intensity of standardized low pressure stimuli by persons with fibromyalgia is consistent with a model of centrally augmented pain processing and that the levels of cortical activity evoked in brain areas involved in pain processing are consistent with the subjects' verbal reports of pain magnitude.

Augmented pain processing in fibromyalgia does not appear to be unique to pain evoked by blunt pressure. Cook and colleagues[10] illustrated a similar result using skin heating stimuli. Heat pain stimuli matched on subjective perceptual intensity and applied to the hand elicited similar patterns of brain activations in nine female fibromyalgia patients and nine gender-matched controls, with the fibromyalgia patients requiring lower temperatures. In contrast, when heat pain stimuli were matched on temperature, significantly greater activations were observed in contralateral insular cortex in the fibromyalgia group. Additionally, the fibromyalgia group displayed significantly greater activity in several regions implicated in pain processing in response to random, nonpainful skin heating.

Stimulus Encoding

To further characterize this exaggerated processing of evoked pain, Grant and coworkers[11] compared the range of BOLD responses elicited in fibromyalgia patients and controls when subjected to a battery of pressure stimuli evoking sensations ranging from faint to moderately intense. Before scanning, the 26 subjects (13 fibromyalgia) underwent psychophysical testing to determine pressures that elicited the following four sensations: (1) nonpainful, (2) faintly painful, (3) very mild, and (4) between slightly and moderately painful pressure. During each 10-minute fMRI scan, subjects experienced 25-second blocks of pressure interleaved with 25 seconds of no pressure, with the four predetermined pressures being presented three times each in random order. Consistent with the aforementioned fMRI studies, the pressures needed to evoke the various subjective levels of pain were lower for subjects with fibromyalgia than for controls, but despite the differences in the range of pressures presented, both groups demonstrated graded BOLD responses in regions of the pain matrix associated with the sensory-discriminative dimension of pain sensation, including the contralateral thalamus, SI, and SII. Controls also exhibited graded responses in two areas associated with affective processing that fibromyalgia subjects did not, namely, the contralateral insula and anterior cingulate cortex

(ACC). It is possible that the fibromyalgia patients did not find the evoked pain stimuli affectively arousing due to affective adaptation caused by their prolonged clinical pain.

Individual Variation Association with Pain Locus of Control

Pain is a multidimensional experience, and a growing body of evidence suggests that, as such, factors beyond the magnitude of painful stimulation influence the perception of pain and any resulting pain behavior. More recent neuroimaging studies have begun to investigate brain regions in which pain-evoked activity is modulated across a population of subjects by subject-specific psychologic variables such as depression, catastrophizing, and perceived control over pain. Farrell and coworkers[12] demonstrated that different beliefs about pain locus of control are associated with different patterns of activation within the pain matrix in response to painful pressure stimuli. Fibromyalgia subjects who believe they have personal control over their pain exhibit greater activation in contralateral SII, whereas fibromyalgia subjects who believe their pain locus of control to be external to themselves exhibit greater responses to evoked pain in the posterior parietal cortex bilaterally, an area involved in sensory integration. These findings suggest that attitudes about pain control may modulate perceived pain by engaging brain regions involved in the interpretation and evaluation of sensory input.

Individual Variation Association with Depression

Depressed mood often accompanies chronic pain, and psychophysical evidence suggests that a negative affect is directly associated with enhanced pain perception in patients with fibromyalgia.[13,14] Using fMRI, Giesecke and colleagues[15] evaluated the effects of symptoms of depression on brain responses to pressure pain in fibromyalgia. Thirty patients with fibromyalgia, seven of whom had previously been diagnosed with major depressive disorder (MDD), and seven control subjects received fMRI scans during alternating pressure and no pressure stimulation blocks using methods similar to the previously described study by Gracely and colleagues.[8] Symptoms of depression were assessed using the Center for Epidemiologic Studies Depression Scale (CES-D). No associations were found between depression and either pressure pain sensitivity or brain activity evoked in regions involved in the sensory discriminative aspect of pain processing. Furthermore, no group differences in brain activity were found among controls, fibromyalgia subjects with MDD, and fibromyalgia subjects without MDD in these same regions; however, CES-D scores were significantly associated with evoked pain activity in the contralateral anterior insula and bilateral amygdala, and only fibromyalgia subjects with MDD exhibited significant activity in these regions. Given that the insula projects to part of the amygdala,[16] and the amygdala is traditionally associated with emotions, these findings suggest that depression modulates evoked pain activity in regions involved in processing affective characteristics of the pain experience.

Individual Variation Association with Catastrophizing

Once thought to be a symptom of depression, catastrophizing is emerging as an independent variable of significance in predicting pain chronicity and the response to pain treatment.[17] Correlation analysis of catastrophizing with brain activity evoked by painful blunt pressure in patients with fibromyalgia revealed significant associations in brain regions related to the anticipation of pain (contralateral medial frontal gyrus, ipsilateral cerebellum) and attention to pain (ACC, bilateral dorsolateral prefrontal cortex), as well as to emotional (ipsilateral claustrum, interconnected to the amygdala) and motor responses (contralateral lentiform nuclei).[18] The deleterious effects of catastrophizing appear to be mediated through a number of separate cognitive mechanisms, and behavioral modification of specific malleable mechanisms, such as interpretation of a perceived threat or distraction therapy, may provide efficacious treatment or prevent the transition from acute to chronic pain in vulnerable individuals.

An important question needing to be addressed is whether augmented central processing of evoked pain is unique to fibromyalgia or is a general consequence of experiencing chronic pain. Jones and Derbyshire[19,20] demonstrated using PET that patients with chronic pain from a known peripheral origin, rheumatoid arthritis, exhibit characteristically distinct brain responses to evoked pain when compared with patients with chronic atypical facial pain, a condition hypothesized to be maintained by aberrant central nervous system sensory processing. Patients who had rheumatoid arthritis were found to have reduced cortical and subcortical responses to painful skin heating when compared with patients with chronic atypical facial pain, although no significant differences were observed in ratings given for the affective components of either the ongoing or the experimental pain experienced by the two patient groups. Giesecke and coworkers[21] directly compared pressure pain sensitivity and brain activity evoked under equal perceived intensity and equal stimulus pressure conditions in fibromyalgia patients, patients with idiopathic chronic low back pain, and healthy controls. Giesecke and colleagues were able to replicate the findings of the initial fMRI study of fibromyalgia tenderness conducted by Gracely and colleagues.[8] Giesecke and colleagues also observed that, despite higher tender point counts in fibromyalgia patients, both patient groups displayed similar pressure pain sensitivities which were significantly lower than those of the healthy controls when evaluated at a site distinct from their regions of pain, namely, the thumb. In addition to displaying similar hyperalgesic responses to pressure pain stimuli, the two patient groups displayed similar patterns of augmented pain processing when compared with controls, suggesting that idiopathic chronic low back pain and fibromyalgia may be maintained by common central mechanisms.

TASK ACTIVATION STUDIES: BRAIN ACTIVITY EVOKED BY A COGNITIVE TASK
Functional Magnetic Resonance Imaging of Cognitive Dysfunction in Fibromyalgia

Patients with fibromyalgia often complain of nonpain symptoms including fatigue and sleep problems. One interesting complaint is of cognitive difficulties referred to as "fibro-fog." Park and coworkers[22] compared fibromyalgia patients (mean age, 47.8 years) with age-matched (mean age, 47.8 years) and older (mean age, 66.9 years) normal control groups on a battery of cognitive tests. The results showed age-related cognitive deficits in the control group, especially in tasks evaluating information processing speed, working memory, free recall memory, and vocabulary fluency. No differences were found in recognition memory and verbal knowledge. The analysis further compared the function of the fibromyalgia patients with that of the two control groups. When comparing the patients with the age-matched control group, the results showed deficits in the patients in working memory, recognition memory, free recall memory, and verbal knowledge, with a marginal deficit in verbal fluency and no difference in information processing speed. Compared to the older control group, patients showed similar performance on working memory, recognition memory, free recall memory, and verbal fluency. The patients differed, and in different directions, from this older group on only two tests. The patients showed decreased verbal knowledge but superior information processing speed; therefore, the cognitive function of patients with fibromyalgia is generally similar to the function of much older persons, especially in terms of memory function. These patients are also worse than older controls on measures of verbal knowledge, which does not usually decline with age. The one area in which a deficit was not found was in information processing speed, which was age appropriate.

These cognitive deficits in fibromyalgia were assessed further in an fMRI BOLD study in which the stimulus presented was a working memory cognitive test rather than painful stimulation. Bangert and colleagues[23] evaluated brain activity during a working memory task in 12 fibromyalgia patients and nine age- and education-matched control subjects. Unlike the study by Park and colleagues[22] that found a deficit in memory performance in the fibromyalgia group, both the patients and healthy controls performed similarly on the tasks; however, the fMRI BOLD analysis showed that the patients had increased activation in a number of brain regions, including bilateral activation in the middle frontal gyrus and activation in the right medial frontal gyrus, superior parietal lobe, and precentral gyrus. These results suggest that the patients were able to produced comparable levels of performance by using more cognitive resources than their pain-free peers.

Functional Magnetic Resonance Imaging Evaluation of Pharmacologic Treatment

The studies described previously used neuroimaging methods to assess the supraspinal correlates of augmented sensitivity to painful stimulation in fibromyalgia and the putative modulation of this sensitivity by emotional and cognitive factors. The functional significance of this increased sensitivity to external painful stimulation is not known. A recent multicenter study has investigated these mechanisms by using fMRI to assess the pharmacologic treatments of fibromyalgia. The noradrenalin serotonin reuptake inhibitor milnacipran has been shown to be effective in relieving the spontaneous pain of fibromyalgia and has recently received approval for the treatment of fibromyalgia in the United States. In a European multicenter trial, 92 female fibromyalgia patients participated in a 13-week, multicenter, double-blind, placebo-controlled, randomized trial assessing the effect of 100 mg of milnacipran twice daily on brain activity evaluated before and after treatment. Patients discontinued all medications that could potentially alter pain perception. In the baseline fMRI session, 2.5-second blunt pressure stimuli were calibrated for each subject to evoke pain rated as 50 mm on a 0- to 100-mm visual analogue scale (VAS). Preliminary results in all subjects showed significant activations in brain regions previously identified in fMRI studies of experimental pain stimuli, including the primary and secondary somatosensory cortices, insular and cingulate cortices, cerebellum, thalamus, and amygdala.[24] Milnacipran (n = 46) reduced VAS ratings of painful pressure in comparison with placebo (n = 46). This effect approached significance for all patients ($P = .055$, one tailed) and was significant in several analyses that considered subgroup membership or influence of baseline pain. The fMRI analyses found different patterns of changed activation in the milnacipran and placebo groups. Milnacipran treatment resulted in increased activation in the caudatus nucleus, anterior insula, anterior cingulum, and amygdala. Placebo treatment resulted in increased activity only in a region of the parietal cortex and in the midinsular cortex. A statistical comparison between the effects of milnacipran and placebo showed increased activity in a large region of the posterior cingulate/precuneus. These preliminary results suggest a pharmacologic effect of milnacipran that is distinctly different from the placebo effect. The exact nature of the effect of milnacipran is not known and could include alteration of pain modulatory systems. In other imaging studies using perceptually equal painful stimuli, patients with fibromyalgia often show suppressed activations when compared with control subjects. The overall findings of increased activity in multiple regions suggest a normalizing effect in which milnacipran exerts a curative action that results in patients responding more similarly to healthy control subjects.

NONTASK ACTIVATION STUDIES

Beyond the Initial Single-photon Emission Computed Tomography Studies: Imaging Spontaneous Pain in Fibromyalgia

All of the previously described studies have examined the responses evoked by painful blunt pressure. Sensitivity to such pressure is a component of the American College of Rheumatology 1990 criteria for fibromyalgia;[1] however, the degree of sensitivity or tenderness varies within fibromyalgia, and patients experience widespread pain both with and without concurrent altered sensitivity to other painful modalities such as heat. The relevance of tenderness to fibromyalgia and chronic widespread pain in general is a current issue of debate.[25] Regardless of the ultimate relevance of tenderness to fibromyalgia, the methods that use task-induced activations to image tenderness cannot be applied directly to the evaluation of widespread spontaneous pain. Possible exceptions include methods that either manipulate the pain or correlate activity with online ratings of fluctuating pain.[26]

Fortunately, several MRI-based methods can be used to evaluate the supraspinal activity related to pain or other nontask-related states. One approach is to evaluate basal regional cerebral blood flow (rCBF) directly with radioactive tracers using PET and SPECT. This evaluation can also be accomplished in MRI by using injected nonradioactive contrast agents by the method of MR perfusion imaging; however, the most appealing method is the use of arterial spin labeling (ASL), which like the BOLD method for task-induced activation, requires no contrast agent of any kind.

Arterial Spin Labeling

Similar to the BOLD method, ASL measures basal rCBF by using magnetized blood as the contrast agent. Blood entering a ROI is tagged by radio frequency (RF) 180-degree inversion pulses, and this effect is compared with the signal from the region in the absence of tagging. The subtraction of the tagged and nontagged image produces a functional image. This approach can be applied throughout the brain to provide a three-dimensional image of basal rCBF. There are several types of ASL methods that vary in the protocol used to tag and assess rCBF. In all methods, the source of the imaged rCBF is mostly from the parenchyma in contrast to the BOLD method which is localized in the draining veins.[27,28] The signal is closer to the neural source, resulting in improved spatial localization.

These assays of rCBF are indirect measures of neural activity that can be compared between populations or within groups over time. The latter permits the assessment of long-duration interventions that cannot be assessed by conventional BOLD techniques. For example, ASL can be used to assess the effects of a slow-acting drug or the influence of a cognitive behavioral treatment program on neural activity in patients with fibromyalgia or other chronic pain conditions.

ASL can also be used to assess task-induced activations much like the BOLD technique. One advantage is a more linear signal in relation to rCBF in comparison with the notable nonlinear characteristics of the BOLD/rCBF function. A second problem with the BOLD method is that it is very susceptible to artifacts present at tissue-air interfaces found in the nose, sinuses, and roof the mouth. ASL is relatively invulnerable to these interface artifacts and can provide superior functional images of brain regions that are difficult to evaluate with BOLD, such as the basal ganglia and orbitofrontal cortex.[29] An additional advantage is that, because of its noise characteristics, ASL is more stable over time, permitting repeat measures of long-duration interventions.

A few studies have applied ASL to evoked and spontaneous pain. In a task design using painful heat to the left hand in 14 healthy control subjects, Owen and coworkers[30] found activations in brain regions previously identified in pain studies, including the bilateral insula, secondary somatosensory cortex and cingulate cortex, and contralateral primary somatosensory cortex and ipsilateral thalamus. In a basal design comparing rCBF in eight patients with fibromyalgia and seven healthy control subjects in our laboratory, we found decreased rCBF in the bilateral thalamus in patients in a comparison with control subjects (L. Hernandez, unpublished observations), a finding observed previously for fibromyalgia[3–5,8] and other painful disorders such as traumatic peripheral neuropathy[6] and metastatic breast cancer.[7]

Structural Changes Evaluated by Voxel-based Morphometry

One method used to quantify focal changes in brain structure associated with neuropathology is voxel-based morphometry (VBM). VBM measures differences in regional concentrations of brain tissue through a voxel-wise comparison of multiple MR images of the brain. Mounting VBM evidence suggests that frequently comorbid chronic pain and stress-related disorders, including chronic low back pain, tension type headache, chronic fatigue syndrome, and posttraumatic stress disorder, are all characterized by regional reductions in gray matter.[31–35] Although fibromyalgia shares many commonalities with these disorders, few studies have investigated possible links between fibromyalgia symptom severity and altered brain morphology. Kuchinad and colleagues[36] discovered that individuals with fibromyalgia exhibit a 3.3 times greater age-associated decrease in gray matter volume when compared with healthy controls. Each year of fibromyalgia was equivalent to 9.5 times the loss of gray matter observed in normal aging. The functional significance of gray matter atrophy in fibromyalgia might include impaired endogenous pain inhibition and deficits in cognitive function as observed by Park and colleagues.[22] In fact, Luerding and colleagues[37] recently demonstrated that the altered brain morphology associated with cognitive impairment in fibromyalgia occurs in brain regions adjacent to and partially overlapping with regions associated with pain modulation. It remains unclear whether prolonged pain experience causes these brain changes or whether altered brain morphology predisposes one to pain. Nevertheless, these findings illustrate the potential of chronic pain to be a neurodegenerative disease.

Structural Changes Evaluated by Diffusion Tensor Imaging

While VBM characterizes macroscopic changes in brain volume, diffusion tensor imaging (DTI) quantifies microstructural organizational changes based on water mobility in brain tissue. Degeneration of white and gray matter would be expected to result in an increase in water motility, expressed as the apparent water diffusion coefficient (ADC), as well as a reduction in the degree of diffusion directionality, or functional anisotropy (FA), due to the loss of myelin and axonal membranes which normally restrict diffusion.[38] Lutz and colleagues[39] conducted a joint VBM-DTI investigation of brain structure in fibromyalgia. Although both methodologies revealed regional brain degeneration in fibromyalgia subjects when compared with healthy controls, only DTI provided evidence that alterations in brain microcircuitry are correlated with fibromyalgia symptom severity, suggesting that DTI might provide a more sensitive measure. Using DTI, Sundgren and colleagues[40] observed reduced FA in the right thalamus of fibromyalgia patients when compared with controls, and the reduction in FA was statistically greater in fibromyalgia individuals with worse clinical pain and an external locus of control, suggesting that it is a clinically relevant finding. The observation of normal ADC values in the right thalamic region of fibromyalgia subjects suggests that abnormalities in FA in this region are more likely the result of neuronal disorganization rather than ongoing axonal degeneration. Unfortunately, DTI is no more able to disclose the neurobiologic basis for the organizational differences it reveals than is VBM.

Neurochemical Changes

Biochemical changes in the brain may define biomarkers that precede structural changes, and one possible explanation for structural changes in chronic pain may be atrophy secondary to excitotoxicity.[32] MR spectroscopy is a noninvasive technique that provides insight into brain biochemistry by measuring regional concentrations or synthesis rates of specific metabolites such as glutamate, aspartate, glycine, and GABA in vivo. Usually, a particular stable metabolite (eg, creatine) is used as a standard, and the concentrations of the test metabolites are expressed as a ratio to this standard. Petrou and colleagues[41] assessed possible correlations between clinical symptoms of fibromyalgia and metabolite ratios in various brain regions within the pain matrix. A significant difference in the variability of choline (Cho)/creatine (Cr) was found between patients and controls in the dorsolateral prefrontal cortex, and variability in this ratio correlated significantly with clinical pain levels at the time of testing, supporting the notion that this covariation is of pathophysiologic significance. To distinguish between cause and effect, the dynamics of metabolite ratios must be studied. Harris and colleagues[42] demonstrated that changing levels of glutamate within the insula following a nonpharmcologic intervention for fibromyalgia are associated with changes in pre- and posttreatment pain thresholds as well as with changes in the BOLD response measured within the insula in patients with fibromyalgia. Glutamate is a major excitatory neurotransmitter known to function in pain pathways. The strategic position of the insula in the bidirectional pathway between the secondary somatosensory cortex (SII) and the amygdala lends it to a regulatory function within the pain matrix. Thus, the observation of these associations with glutamate level in the insula is not surprising; however, the findings illustrate the potential for glutamate to serve as a biomarker of disease severity in fibromyalgia.

Functional Connectivity Magnetic Resonance Imaging

A major focus of neuroscience is the evaluation of interconnectivity of neuronal processing units on scales ranging from synaptic connections between individual neurons to long range connections between brain regions. These interconnections are established at both the structural (anatomic) and functional level, and one of the advantages of fMRI is the potential to evaluate interconnections and causal action. One method that has gained considerable attention evaluates the correlations of spontaneous fMRI fluctuations (<0.08 Hz), usually at rest in the absence of stimulation. Simultaneous assessment of EKG and respiration permit the analytic compensation for cardiovascular and respiratory movement. In seeded analyses, brain interconnections are evaluated using a particular locus (voxel or ROI) as the independent reference signal and displaying the regions "connected" to the seeded region. Multiple brain networks are displayed by varying the seeded location. These analyses are usually based on a priori hypotheses and the choice of seed location. Alternatively, non-seeded analyses can discover networks without prior assumptions or placement of seeds. One such example is the use of self-organizing maps that use neural network approaches to find networks related to a task[43,44] or that are active during the resting state.[45]

Functional Connectivity Magnetic Resonance Imaging Analysis of the Default Mode

Analyses of connectivity during the resting state have been used to define the "default mode" of cognitive processing, that is, the normal activity present when not engaged in a task. Studies in healthy subjects have been used to define this network, whereas comparisons between control and affected populations have demonstrated baseline differences in default mode processing. Using a seed in posterior cingulate cortex, our lab compared resting state activity in 20 subjects (10 FM) and found statistically significant increases in activity in the region of the insula/orbital cortex in FM subjects, a region that is hypothesized to be active in the pain processing network and is active in many pain neuroimaging experiments.[46]

The default mode may explain many findings of task-induced deactivations (TIDs), which are regions of deactivations during a task in comparison with a nontask control condition. TIDs may actually represent the effects of default mode activation in the control condition that is not present during the task.

We have used this method in our laboratory to compare the effects of painful pressure in 13 control patients and 22 patients with fibromyalgia.[47] The fibromyalgia group showed a prominent TID in the medial frontal cortex (while no such effect was observed in healthy control subjects). The decrease in this activity during painful pressure was associated with the magnitude of the pressure. This result suggested the pain evoked by the pressure was sufficient to disrupt default-mode spontaneous thought (associated with medial frontal cortical activity) in the fibromyalgia group. In contrast, this same pressure applied to healthy control subjects did not evoke a level of pain sufficient to disrupt default-mode spontaneous thought. The conventional method of demonstrating increased pressure pain sensitivity in fibromyalgia has been to show, in comparison with control subjects, an increased activation to similar stimulus pressures. This result suggests an alternative method based on disruption of ongoing activity. This method is similar to the animal model of response suppression and may provide a more sensitive indicator of augmented pressure pain sensitivity in fibromyalgia or related disorders.

Establishing Effective Connectivity with Structural Equation Modeling

The functional connectivity method reveals brain regions whose activity covaries but does not establish effective connectivity, defined as the causal action of one brain region on another. The causal direction of the connection can be ascertained by other procedures such as structural equation modeling. Labus and coworkers[48] have applied these methods to functional images of 46 patients (22 men) with irritable bowel syndrome using PET. The analysis revealed that the sex-related differences in brain activation were mediated predominantly by emotional-arousal networks rather than networks implicated in visceral afferent processing.

Positron Emission Tomography

The PET method described previously produced activation maps using injections of ^{15}O radioactive water ($H_2^{15}O$) as a tracer. This method preceded the widespread use of fMRI and was the standard for many years. The current popularity of fMRI is likely due to several factors, including the lack of injection of radioactive tracers, the lack of a needed cyclotron to make the tracers, and increased spatial and temporal resolution. Nevertheless, PET retains several advantages when compared with fMRI. PET measures blood flow directly, and every measurement is an absolute measurement rather than a relative measurement. Baseline assessments can be compared between groups, and the effects of long-lasting interventions can be easily quantified.

PET has been used to quantify brain activity associated with pain stimulation in a large number of studies and forms the scientific background for the current application of fMRI methods. Similarly, several PET activation studies preceded fMRI neuroimaging of fibromyalgia, and PET continues to be used to address questions that cannot be answered using fMRI.

Positron Emission Tomography Studies of Nonpharmacologic Treatment and Basal Differences Between Fibromyalgia and Control Subjects

In more conventional activation studies, Wik and coworkers[49,50] used PET to compare the resting state of eight fibromyalgia patients and eight control subjects and to assess the effects of hypnosis on FM patients. As with fMRI, evaluation of rCBF provides an inference of neuronal brain activity. The PET method using [18F]fluorodeoxyglucose (FDG) avoids this inference by directly assessing glucose metabolism, and this method has been used in a number of studies of fibromyalgia. Yunnus and coworkers[51] used FDG to assess glucose metabolism in 12 fibromyalgia patients and seven control subjects and found no difference in the resting state between the patient and control groups. Using a similar FDG approach, Walitt and coworkers[52] found that improvement in a comprehensive treatment program was associated with a trend for significant increases in brain metabolism in limbic structures.

Positron Emission Tomography Ligand Binding

PET methods include one more procedure that cannot be performed by fMRI. Using ligand-binding techniques, PET can be used to assess the availability of specific receptors across groups and the change in this availability over time. Of particular note for pain studies, one technique uses a radiolabeled opioid, [11C]carfentanil, to assess availability of the mu opioid receptor (MOR). Harris and coworkers[53] used this approach to compare MOR binding in 17 patients with fibromyalgia and 17 control subjects. The results were expressed by the MOR binding potential, which is related to receptor function and inversely related to receptor occupancy by endogenous opioids. The analysis found significantly reduced overall MOR binding potential in the patient group compared to controls, and after controlling for this overall difference, significant regional reductions in MOR binding potential were observed in the right and left nucleus accumbens and the left amygdala of the FM group. In addition, a trend towards reduced MOR binding potential in the right dorsal ACC of FM subjects was also observed. This result is consistent with two mechanisms that act singly or jointly. The reduced MOR binding potential could reflect occupancy by endogenous opioids released as a consequence of the ongoing pain in fibromyalgia. The reduced MOR binding potential could also reflect receptor down-regulation that could also result from persistent occupancy from endogenous opioids. This pattern of reduced binding potential could reflect a generalized effect of chronic pain or an effect specific to fibromyalgia. A comparison with other studies of opioid binding potential in chronic pain states reveals different patterns for rheumatoid arthritis[54] and neuropathic pain,[55,56] suggesting that overall reduced opioid binding potential may be associated with chronic pain, but the distribution of the reduced opioid binding potential may be specific to different pain syndromes.

In addition to these group results, the study by Harris and colleagues[53] examined individual differences in MOR binding potential in the group with fibromyalgia. A regression analysis showed that individual MOR binding potential in the left nucleus accumbens was negatively associated with affective pain ratings on the short form of the McGill Pain Questionnaire, and that the MOR binding potential in the left amygdala was negatively associated with depression scores from the CES-D depression scale. These results support the group results and provide preliminary evidence for the application of these methods to individual cases.

SUMMARY

Since the initial application of PET and SPECT to patients with fibromyalgia, three groups of studies have applied a wide array of neuroimaging techniques to evaluate this disorder. One group has evaluated the hallmark of tenderness in fibromyalgia by using (primarily) fMRI BOLD activation studies to demonstrate augmented sensitivity to painful pressure and the association of this augmentation with variables such as depression and catastrophizing. A second emerging group of studies has evaluated the symptoms of cognitive dysfunction using the fMRI BOLD method. The third group has provided information about differences in this group that may relate to underlying mechanisms and the primary symptom of widespread pain. Using a wide array of techniques, these studies have found differences in opioid receptor binding, in the concentration of metabolites associated with neural processing in pain-related regions, in functional brain networks, and in regional brain volume and white matter tracks. The initial findings of differences in brain activity using SPECT have been replicated using varied techniques such as PET and ASL. A common theme of all of these methods is that they provide information that may be pertinent to the otherwise unobservable and poorly treated symptoms of persistent widespread chronic pain.

REFERENCES

1. Wolfe F, Smthye HA, Yunus MB, et al. The American College of Rheumatology 1990 Criteria for the Classification of Fibromyalgia. Report of the Multicenter Criteria Committee. Arthritis Rheum 1990;33:160–72.
2. Petzke F, Clauw DJ, Ambrose K, et al. Increased pain sensitivity in fibromyalgia: effects of stimulus type and mode of presentation. Pain 2003;105(3):403–13.
3. Mountz JM, Bradley LA, Modell JG, et al. Fibromyalgia in women: abnormalities of regional cerebral blood flow in the thalamus and the caudate nucleus are associated with low pain threshold levels. Arthritis Rheum 1995;38(7):926–38.
4. Kwiatek R, Barnden L, Tedman R, et al. Regional cerebral blood flow in fibromyalgia: single-photon emission computed tomography evidence of reduction in the pontine tegmentum and thalami. Arthritis Rheum 2000;43(12):2823–33.
5. Bradley LA, Sotolongo A, Alberts KR, et al. Abnormal regional cerebral blood flow in the caudate nucleus among fibromyalgia patients and non-patients is associated with insidious symptom onset. J Muscoskel Pain 1999;7:285–92.
6. Iadarola MJ, Max MB, Berman KF, et al. Unilateral decrease in thalamic activity observed with positron emission tomography in patients with chronic neuropathic pain. Pain 1995;63(1):55–64.
7. Di Piero V, Jones AK, Iannotti F, et al. Chronic pain: a PET study of the central effects of percutaneous high cervical cordotomy. Pain 1991;46(1):9–12.
8. Gracely RH, Petzke F, Wolf JM, et al. Functional magnetic resonance imaging evidence of augmented pain processing in fibromyalgia. Arthritis Rheum 2002; 46(5):1333–43.
9. Gracely RH, Dubner R, McGrath PA. Narcotic analgesia: fentanyl reduces the intensity but not the unpleasantness of painful tooth pulp sensations. Science 1979;203(4386):1261–3.

10. Cook DB, Lange G, Ciccone DS, et al. Functional imaging of pain in patients with primary fibromyalgia. J Rheumatol 2004;31(2):364–78.
11. Grant MA, Farrell MJ, Kumar R, et al. fMRI evaluation of pain intensity coding in fibromyalgia patients and controls. Arthritis Rheum 2001;44(Suppl 9):S394 [abstract].
12. Farrell MJ, VanMeter JW, Petzke F, et al. Supraspinal activity associated with painful pressure in fibromyalgia is associated with beliefs about locus of pain control. Arthritis Rheum 2001;44(Suppl 9):S394 [abstract].
13. Geisser ME, Casey KL, Brucksch CB, et al. Perception of noxious and innocuous heat stimulation among healthy women and women with fibromyalgia: association with mood, somatic focus, and catastrophizing. Pain 2003;102(3):243–50.
14. Staud R, Robinson ME, Vierck CJ Jr, et al. Ratings of experimental pain and pain-related negative affect predict clinical pain in patients with fibromyalgia syndrome. Pain 2003;105(1–2):215–22.
15. Giesecke T, Gracely RH, Williams DA, et al. The relationship between depression, clinical pain, and experimental pain in a chronic pain cohort. Arthritis Rheum 2005;52(5):1577–84.
16. Augustine JR. Circuitry and functional aspects of the insular lobe in primates including humans. Brain Res Brain Res Rev 1996;22(3):229–44.
17. Burton AK, Tillotson KM, Main CJ, et al. Psychosocial predictors of outcome in acute and subchronic low back trouble. Spine 1995;20(6):722–8.
18. Gracely RH, Geisser ME, Giesecke T, et al. Pain catastrophizing and neural responses to pain among persons with fibromyalgia. Brain 2004;127(Pt 4): 835–43.
19. Derbyshire SW, Jones AK, Devani P, et al. Cerebral responses to pain in patients with atypical facial pain measured by positron emission tomography. J Neurol Neurosurg Psychiatry 1994;57(10):1166–72.
20. Jones AK, Derbyshire SW. Reduced cortical responses to noxious heat in patients with rheumatoid arthritis. Ann Rheum Dis 1997;56(10):601–7.
21. Giesecke T, Gracely RH, Grant MA, et al. Evidence of augmented central pain processing in idiopathic chronic low back pain. Arthritis Rheum 2004;50(2): 613–23.
22. Park DC, Glass JM, Minear M, et al. Cognitive function in fibromyalgia patients. Arthritis Rheum 2001;44(9):2125–33.
23. Bangert AS, Glass JM, Welsh RC, et al. Functional magnetic resonance imaging of working memory in fibromyalgia. Arthritis Rheum 2003;48:S90 [abstract].
24. Jensen KB, Kosek E, Petzke F, et al. Evidence of dysfunctional pain inhibition in fibromyalgia reflected in rACC during provoked pain. Pain 2009;10.1016/j.pain.2009.03.018.
25. Gracely RH. A pain psychologist's view of tenderness in fibromyalgia. J Rheumatol 2007;34(5):912–3.
26. Apkarian AV, Krauss BR, Fredrickson BE, et al. Imaging the pain of low back pain: functional magnetic resonance imaging in combination with monitoring subjective pain perception allows the study of clinical pain states. Neurosci Lett 2001; 299(1–2):57–60.
27. Duong TQ, Yacoub E, Adriany G, et al. High-resolution, spin-echo BOLD, and CBF fMRI at 4 and 7 T. Magn Reson Med 2002;48(4):589–93.
28. Pfeuffer J, Adriany G, Shmuel A, et al. Perfusion-based high-resolution functional imaging in the human brain at 7 Tesla. Magn Reson Med 2002;47(5):903–11.
29. Hernandez-Garcia L. Arterial spin labeling for quantitative functional MRI. Conf Proc IEEE Eng Med Biol Soc 2004;7:5230–3.

30. Owen DG, Bureau Y, Thomas AW, et al. Quantification of pain-induced changes in cerebral blood flow by perfusion MRI. Pain 2008;136(1–2):85–96.
31. Villarreal G, Hamilton DA, Petropoulos H, et al. Reduced hippocampal volume and total white matter volume in posttraumatic stress disorder. Biol Psychiatry 2002;52(2):119–25.
32. Apkarian AV, Sosa Y, Sonty S, et al. Chronic back pain is associated with decreased prefrontal and thalamic gray matter density. J Neurosci 2004;24(46):10410–5.
33. Schmidt-Wilcke T, Leinisch E, Straube A, et al. Gray matter decrease in patients with chronic tension type headache. Neurology 2005;65(9):1483–6.
34. de Lange FP, Kalkman JS, Bleijenberg G, et al. Gray matter volume reduction in the chronic fatigue syndrome. Neuroimage 2005;26(3):777–81.
35. Chen S, Xia W, Li L, et al. Gray matter density reduction in the insula in fire survivors with posttraumatic stress disorder: a voxel-based morphometric study. Psychiatry Res 2006;146(1):65–72.
36. Kuchinad A, Schweinhardt P, Seminowicz DA, et al. Accelerated brain gray matter loss in fibromyalgia patients: premature aging of the brain? J Neurosci 2007;27(15):4004–7.
37. Luerding R, Weigand T, Bogdahn U, et al. Working memory performance is correlated with local brain morphology in the medial frontal and anterior cingulate cortex in fibromyalgia patients: structural correlates of pain-cognition interaction. Brain 2008;131(Pt 12):3222–31.
38. Basser PJ, Pierpaoli C. Microstructural and physiological features of tissues elucidated by quantitative diffusion-tensor MRI. J Magn Reson B 1996;111(3):209–19.
39. Lutz J, Jager L, de Quervain D, et al. White and gray matter abnormalities in the brain of patients with fibromyalgia: a diffusion-tensor and volumetric imaging study. Arthritis Rheum 2008;58(12):3960–9.
40. Sundgren PC, Petrou M, Harris RE, et al. Diffusion-weighted and diffusion-tensor imaging in fibromyalgia patients: a prospective study of whole brain diffusivity, apparent diffusion coefficient, and fraction anisotropy in different regions of the brain and correlation with symptom severity. Acad Radiol 2007;14(7):839–46.
41. Petrou M, Harris RE, Foerster BR, et al. Proton MR spectroscopy in the evaluation of cerebral metabolism in patients with fibromyalgia: comparison with healthy controls and correlation with symptom severity. AJNR Am J Neuroradiol 2008;29(5):913–8.
42. Harris RE, Sundgren PC, Pang Y, et al. Dynamic levels of glutamate within the insula are associated with improvements in multiple pain domains in fibromyalgia. Arthritis Rheum 2008;58(3):903–7.
43. Fischer H, Hennig J. Neural network-based analysis of MR time series. Magn Reson Med 1999;41(1):124–31.
44. Ngan SC, Hu X. Analysis of functional magnetic resonance imaging data using self-organizing mapping with spatial connectivity. Magn Reson Med 1999;41(5):939–46.
45. Peltier SJ, Polk TA, Noll DC. Detecting low-frequency functional connectivity in fMRI using a self-organizing map (SOM) algorithm. Hum Brain Mapp 2003;20(4):220–6.
46. Welsh RC, Krishnan S, Patel R, et al. Altered pain functional connectivity (fcMRI) at rest in fibromyalgia. Arthritis Rheum 2006;54(9):S126 [abstract].
47. Patel R, Glass JM, Clauw DJ, et al. Mechanisms of task induced deactivation in fibromyalgia. In: Flor H, Kalso E, Dostrovsky J, editors. Proceedings of the 11th World Congress on Pain. Sydney, Australia: IASP Press; 2005. p. 1259-P129, 450 [abstract].

48. Labus JS, Naliboff BN, Fallon J, et al. Sex differences in brain activity during aversive visceral stimulation and its expectation in patients with chronic abdominal pain: a network analysis. Neuroimage 2008;41(3):1032–43.
49. Wik G, Fischer H, Bragee B, et al. Functional anatomy of hypnotic analgesia: a PET study of patients with fibromyalgia. Eur J Pain 1999;3(1):7–12.
50. Wik G, Fischer H, Bragee B, et al. Retrosplenial cortical activation in the fibromyalgia syndrome. Neuroreport 2003;14(4):619–21.
51. Yunus MB, Young CS, Saeed SA, et al. Positron emission tomography in patients with fibromyalgia syndrome and healthy controls. Arthritis Rheum 2004;51(4):513–8.
52. Walitt B, Roebuck-Spencer T, Esposito G, et al. The effects of multidisciplinary therapy on positron emission tomography of the brain in fibromyalgia: a pilot study. Rheumatol Int 2007;27(11):1019–24.
53. Harris RE, Clauw DJ, Scott DJ, et al. Decreased central mu-opioid receptor availability in fibromyalgia. J Neurosci 2007;27(37):10000–6.
54. Jones AK, Cunningham VJ, Ha-Kawa S, et al. Changes in central opioid receptor binding in relation to inflammation and pain in patients with rheumatoid arthritis. Br J Rheumatol 1994;33(10):909–16.
55. Jones AK, Watabe H, Cunningham VJ, et al. Cerebral decreases in opioid receptor binding in patients with central neuropathic pain measured by [111C]diprenorphine binding and PET. Eur J Pain 2004;8(5):479–85.
56. Willoch F, Schindler F, Wester HJ, et al. Central post stroke pain and reduced opioid receptor binding within pain processing circuitries: a [11C]diprenorphine PET study. Pain 2004;108(3):213–20.

Key Symptom Domains to Be Assessed in Fibromyalgia (Outcome Measures in Rheumatoid Arthritis Clinical Trials)

Ernest H. Choy, MD, FRCP[a],*, Philip J. Mease, MD[b,c]

KEYWORDS

- Fibromyalgia • Domains • Core data set
- Assessment • Clinical trials

Fibromyalgia (FM) affects 2% of the population.[1–3] The dominant symptom is chronic widespread pain with tenderness reflecting hyperalgesia and allodynia.[4] The American College of Rheumatology (ACR) classification criteria in 1990 stipulated the presence of chronic widespread pain for at least 3 months and the presence of at least 11 of 18 tender points.[5] The cost to health care providers and society associated with FM are high,[6] although constructive diagnosis and management can reduce health care utilization.[7] Although pain is the dominant symptom in FM, there are numerous associated symptoms, including fatigue, morning stiffness, depression, anxiety, paraesthesia, headache, and nonrestorative sleep.[8]

Recent research has advanced our understanding of the pathophysiology of FM. It has also highlighted possible therapeutic strategies that may be effective to advance current management. Consequently, the number of clinical trials in FM has greatly increased in the past decade. With the approval of pregabalin, duloxetine, and milnacipran for treatment of FM by the US Food and Drug Administration, the number of clinical trials in FM is likely to increase. Hitherto, clinical trials in FM have used different outcome instruments assessing different symptom domains. Development of a consensus on a core set of outcome measures that should be assessed and reported in all clinical trials is needed to facilitate interpretation, pooling, and

[a] Sir Alfred Baring Garrod Clinical Trials Unit, Academic Department Rheumatology, Weston Education Centre, King's College London, Cutcombe Road, London SE5 9RJ, UK
[b] Division of Rheumatology Research, Swedish Medical Center, Seattle, WA 98104, USA
[c] University of Washington, Seattle, WA 98104, USA
* Corresponding author.
E-mail address: ernest.choy@kcl.ac.uk (E.H. Choy).

Rheum Dis Clin N Am 35 (2009) 329–337
doi:10.1016/j.rdc.2009.05.002
0889-857X/09/$ – see front matter © 2009 Elsevier Inc. All rights reserved.

comparison of results. This aligns with the key objective of the Outcome Measures in Rheumatoid Arthritis Clinical Trials (OMERACT) initiative to improve outcome measurement in rheumatic diseases through a data-driven interactive consensus process.

OUTCOME MEASURES IN RHEUMATOID ARTHRITIS CLINICAL TRIALS

The acronym OMERACT was coined at the first OMERACT conference in 1992 when the main focus was rheumatoid arthritis. Since then, the OMERACT initiative has facilitated international networks and working groups to improve outcome measurement in many rheumatic diseases. The key outcome for OMERACT is to reach consensus over what should be measured and how measurement should be performed in clinical trials for each clinical indication. Specific domains are formulated for the indication in question. In each domain, measures are collected and tested for their applicability: truth, discrimination, and feasibility. The domains and the applicable measures form the basis for the consensus guidelines (ie, a core data set). An example is the core data set in rheumatoid arthritis, which includes pain, patient global assessment, physical disability, swollen joints, tender joints, acute-phase reactants, and physician global assessment.[9] The OMERACT process is data driven. Truth should be established by the demonstration of face, construct, content, and criterion validity. The discrimination power of an instrument can be assessed by its sensitivity to change. Feasibility can be determined by the ease of use of instruments in most clinical trials. Literature reviews and validation studies are usually performed by working groups. The formulation and selection of the domains are made by larger committees, and the presentation of evidence and final selection occur at the OMERACT biennial conference. Here, plenary presentations alternate with small group sessions in which participants express their views and preferences. These views are brought back to the plenary session, where a final consensus is formulated, with the help of interactive voting. When data-driven decisions cannot be made, recommendations on a research agenda are produced. The result of this research should help to refine OMERACT guidelines.

DEVELOPMENT OF CORE OUTCOME DOMAINS THROUGH OUTCOME MEASURES IN RHEUMATOID ARTHRITIS CLINICAL TRIALS

The OMERACT process to establish a core data set for FM was initiated in 2004 and developed over 4 years through patient focus groups, physician and patient Delphi processes, systematic review, and data mining of clinical trials in FM.[10–12] The objective of these work streams was to generate the necessary data and analyses to satisfy the OMERACT filters of truth, discrimination, and feasibility.

Patient focus groups were used to screen for possible outcome domains. The face validity of these domains was confirmed by physician and patient Delphi processes. Construct validity refers to evidence supporting whether a given instrument actually assesses the topic it purports to measure. Although almost all the instruments used in clinical trials of FM were developed and validated in other medical conditions, it cannot be assumed that these "adopted" instruments actually measure what they purport to assess. For example, a scale claiming to measure fatigue developed and validated in the context of sports medicine may not be measuring the same type of fatigue affecting individuals who have FM. Thus, despite the common name "fatigue," evidence would be needed to support a claim that the same fatigue construct was being assessed by this instrument in both populations. Support for construct validity in measurement of FM (ie, whether the instrument is really measuring what it is supposed to measure) has not been established. An example is the Medical Outcome Study Sleep Questionnaire, which is a validated questionnaire developed to assess quality of sleep in patients who have primary sleep disorders. It has been used in several clinical trials in FM, but its validity and performance in FM have not been examined systematically. The construct validity of the instruments is often demonstrated by convergent and divergent relations of similar and dissimilar instruments. Instruments measuring similar constructs would be expected to have the strongest relations (positive or negative depending on the direction of the scale), suggesting convergence, whereas unrelated constructs would be expected to demonstrate weaker relations, suggesting divergence. For FM, correlation matrices containing all the outcome measures were used to demonstrate construct validity. Content validity refers to the extent to which a measure or group of measures is able capture the relevant facets of a given condition. Patient global impression of change was used as a surrogate of overall improvement, and multivariate regression analysis was used to demonstrate the content validity.

Patient Focus Group

Six patient focus groups were conducted by one experienced researcher in three centers in the United States.[10] All patients fulfilled the ACR classification criteria. Semistructured guided discussions on topics related to general and treatment-related FM experiences were held. In total, 48 female patients participated in these focus groups. Overall, patients reported delay in the diagnosis of FM, but most felt relief when the diagnosis was made. The impact of FM on daily life was found to be substantial and similar across all focus groups. The key domains most frequently identified as having the greatest impact on the patients' lives were pain, fatigue, disturbed sleep, depression, anxiety, and cognitive impairment.

Physician and Patient Delphi Exercise

Remarkable consensus regarding the relevant domains for FM is supported by a Delphi exercise by clinicians or researchers in patient focus groups,[10] in a Delphi exercise conducted in patients who had FM,[11] and through voting at OMERACT conferences 7 and 8.[12] Each of these studies provided empiric support for the selection outcome domains that should be considered for inclusion in the core data set.[12,13] From these works, the relevant domains for FM seem to be pain, patient global assessment, fatigue, health-related quality of life (HRQoL), multidimensional function, sleep, depression, physical function, tenderness, dyscognition (cognitive dysfunction), and anxiety.

Systematic Review

The feasibility and discriminatory power of specific outcome instruments used to assess different domains were examined by a systematic review of instruments that have been used in clinical trials of FM.[14] A literature search using the key words "fibromyalgia," "treatment or management," and "trial" for all publications until the end of December 2007 was carried out using Medline, PubMed, EMBASE, PsycINFO, CINAHL, Web of Sciences, Cochrane Central Register of Controlled Trials, and Cochrane Database of Systematic Reviews. Additionally, a manual search of the bibliographies of trials identified was undertaken. For non-English publications, whenever possible, English translations were obtained or assessment and data extraction were performed by native speakers of the respective languages. Studies were only included if the ACR 1990 classification criteria were used to define FM. Studies that included patients who had other diseases, such as chronic fatigue syndrome, were excluded unless patients who had ACR criteria-defined FM were separated for analysis and the result was reported. Only clinical trials were included. Reviews were examined only to ensure that all clinical trials had been identified. Information on intervention, randomization, blinding, outcome measures, and results were extracted. Outcome measures or instruments were mapped to relevant domains identified through patient focus groups and Delphi processes. Multidimensional instruments were often listed under more than one domain because of their subscales being used for different purposes. The discriminatory power of an instrument was assessed by its effect size calculated from Rosnow and Rosenthal's modified version of Cohen's d method.

One hundred eighty-five trials were identified; outcome measures were mapped into 15 domains, of which 10 were identified by patient focus groups and Delphi processes as important and five were not. The 10 key domains were pain, depression, fatigue, sleep, patient global impression, multidimensional function, HRQoL, morning stiffness, clinician global assessment, and anxiety. Dyscognition was the only key domain identified by patient focus groups and Delphi processes, but it was rarely assessed in clinical trials. In the few trials that assessed dyscognition, data were not reported in most. Numerous instruments had been used to assess these domains. For domains like pain, almost 50 different instruments had been used.

For pain, visual analog scales are commonly used, although phrases used to anchor the ends of the scale vary. A visual analog scale has an effect size of 0.7, suggesting that it is moderately to highly sensitive to change. Tenderness or tender point count (TPC) was grouped under pain for the systematic review. Despite controversy regarding its usefulness in clinical trials and for diagnosis of FM,[15,16] pressure pain threshold as measured by dolorimetry and TPC was moderately sensitive to change in trials of pharmacologic intervention.

Patient global assessment is commonly assessed by Likert or visual analog scales. They are highly sensitive to change. Other instruments were less extensively studied.

There are two broad categories of instruments that assess function in FM. One group, such as the Health Assessment Questionnaire, only assesses physical function, and the other group, such as the Fibromyalgia Impact Questionnaire, assesses multidimensional function.

The Fibromyalgia Impact Questionnaire is a multidimensional, disease-specific, 20-question, self-report questionnaire that assesses the overall symptomatology in patients who have FM. It is the only multidimensional instrument that has been developed and validated for FM. It has 10 items. The first item contains 11 questions related to physical function measured on a four-point Likert scale. The other items include pain, fatigue, morning tiredness or sleep, stiffness, anxiety, and depression. The Fibromyalgia Impact Questionnaire total score is moderately sensitive to change.

The Short Form 36 (SF-36) health survey is one of the most common generic health status instruments used in clinical trials. It is a generic health status instrument that has been validated in a broad range of diseases. It has eight domains: physical functioning, role limitations because of physical problems, bodily pain, general health perceptions, energy/vitality, social functioning, role limitations attributable to emotional problems, and mental health. These can be combined into two summary scores: a physical component score and a mental component score. It has been used to assess HRQoL in FM, although it has been used mainly in clinical trials of pharmacologic interventions. The physical and mental component scores, in addition to the individual domain, have been reported and seem to be moderately sensitive to change.

Several validated instruments for assessing depression, such as the Hamilton Depression Scale, Centre for Epidemiologic Studies Depression Scale, and Beck's Depression Inventory, have been adopted to assess depression in FM. The effect sizes of these are small to moderate. The result is biased by the design of recent trials because they have excluded patients with significant depression. Consequently, baseline depression scores in these studies were normal or low, and hence underestimated the discriminatory power of these instruments in FM.

For fatigue, visual analog and Likert scales were often used. They seem to be at least moderately sensitive to change. Recent studies have adopted multidimensional fatigue instruments, such as the multidimensional fatigue inventory, in addition to using the vitality domain of the SF-36 or the fatigue subscale of the Fibromyalgia Impact Questionnaire.

A visual analog scale and the sleep subscale of the Fibromyalgia Impact Questionnaire have been used to assess the quality of sleep in FM. Both instruments have effect sizes of approximately 0.5, indicating that they are moderately sensitive to change. Recent studies have also adopted such instruments as the Medical Outcome Sleep Index and Jenkins Sleep Scale.

Anxiety has been assessed by a visual analog scale and the State-Trait Anxiety Inventory. Both were sensitive in trials of nonpharmacologic interventions. Their use in trials of pharmacologic interventions is limited, however.

Morning stiffness is one of the items in the Fibromyalgia Impact Questionnaire. In addition, visual analog and Likert scales have been used in clinical trials to assess severity of morning stiffness. These instruments are moderately sensitive to change.

The clinician's global impression of change was a common end point in FM studies; however, in recent years, this outcome assessment has been dropped in favor of reliance on the patient as the best reporter of change in disease status.

Data Mining of Clinical Trials

To demonstrate the content, construct, and criterion validity of the core data set, data from randomized control trials in FM were analyzed. Four pharmaceutical companies, Eli Lilly (Indianapolis, Indiana), Forest Laboratories (Jersey City, New Jersey), Jazz Pharmaceuticals (Palo Alto, California), and Pfizer (New York, New York), agreed to support the OMERACT process by allowing data from their randomized controlled trials in FM to be analyzed. Data from 10 randomized clinical trials of four compounds (milnacipran, duloxetine, pregabalin, and sodium oxybate) were included. Milnacipran and duloxetine are serotonin and norepinephrine reuptake inhibitors, whereas pregabalin is an alpha-2-delta calcium channel antagonist. Sodium oxybate is the sodium salt of gamma-hydroxybutyrate, which is a central nervous system depressant and a sleep modifier. Because FM is a heterogeneous condition, including clinical trials of different medications with different modes of action is important; agents acting on different pathways may have a dissimilar impact on individual domains. For the analysis, data from clinical trials of the same medication were pooled together. All the outcome measures used in the clinical trials were mapped onto one or more of the following domains: pain, patient global assessment, fatigue, HRQoL, multidimensional function, sleep, depression, physical function, tenderness, dyscognition, and anxiety. For outcome measures, which have subscales, such as the SF-36 and Fibromyalgia Impact Questionnaire, the individual subscales and component scores were mapped and included in the analyses separately.

Not all the domains were measured in all the clinical trials. Although some domains, such as pain, mood, and fatigue, were assessed in all trials, other domains, such as stiffness and tenderness, were less consistently assessed, and dyscognition was evaluated in trials of only one compound. When instruments were mapped to different domains, there was a large overlap between HRQoL and multidimensional function, which was assessed by the SF-36 or Fibromyalgia Impact Questionnaire in all the trials. In trials of one medication, the EuroQol-5D was also used. Given the overlap, HRQoL and multidimensional function were collapsed into one domain: multidimensional function.

Correlation matrices were constructed using Pearson and Spearman correlation coefficients to demonstrate content validity. The mean correlation coefficient of outcome measures mapping to the same domain (intradomain correlation coefficient) was used as an indicator of convergent validity. The mean correlation coefficient of outcome measures of different domains (interdomain correlation coefficient) was used as an indicator of divergent validity. In general, instruments for pain, tenderness, fatigue, depression, and multidimensional function demonstrated good convergent and divergent relations, with the mean intradomain correlation coefficient being greater than the mean interdomain correlation coefficient. For multidimensional function and sleep, the difference between the mean intradomain and interdomain correlation coefficients was small. For multidimensional function, this was expected, given the breadth of this construct. For sleep, lack of separation was somewhat unexpected. This could be attributable to the treatment failing to improve sleep or to limitations of each of the instruments not being able to assess the facets of sleep that are of importance to individuals who have FM. Further analyses showed that the Medical Outcome Study Sleep Index, including such items as snoring and waking up with shortness of breath, was relevant for some sleep disorders but less relevant in FM. This was confirmed by examining the correlation coefficients of the snoring and waking up with shortness of breath items with the Patient Global Impression of Change, which were 0.02 and 0.18, respectively. Hence, the discriminatory power of the Medical Outcome Study Sleep Indices was reduced. In some studies, a patient global rating of sleep quality based on a Likert scale was also used. It also showed a moderate correlation with the Patient Global Impression of Change (correlation coefficient, $r = 0.4$), as did the sleep disturbance item of the Medical Outcome Study Sleep Index ($r = 0.4$. These data showed that subscales may be preferred to the overall indices on some sleep instruments adopted from other medical conditions.

Initially, measures of tenderness were mapped to the pain domain. The instruments used included TPC and dolorimetry. The correlation coefficient between tenderness and self-reported pain scale was at best moderate (≤ 0.4), however, whereas the correlation between TPC and dolorimetry correlation was high $r = 0.59$, suggesting that tenderness and spontaneous self-report of pain may not be measuring the same construct in FM and should be treated separately.

For stiffness, dyscognition, and anxiety, convergent and divergent validities could not be determined because these domains were measured by only one instrument in these trials.

Univariate analysis showed that correlations among instruments of different domains with the Patient Global Impression of Change were moderate to high. For depression, the mean correlation coefficient with the Patient Global Impression of Change was less than 0.5; however, in all the clinical trials included in this analysis, patients with severe comorbid depression were excluded. In addition, patients with moderate depression were excluded in trials of three compounds. Consequently, baseline depression scores were low, reducing the effect size of these change scores.

Multivariate analyses using the Patient Global Impression of Change as a surrogate for disease status and instruments assessing different domains as independent variables were also carried out. The overall R^2 values from multivariate analyses were taken as the adequacy of the domains and associated instruments to evaluate overall improvement in these clinical trials of FM—a demonstration of criterion and content validity. Regression analyses were also performed to assess whether there is any significant overlap between domains and instruments. Multivariate analyses showed moderate to high R^2 values: between 0.4 and 0.67. R^2 value was related to the number of domains assessed. In studies in which some of the potential domains were not assessed, such as tenderness, the R^2 value was also lower, suggesting that missing key domains affect the overall coverage of content relevant to the condition of FM. In all the regression analyses, pain, fatigue, physical function, multidimensional function, and depression were retained in all the clinical trials of all four compounds. Tenderness was retained in all the clinical trials of the three compounds in which it was assessed, which further supports the inclusion of tenderness as a separate domain in the core data set. Sleep was retained in two of three possible clinical trial groups. Stiffness was retained in two of four groups, and dyscognition was not retained in these regression analyses.

FINAL OUTCOME MEASURES IN RHEUMATOID ARTHRITIS CLINICAL TRIALS RECOMMENDATION ON CORE DATA SET FOR FIBROMYALGIA

The results from the data-mining exercise support including pain, fatigue, and multidimensional function as domains in a core data set for clinical trials in FM. Although adopted from other medical conditions, instruments used to assess these domains demonstrate face, construct, content, and criterion validity in FM. The analysis also suggested the inclusion of tenderness as a separate domain from pain. Physiologically, this would be logical because spontaneous and evoked pain involve different pathways. Furthermore, it mirrors the need to assess patient-reported pain and tender joint count in rheumatoid and psoriatic arthritis. Although TPC and dolorimetry have deficiencies and can be improved, they are feasible, and current analyses showed that they contribute significantly to the content validity when added to the core data set.

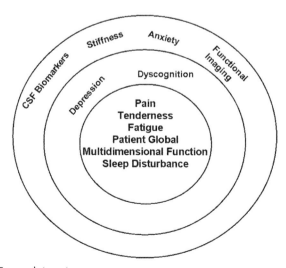

Fig. 1. OMERACT core data set.

"Nonrestorative" sleep in FM is common and thought to be of pathogenic importance in FM. Moldofsky and colleagues[17] showed that symptoms similar to FM could be induced in healthy normal volunteers by disturbing the quality of sleep. Patients and clinicians agree that it should be included in the core data set. Adopting validated instruments for assessing primary sleep disorder may not be ideal, however. Using subscales, such as the sleep disturbance subscale of the Medical Outcome Sleep Index, may be preferable. Because sleep was retained in regression analyses in all but one group, there is a strong argument for including some element of sleep in the core data set.

Although depression is a common symptom in FM and is rated as important by patients and clinicians, the exclusion of patients with moderate and severe depression in most clinical trials makes it unlikely that any instrument used to measure depression would be extremely sensitive to change. Given that this exclusion criterion is common in FM clinical trials, it seems unnecessary to stipulate the inclusion of depression in the core data set. Nonetheless, the assessment of depression in FM is recommended in many clinical trials.

Assessment of dyscognition was rated as important by patients and clinicians. There are limited data on how it should be assessed, however. A small number of trials have used the Multiple Ability Self-Report Questionnaire, but there is insufficient evidence to support its inclusion into the core data set, although assessment of dyscognition is recommended in clinical trials of FM.

For anxiety, morning stiffness, imaging, and biomarkers, evidence was limited. They were included in the research agenda for future OMERACT meetings.

Fig. 1 summarizes the final OMERACT recommendation. Pain, tenderness, fatigue, patient global assessment, multidimensional function, and sleep are included in the FM core data set. Depression and dyscognition are in the middle circle, indicating that they are recommended but not mandated. Anxiety, morning stiffness, imaging, and biomarkers are included in the research agenda.

REFERENCES

1. Wolfe F, Ross K, Anderson J, et al. The prevalence and characteristics of fibromyalgia in the general population. Arthritis Rheum 1995;38:19–28.
2. White KP, Speechley M, Harth M, et al. The London Fibromyalgia Epidemiology Study: the prevalence of fibromyalgia syndrome in London, Ontario. J Rheumatol 1999;26:1570–6.
3. Branco JC, Bannwarth B, Failde I, et al. Prevalence of fibromyalgia: a survey in five European countries. Semin Arthritis Rheum 2009, in press.
4. Staud R, Rodriguez ME. Mechanisms of disease: pain in fibromyalgia syndrome. Nat Clin Pract Rheumatol 2006;2:90–8.
5. Wolfe F, Smythe HA, Yunus MB, et al. The American College of Rheumatology 1990 criteria for the classification of fibromyalgia. Arthritis Rheum 1990;33:160–72.
6. Boonen A, van den Heuvel R, van Tubergen A, et al. Large differences in cost of illness and well-being between patients with fibromyalgia, chronic low back pain, or ankylosing spondylitis. Ann Rheum Dis 2005;64:396–402.
7. Hughes G, Martinez C, Myon E, et al. The impact of a diagnosis of fibromyalgia on health care resource use by primary care patients in the UK: an observational study based on clinical practice. Arthritis Rheum 2006;54:177–83.
8. Buskila D. Fibromyalgia, chronic fatigue syndrome, and myofascial pain syndrome. Curr Opin Rheumatol 2001;13:117–27.

9. Boers M, Tugwell P, Felson DT, et al. World Health Organization and International League of Associations for Rheumatology core endpoints for symptom modifying antirheumatic drugs in rheumatoid arthritis clinical trials. J Rheumatol Suppl 1994; 41:86–9.

10. Arnold LM, Crofford LJ, Mease PJ, et al. Patient perspectives on the impact of fibromyalgia. Patient Educ Couns 2008;73:114–20.

11. Mease PJ, Arnold LM, Crofford LJ, et al. Identifying the clinical domains of fibromyalgia: contributions from clinician and patient Delphi exercises. Arthritis Rheum 2008;59:952–60.

12. Mease P, Arnold LM, Bennett R, et al. Fibromyalgia syndrome. J Rheumatol 2007; 34:1415–25.

13. Mease PJ, Clauw DJ, Arnold LM, et al. Fibromyalgia syndrome. J Rheumatol 2005;32:2270–7.

14. Carville SF, Choy EH. Systematic review of discriminating power of outcome measures used in clinical trials of fibromyalgia. J Rheumatol 2008;35:2094–105.

15. Katz RS, Wolfe F, Michaud K. Fibromyalgia diagnosis: a comparison of clinical, survey, and American College of Rheumatology criteria. Arthritis Rheum 2006; 54:169–76.

16. Wolfe F. The relation between tender points and fibromyalgia symptom variables: evidence that fibromyalgia is not a discrete disorder in the clinic. Ann Rheum Dis 1997;56:268–71.

17. Moldofsky H, Scarisbrick P, England R, et al. Musculoskeletal symptoms and non-REM sleep disturbance in patients with "fibrositis syndrome" and healthy subjects. Psychosom Med 1975;37:341–51.

Advances in the Assessment of Fibromyalgia

David A. Williams, PhD[a],*, Stephen Schilling, PhD[b]

KEYWORDS

- Chronic fatigue • Fibromyalgia • Pain • Questionnaire
- Co-morbidities

Fibromyalgia (FM) is a manifestation of chronic widespread pain (CWP) and tenderness with a prevalence of 2% in the general population.[1] Clinically, patients who have FM present with a variety of physical symptoms that include widespread pain and tenderness but also fatigue, sleep disturbance, decrements in physical functioning, mood disturbances, and problems with cognition, such as memory problems, concentration difficulties, and diminished mental clarity.[2,3] FM occurs more frequently in females[1] and is associated with overall diminished quality of life,[4] diminished functional status,[5] and higher-than-expected healthcare utilization.[6]

Emerging insights into the pathophysiology of FM suggest that it is a disorder of central sensory processing, often comprising a genetic predisposition and exposure to stressors of a physical or psychological nature.[7-9] In part, the augmented experience of pain in individuals who have FM is thought to be associated with either (1) excessive spinal facilitation of afferent nociceptive signaling to higher cortical pain processing regions or (2) deficiencies in descending cortical mechanisms responsible for dampening nociception.[10,11] As such, recent clinical trials have explored the use of pharmacological compounds targeting one or both of these mechanisms with measured success.[12-15] Pharmacological compounds, however, are neither curative nor address all aspects of this condition and, as such, nonpharmacological approaches continue to play an important role in the comprehensive management of FM.[16]

This article was supported in part by NIAMS/NIH grant U01AR55069.

[a] Department of Anesthesiology, Chronic Pain & Fatigue Research Center, University of Michigan, 24 Frank Lloyd Wright Drive, Lobby M, Ann Arbor, MI 48106, USA
[b] English Language Institute Testing, University of Michigan, 500 East Washington Street, Ann Arbor, MI 48104 USA
* Corresponding author.
E-mail address: daveawms@umich.edu (D.A. Williams).

Despite attempts to identify sensitive and specific biomarkers for FM, patients' self-reporting remains the best clinical approach to understanding the experience of FM for most individuals. This article provides a brief review of several topics pertinent to understanding current practices in the assessment of FM, including (1) viewing FM as a member of a larger chronic illness continuum, (2) understanding the value of patient-reported outcomes, (3) identifying the relevant domains of assessment for FM and how to assess them, and (4) reviewing emerging trends in the future of multi-dimensional assessment.

FIBROMYALGIA AS PART OF A LARGER CHRONIC ILLNESS CONTINUUM

What is now termed "fibromyalgia" was earlier called "fibrositis." The change in nomenclature occurred in the mid-1970s[17] to reflect the lack of evidence for any inflammation in the connective tissues of individuals presenting with this condition. Researchers needed a means of quantifying the pain experience in these patients and as such, chose to quantify tender points (regions of extreme tenderness). With this choice, FM became a condition of both pain and tenderness—two constructs that may or may not be synonymous.[18]

Many researchers within the field of chronic pain believe that chronic pain itself is a disease. The underlying mechanisms of this disease may in fact be similar across many pain conditions previously considered idiopathic or functional pain syndromes and operate similarly regardless of whether the pain is present throughout the body, as with FM, or localized to specific regions (eg, low back, bowel, or bladder). Although treated as separate conditions, disorders such as FM, irritable bowel syndrome (IBS), temporomandibular joint disorder (TMDJ), and vulvodynia may in fact share more commonalities than differences in their etiologies. Such similarities, however, are usually masked due to these conditions being represented in separate clinics, and evaluated by separate medical subspecialties and separate teams of researchers. When comorbidities of these conditions are assessed, having more than one of these conditions at a given time is quite common.[19] Appendix 1 offers a symptom checklist and diagnostic module research tool for identifying comorbidities in this spectrum of illness. The tool has two parts: (1) a self-reported symptom checklist that serves as a screening tool for conditions in this spectrum of illness, and (2) the specific diagnostic criteria for the various comorbidities that can be assessed via interview between patient and clinical staff. Greater endorsement of symptoms on this checklist has been associated with more profound overall severity and impact of illness within this spectrum, helping to underscore the interrelatedness of symptoms within these conditions.[20]

THE VALUE OF PATIENT-REPORTED OUTCOMES

The adoption of the tender point count was an attempt to objectify the pain report of patients who have FM. The biomedical community has historically relied upon and valued objective measures of physiological activity or structure to assess the health of patients (eg, lab values, radiographic images, biomarkers, etc.). Although these measures can be remarkably accurate for measuring specific physiological constructs (eg, bone healing, blood flow), they cannot capture the more subjective perceptions of patients' health, well-being, and health-related quality of life (HRQoL) thought to drive much of the variance in outcomes and health care utilization in chronic illnesses.[21,22]

For example, if a patient who had intermittent but chronic headaches attended an office visit where she was evaluated as being physically normal, it would be incorrect to infer this patient had a good HRQoL.

For many medical conditions, objective physical measures or measures of functional capacity correlate only modestly with patient-reported measures of symptoms or HRQoL (eg, rarely above 0.40 and more typically below 0.20).[23] In a study of subjects who have FM, functional status was assessed by actigraphy and by self-report. The self-report data revealed far worse functional status than did the actigraphy monitoring.[24] Substantial differences between objective methods, such as neurological assessment, and self-report have been identified in the measurement of cognitive status;[25] measures of sleep quality differ markedly depending upon whether measured by self-report or by polysomnography (correlations only between 0.06–0.32);[26] and self-reported clinical pain is only modestly associated with more objective evoked pain ratings of tenderness derived from heat, dolorimeter, and pressure.[27]

It is tempting to conclude that the objective clinical measures present only facts, whereas the subjective patient-reported measures represent inaccuracies (eg, noise, bias, psychological factors, error) but this would be a mistake. Both are linked to clinically relevant outcomes, yet the low-to-modest relationship between these two types of measures suggests that they are capturing unique information related to health, and so both are necessary to understand the clinical picture of a given patient.[23]

CAN THE DISORDER BE MEASURED SEPARATELY FROM QUALITY OF LIFE?

In chronic illnesses, by definition, there is no cure available; thus, interventions for chronic illnesses at best serve to manage the condition while it persists within the individual. Chronic illness management interventions seek to arrest progression, palliate symptoms, elicit patients' involvement in self-care, reduce symptoms, improve function, and help to restore the dignity of the individual living with the illness. For chronic illnesses, there can not be a single biomarker that captures all of these matters or that adequately measures the totality of the illness process and its impact on the individual. To state that measuring the cardinal symptom of the illness is paramount and that HRQoL is secondary misses the fact that, with chronicity, matters of HRQoL become inseparably fused with the chronic illness itself and must be meaningfully assessed and included in a comprehensive management plan for the individual.

In general terms, HRQoL is thought to encompass a number of primary domains (ie, physical functioning, psychological functioning, social functioning, overall life satisfaction/wellbeing, perceptions of health status) and secondary domains (ie, neuropsychological functioning, personal productivity, intimacy and sexual functioning, sleep quality, pain, symptoms of illness, spirituality).[28] Whereas it can be seen how the treatment of a finger laceration within the biomedical model might not need to fully consider HRQoL domains, it is nearly impossible to consider the experience of a condition like FM in the absence of most of these domains.

IDENTIFYING RELEVANT DOMAINS OF ASSESSMENT FOR FIBROMYALGIA

The Outcome Measures in Rheumatology Clinical Trials (OMERACT) network has helped to resolve problems in outcomes measurement by establishing core data sets that should be collected and reported in clinical trials involving rheumatological conditions.[29] One task force within OMERACT has focused upon domains of relevance to FM. With initial work dating back to 2004, two Delphi studies have been conducted in an attempt to establish consensus regarding the clinical domains on which FM has an impact. These two studies, one conducted within subjects with FM[3,30] and the other with clinicians,[3,31] revealed remarkable consensus regarding the need to assess multiple domains in FM, including pain, fatigue, functional status, sleep, mood, tenderness, stiffness, and problems with concentration/memory (ie, dyscognition).

The Initiative on Methods, Measurement, and Pain Assessment in Clinical Trials (IMMPACT) is a second organization focused upon identifying the domains that should be assessed in research involving chronic pain in general. This group identifies four core areas for assessment: (1) pain intensity, (2) physical functioning, (3) emotional functioning, and (4) overall improvement/wellbeing.[32] The remarkable agreement between these two independent groups regarding thorough assessment of individuals having painful conditions proves that assessment of pain intensity alone is largely insufficient for chronic pain conditions like FM.

Whereas OMERACT and IMMPACT offer guidance as to the domains of relevance for chronic pain conditions, the actual assessment of those domains has been done with a variety of instruments.[33–35] The next section reviews some of the more commonly used assessment instruments associated with the domains of relevance for FM.

Pain in FM is most commonly assessed using either the McGill Pain Questionnaire,[36,37] or the Brief Pain Inventory (BPI).[38] These measures have been found to be relatively good generic instruments for the assessment of pain and its various parameters (eg, quality, quantity, spatial location, temporal occurrence, affect, and behavioral impact). Because the pain associated with FM is similar to other forms of chronic pain, these instruments are likely to perform well.[39–41]

Eighty-one percent of patients who have FM also report having fatigue.[18] Multiple measures have been used in the assessment of fatigue. Some measures are unidimensional visual analogue scales (VAS), whereas others attempt to assess multiple dimensions of fatigue involving physical fatigue, mental fatigue, motivation, and so forth. Examples of multidimensional fatigue instruments include the Multidimensional Assessment of Fatigue,[42] the fatigue subscale of the Profile of Mood States,[43] the Profile of Fatigue-Related Symptoms,[44] the Fatigue Severity Scale,[45] and the Multidimensional Fatigue Inventory.[46] Many of these instruments were originally developed in the realm of cancer research and were then applied to FM after being used in at least one study involving a rheumatologic population.

Sleep disturbances affect 75% of patients with FM.[18] Like fatigue measures, there are both unidimensional VAS scales (eg, sleep quality, difficulty falling asleep, difficulty staying asleep, or impact of sleep) and multidimensional scales. Examples of multidimensional scales include the Medical Outcomes Study sleep scale,[47] the Pittsburgh Sleep Quality Index,[48] and the Sleep Assessment Questionnaire.[49] Also like the fatigue measures, many of the measures of sleep were borrowed from other clinical populations with little validation occurring specifically in FM.

A patient need not be psychiatrically ill in order to have matters of affect influence pain and wellbeing. Many measures of affect have been used in the assessment of FM and a sampling is listed below. Depressive symptoms are often assessed by the Beck Depression Inventory,[50] a widely used instrument in mental health research. The Center for Epidemiological Studies Depression Scale[51] and the Patient Health

Questionnaire[52] are instruments that are often used to detect depressive symptoms in the general population. Measures of anxiety include the Beck Anxiety Inventory[53] and the State Trait Anxiety Inventory.[54] The Hospital Anxiety and Depression Scale[55] is a single instrument that captures both depressive and anxiety symptoms. More general measures of multiple moods include the Profile of Mood States,[43] and the Positive and Negative Affect Scale.[56]

Patients who have FM often complain of dyscognition or "fibro-fog." No clear definition exists for fibro-fog; however, it tends to refer to a composite experience involving slowing of information processing; difficulties in multitasking, particularly under distracting conditions; failures of memory, poor concentration and clarity of thought, and perceived deficits in executive function. Despite its importance, to date there is no simple measure of dyscognition available for patients who have FM.[57] One measure that does tap a number of domains of perceived cognitive difficulties is the Multiple Ability Self-Report Questionnaire (MASQ).[58] This brief questionnaire is comprised of five cognitive domains: language ability, visuoperceptual ability, verbal memory, visual memory, and attention/concentration. Whereas the MASQ is a self-report measure of perceived cognitive difficulty, other more objective neuropsychological batteries of cognitive performance may be able to offer additional insight into the nature of "fibro-fog" within individuals.

In the context of functional status, patients who have FM often complain of stiffness. To date, there are only a few measures of stiffness. These include the WOMAC,[59] a 24-item questionnaire addressing stiffness in the context of arthritis, and a single-item VAS in the Fibromyalgia Impact Questionnaire,[60] one of the few disease-specific measures of FM.

Other measures of functional status include the Stanford Health Assessment Questionnaire,[61] which has been adapted into an FM-specific functional assessment tool,[62] and the Medical Outcomes Short Form, SF-36,[63] perhaps the most commonly used measure of functional status and HRQoL in clinical outcomes research.

As is evident from the text above, the assessment of multiple domains can require a great deal of time and effort on the part of the patient. For both clinical and research purposes, it is preferable to use assessment instruments possessing strong support of validity in each domain for specific chronic illnesses. In the case of FM, early work in this area required that instruments be borrowed from other diseases, given that the research criteria for FM were established only as recently as 1990 and consensus as to domains of relevance is still emerging. Clearly, sufficient time has not passed to develop new disease-specific measures for each of the relevant domains in FM or to conduct studies supporting the valid use of existing, that is, legacy instruments specifically in the context of FM.

MOVING BEYOND LEGACY MEASURES

Even when disease-specific measures exist, we can not be certain that sufficient methodological rigor has accompanied their development. The institutes, agencies, and centers that comprise the US Department of Health and Human Services has recognized that health outcomes research in general is hampered by three broad problems: (1) a reliance upon legacy instruments developed within disease-specific silos having variable psychometric properties or relevance to HRQoL, (2) an inability to compare outcomes across disease states due to different measures and scaling being used, and (3) inefficiencies in assessing multiple domains of clinical relevance. In order to address these problems, NIH launched a Roadmap initiative known as PROMIS

(Patient-Reported Outcomes Measurement Information System), a large-scale assessment infrastructure to develop brief yet valid assessments of multiple domains of quality of life.[64]

In the development of PROMIS, domains of quality of life were identified that reflected many of the domains described earlier; initially, these included (1) physical functioning, (2) fatigue, (3) pain, (4) emotional distress, (5) social role participation, and several global items.[65] Rather than relying upon classical approaches of test construction in which reliability and validity depends heavily upon completion of each item within the test, PROMIS borrowed methods used successfully in educational testing: item response theory (IRT) and computer adaptive testing (CAT). These methods use large item banks representing aspects of a given domain, such as pain or fatigue. Each item within the item bank is analyzed and calibrated along the domain of interest using factor analytic methods and IRT. The possession of the performance characteristics of each item permits the development and use of CAT. Whereas in classically constructed tests all items on the test would need to be administered to an individual in order to obtain a valid score, CAT only delivers a few items from the overall item bank representing the domain of interest. It does this by first delivering a seed item and then, depending upon the response to the seed, returns to the item bank to select the next item that provides the most relevant additional information about the domain. For example, if assessing physical functioning, a patient might be asked about getting out of bed, walking, climbing stairs, and running. Under a classically developed test, all items would need to be administered even if the patient indicated that s/he could not get out of bed. Under CAT, only items that add precision to the measurement of the domain for that individual are needed. Although each individual taking the CAT would receive different items, all items within the bank reflect aspects of a common domain.

In the development of PROMIS, an item library was created by assembling the many existing legacy questionnaires purporting to measure each domain. The entire item library contained over 10,000 entries and, as might be expected, there were many redundancies. A qualitative process known as "binning and winnowing" was used to refine the library, as were patient focus groups, expert consultation, the rewriting of items, cognitive interviewing, and standardization of the item stems and response sets.[65]

Each item bank was field tested in thousands of individuals in order to conduct the psychometric evaluation of the banks. Quantitative evaluation included traditional descriptive statistics (ie, item analysis and scale analysis), evaluation of the assumptions of IRT (ie, unidimensionality, local independence, and monotonacity), fitting of the IRT model to the data (ie, estimation of IRT model parameters, examination of model fit, evaluation of item and scale properties), evaluation of differential item functioning among demographic and clinical groups, and item calibration for item banking (ie, standardized theta metric for United States population and clinical groups, and identifying discrimination and threshold parameters for use in CAT algorithms).[66] In addition to the use of CAT, static short forms containing highly relevant items for specific clinical populations have also been developed and evaluated.

PROMIS can be used clinically or for research purposes for the efficient and generic measurement of patient-reported outcomes across a wide range of chronic diseases and dimensions.[67] The benefit of this system is the ability to assess multiple domains using fewer items (ie, less patient burden) with greater precision (ie, increased power for clinical trials with fewer subjects). Whereas PROMIS was established for the general assessment of chronic illnesses; greater precision can be attained when the item banks are further calibrated to be used with specific illnesses. Currently, a disease-specific calibration of PROMIS item banks for use in FM is underway as a cooperative agreement between the University of Michigan and NIAMS/NIH. In this study, the existing item banks within PROMIS are being calibrated in field tests requiring thousands of individuals who have FM so that CATs can be developed with algorithms specific to FM.

FUTURE ASSESSMENT IN FIBROMYALGIA

With assessment tools like those of PROMIS, both researchers and clinicians will be able to evaluate the multiple domains of relevance to individuals suffering with FM and related conditions with greater precision and efficiency. Still lacking for PROMIS and for the field of FM research generally, however, are consensual demarcations indicative of clinically meaningful change in each of the domains or composites of domains. Work in this area is being advanced by investigators led by Dr. Lesley Arnold at the University of Cincinnati in conjunction with NIAMS/NIH and by other collaborators within OMERACT specifically for FM and by IMMPACT for general chronic pain.[32] As interventions for FM become more specialized by targeting various aspects of FM, (eg, pain, function, sleep, fatigue, etc.), it is likely that more specialized assessment tools will be needed. The development of high quality assessment instruments for FM is recognized by academia and by industry as a high priority research agenda item. As FM appears to represent one of several conditions within a broader sphere of central pain disorders, it is likely that advances in the assessment of FM will translate into benefits for other chronic pain conditions as well.

REFERENCES

1. Wolfe F, Ross K, Anderson J, et al. The prevalence and characteristics of fibromyalgia in the general population. Arthritis Rheum 1995;38:19–28.
2. Bennett RM, Jones J, Turk DC, et al. An internet survey of 2,596 people with fibromyalgia. BMC Musculoskelet Disord 2007;8:27–38.
3. Mease PJ, Arnold LM, Crofford LJ, et al. Identifying the clinical domains of fibromyalgia: contributions from clinician and patient Delphi exercises. Arthritis Rheum 2008;59:952–60.
4. Forseth KO, Gran JT. Management of fibromyalgia: what are the best treatment choices? Drugs 2002;62:577–92.
5. Hoffman DL, Dukes EM. The health status burden of people with fibromyalgia: a review of studies that assessed health status with the SF-36 or the SF-12. Int J Clin Pract 2008;62:115–26.
6. Berger A, Dukes E, Martin S, et al. Characteristics and healthcare costs of patients with fibromyalgia syndrome. Int J Clin Pract 2007;61:1498–508.
7. Ablin J, Neumann L, Buskila D. Pathogenesis of fibromyalgia—a review. Joint Bone Spine 2008;75:273–9.
8. Staud R, Rodriguez ME. Mechanisms of disease: pain in fibromyalgia syndrome. Nat Clin Pract Rheumatol 2006;2:90–8.
9. Dadabhoy D, Clauw DJ. Fibromyalgia: progress in diagnosis and treatment. Curr Pain Headache Rep 2005;9:399–404.

10. Yoshimura M, Furue H. Mechanisms for the anti-nociceptive actions of the descending noradrenergic and serotonergic systems in the spinal cord. J Pharmacol Sci 2006;101:107–17.

11. Staud R, Spaeth M. Psychophysical and neurochemical abnormalities of pain processing in fibromyalgia. CNS Spectr 2008;13:12–7.

12. Mease PJ, Russell IJ, Kajdasz DK, et al. Long-term safety, tolerability, and efficacy of duloxetine in the treatment of fibromyalgia. Semin Arthritis Rheum 2009; [Epub ahead of print].

13. Arnold LM, Russell IJ, Diri EW, et al. A 14-week, randomized, double-blinded, placebo-controlled monotherapy trial of pregabalin in patients with fibromyalgia. J Pain 2008;9:792–805.

14. Mease PJ, Clauw DJ, Gendreau RM, et al. The efficacy and safety of milnacipran for treatment of fibromyalgia. a randomized, double-blind, placebo-controlled trial. J Rheumatol 2009;36:398–409.

15. Clauw DJ, Mease P, Palmer RH, et al. Milnacipran for the treatment of fibromyalgia in adults: a 15-week, multicenter, randomized, double-blind, placebo-controlled, multiple-dose clinical trial. Clin Ther 2008;30:1988–2004.

16. Goldenberg DL, Burckhardt C, Crofford L. Management of fibromyalgia syndrome. JAMA 2004;292:2388–95.

17. Smythe HA, Moldofsky H. Two contributions to understanding of the "fibrositis" syndrome. Bull Rheum Dis 1977;28:928–31.

18. Wolfe F, Smythe HA, Yunus MB, et al. The American college of rheumatology 1990 criteria for the classification of fibromyalgia: report of the multicenter criteria committee. Arthritis Rheum 1990;33:160–72.

19. Clauw DJ, Chrousos GP. Chronic pain and fatigue syndromes: overlapping clinical and neuroendocrine features and potential pathogenic mechanisms. Neuroimmunomodulation 1997;4:134–53.

20. Geisser ME, Strader DC, Petzke F, et al. Comorbid somatic symptoms and functional status in patients with fibromyalgia and chronic fatigue syndrome: sensory amplification as a common mechanism. Psychosomatics 2008;49:235–42.

21. Jiang Y, Hesser JE. Patterns of health-related quality of life and patterns associated with health risks among Rhode Island adults. Health Qual Life Outcomes 2008;6:1–11.

22. Dominick KL, Ahern FM, Gold CH, et al. Health-related quality of life and health service use among older adults with osteoarthritis. Arthritis Rheum 2004;51:326–31.

23. Hahn EA, Cella D, Chassany O, et al. Precision of health-related quality-of-life data compared with other clinical measures. Mayo Clin Proc 2007;82:1244–54.

24. Kop WJ, Lyden A, Berlin AA, et al. Ambulatory monitoring of physical activity and symptoms in fibromyalgia and chronic fatigue syndrome. Arthritis Rheum 2005;52:296–303.

25. Snitz BE, Morrow LA, Rodriguez EG, et al. Subjective memory complaints and concurrent memory performance in older patients of primary care providers. J Int Neuropsychol Soc 2008;14:1004–13.

26. Unruh ML, Redline S, An MW, et al. Subjective and objective sleep quality and aging in the sleep heart health study. J Am Geriatr Soc 2008;56:1218–27.

27. Geisser ME, Gracely RH, Giesecke T, et al. The association between experimental and clinical pain measures among persons with fibromyalgia and chronic fatigue syndrome. Eur J Pain 2007;11:202–7.

28. Naughton MJ, Shumaker SA. The case for domains of function in quality of life assessment. Qual Life Res 2003;12(Suppl 1):73–80.
29. Tugwell P, Boers M, Brooks P, et al. OMERACT: an international initiative to improve outcome measurement in rheumatology. Trials 2007;8:38.
30. Arnold LM, Crofford LJ, Mease PJ, et al. Patient perspectives on the impact of fibromyalgia. Patient Educ Couns 2008;73:114–20.
31. Mease PJ, Clauw DJ, Arnold LM, et al. Fibromyalgia syndrome. J Rheumatol 2005;32:2270–7.
32. Dworkin RH, Turk DC, Wyrwich KW, et al. Interpreting the clinical importance of treatment outcomes in chronic pain clinical trials: IMMPACT recommendations. J Pain 2008;9:105–21.
33. Mease P. Fibromyalgia syndrome: review of clinical presentation, pathogenesis, outcome measures, and treatment. J Rheumatol Suppl 2005;75:6–21.
34. Arnold LM, Keck PEJ, Welge JA. Antidepressant treatment of fibromyalgia. A meta-analysis and review. Psychosomatics 2000;41:104–13.
35. Offenbacher M, Cieza A, Brockow T, et al. Are the contents of treatment outcomes in fibromyalgia trials represented in the International Classification of Functioning, Disability, and Health? Clin J Pain 2007;23:691–701.
36. Melzack R. The McGill pain questionnaire: major properties and scoring methods. Pain 1975;1:277–99.
37. Melzack R. The short-form McGill pain questionnaire. Pain 1987;30:191–7.
38. Keller S, Bann CM, Dodd SL, et al. Validity of the brief pain inventory for use in documenting the outcomes of patients with noncancer pain. Clin J Pain 2004; 20:309–18.
39. Dworkin RH, Turk DC, Farrar JT, et al. Core outcome measures for chronic pain clinical trials: IMMPACT recommendations. Pain 2005;113:9–19.
40. Jensen MP, Miller L, Fisher LD. Assessment of pain during medical procedures: a comparison of three scales. Clin J Pain 1998;14:343–9.
41. Jensen MP, McFarland CA. Increasing the reliability and validity of pain intensity measurement in chronic pain patients. Pain 1993;55:195–203.
42. Belza BL, Henke CJ, Yelin EH, et al. Correlates of fatigue in older adults with rheumatoid arthritis. Nurs Res 1993;42:93–9.
43. McNair D, Lorr M, Droppleman L. Manual for the profile of mood states. San Diego (CA): Educational Testing Service; 1971.
44. Ray C, Weir W, Phillips S, et al. Development of a measure of symptoms in chronic fatigue syndrome: the profile of fatigue related symptoms (PFRS). Psychol Health 1992;7:27–43.
45. Krupp LB, LaRocca NG, Muir-Nash J, et al. The fatigue severity scale. Application to patients with multiple sclerosis and systemic lupus erythematosus. Arch Neurol 1989;46:1121–3.
46. Smets EM, Garssen B, Bonke B, et al. The multidimensional fatigue inventory (MFI) psychometric qualities of an instrument to assess fatigue. J Psychosom Res 1995;39:315–25.
47. Hays RD, Stewart A. Sleep measures. In: Stewart AL, Ware JE, editors. Measuring functioning and well-being: the medical outcomes study approach. Durham: Duke University Press; 1992. p. 235–59.
48. Buysse DJ, Reynolds CF III, Monk TH, et al. The Pittsburgh sleep quality index: a new instrument for psychiatric practice and research. Psychiatry Res 1989; 28:193–213.

49. Cesta A, Moldofsky H, Sammut C. The sensitivity and specificity of the sleep assessment questionnaire (SAQ) as a measure of nonrestorative sleep [abstract]. Sleep 1999;22:14.
50. Beck AT, Steer RA, Brown GK. Manual for the Beck depression inventory-II. San Antonio (TX): Psychological Corporation; 1996.
51. Radloff LS. The CES-D Scale: a self-report depression scale for research in the general population. Appl Psychol Meas 1977;1:385–401.
52. Kroenke K, Spitzer RL, Williams JB. The PHQ-9: validity of a brief depression severity measure. J Gen Intern Med 2001;16:606–13.
53. Beck AT, Steer RA. Beck anxiety inventory: manual. 2nd edition. San Antonio: The Psychological Corporation, Harcourt Brace Jovanovich, Inc.; 1990.
54. Spielberger CD, Gorsuch RL, Lushene R. Manual for the state-trait anxiety inventory: (STAI) (Self-Evaluation Questionnaire). Palo Alto (CA): Consulting Psychologists Press; 1979.
55. Zigmond AS, Snaith RP. The hospital anxiety and depression scale. Acta Psychiatr Scand 1983;67:361–70.
56. Watson D, Clark LA, Tellegen A. Development and validation of brief measures of positive and negative affect: the PANAS scales. J Pers Soc Psychol 1988;54:1063–70.
57. Silverman SL, Martin SA. Assessment tools and outcome measures used in the investigation of fibromyalgia. In: Wallace DJ, Clauw DJ, editors. Fibromyalgia & other central pain syndromes. Philadelphia: Lippincott Williams & Wilkins; 2005. p. 309–19.
58. Seidenberg M, Haltiner A, Taylor MA, et al. Development and validation of a multiple ability self-report questionnaire. J Clin Exp Neuropsychol 1994;16:93–104.
59. Bellamy N, Buchanan WW, Goldsmith CH, et al. Validation study of WOMAC: a health status instrument for measuring clinically important patient relevant outcomes to antirheumatic drug therapy in patients with osteoarthritis of the hip or knee. J Rheumatol 1988;15:1833–40.
60. Burckhardt CS, Clark SR, Bennett RM. The fibromyalgia impact questionnaire: development and validation. J Rheumatol 1991;18:728–33.
61. Fries JF, Spitz P, Kraines RG, et al. Measurement of patient outcome in arthritis. Arthritis Rheum 1980;23:137–45.
62. Wolfe F, Hawley DJ, Goldenberg DL, et al. The assessment of functional impairment in fibromyalgia (FM): Rasch analyses of 5 functional scales and the development of the FM Health Assessment Questionnaire. J Rheumatol 2000;27:1989–99.
63. Ware JE, Snow K, Kosinski M. SF-36® health survey: manual and interpretation guide. Lincoln (RI): QualityMetric, Inc.; 2000.
64. Reeve BB, Burke LB, Chiang YP, et al. Enhancing measurement in health outcomes research supported by agencies within the US Department of Health and Human Services. Qual Life Res 2007;16(Suppl 1):175–86.
65. Cella D, Yount S, Rothrock N, et al. The patient-reported outcomes measurement information system (PROMIS): progress of an NIH Roadmap cooperative group during its first two years. Med Care 2007;45:S3–11.
66. Reeve BB, Hays RD, Bjorner JB, et al. Psychometric evaluation and calibration of health-related quality of life item banks: plans for the patient-reported outcomes measurement information system (PROMIS). Med Care 2007;45:S22–31.
67. Fries JF, Bruce B, Cella D. The promise of PROMIS: using item response theory to improve assessment of patient-reported outcomes. Clin Exp Rheumatol 2005;23:S53–7.

APPENDIX 1

The Complex Medical Symptoms Inventory (CMSI) is a diagnostic tool to assist in identifying the presence of conditions that commonly accompany FM. The tool consists of two parts: (1) a symptom checklist that serves as a screener and (2) the published diagnostic criteria for several of the more common conditions within this spectrum of illnesses. The latter is to be administered by staff interview.

Complex Medical Symptoms Inventory

Instructions: Please read the following list of symptoms. If you have had any of these symptoms **for at least three (3) months in the past year,** or **for a 3-month period during your lifetime,** please mark the appropriate box.

	Symptom	3 Months During the Last Year (12 Months)	3 Months During Your Lifetime	*For Staff Use Only*
1	Muscle or joint pain			☐ M:FM ☐ M:CFS
2	Morning stiffness			
3	Muscle spasms			
4	Persistent fatigue not relieved with rest			☐ M:CFS
5	Extreme fatigue following exercise or mild exertion			
6	Recurrent fevers			
7	Dry eyes			
8	Dry mouth			
9	Fingers turn blue and/or white in the cold			
10	Numbness or tingling in arms or legs			
11	Shortness of breath during normal activity			
12	Impaired memory, concentration, or attention			
13	Chest pain			
14	Palpitations			
15	Rapid heart rate			
16	Heartburn			
17	Vomiting			
18	Nausea			
19	Abdominal pain or discomfort			☐ M:IBS
20	Problems with balance			
21	Dizziness			
22	Ringing in ears			
23	Ear pain			☐ M:TMDJ
24	Sensation of ear blockage or fullness			

(continued on next page)

	Symptom	3 Months During the Last Year (12 Months)	3 Months During Your Lifetime	For Staff Use Only
25	Sinus pressure			
26	Pelvic/bladder discomfort (pain or pressure)			
27	Urinary urgency			
28	Urinary frequency, >8/day during waking hours			
29	Frequent nocturia (nighttime urination), 3/night			
30	Sensation of bladder fullness after urination			
31	Jaw and/or face pain			☐ M:TMDJ
32	Temple pain			
33	Pulsating and/or one-sided headache pain or migraines			☐ M:MI
34	Pressing/tightening headache pain or tension headaches			
35	Sensitivity to certain chemicals, such as perfumes, laundry detergents, gasoline, and others			
36	Sensitivity to sound			
37	Sensitivity to odors			
38	Body feeling tender			
39	Frequent sensitivity to bright lights			
FEMALES ONLY:				
40	Constant burning or raw feeling at opening of vagina			☐ M:VDYN
41	Itching at opening of vagina			

Module	Diagnosis Criteria Citation	Symptom Question	Supporting Symptoms/ Qualifiers	Physical Exam	Notes
M: FM	**Fibromyalgia** Wolfe F. The 1990 ACR criteria for the classification of fibromyalgia. Report of multicenter criteria committee. Arthritis Rheum, 1990;33:160–172.	(Sx 1) Muscle or joint pain	Pain must be present in all four quadrants, including the axial skeleton	Tender point 11/18 TP to 4 kg of digital pressure	N/A
[ ] Yes [ ] No		1A	Pain in upper right quadrant*		
[ ] Yes [ ] No		1B	Pain in upper left quadrant*		
[ ] Yes [ ] No		1C	Pain in lower right quadrant*		
[ ] Yes [ ] No		1D	Pain in lower left quadrant*		
[ ] Yes [ ] No		1E	Pain in the axial skeleton (neck, chest, back, buttocks)*		
[ ] Yes [ ] No		1F	11/18 tender points (#TP =_____)		
[ ] Yes [ ] No		M:FM	**Diagnosis: YES to 1A-1F**		

*Can refer to body map on BPI for pain location.

Module	Diagnosis Criteria Citation	Symptom Question	Supporting Symptoms/ Qualifiers	Physical Exam	Notes
M: CFS	**Chronic fatigue syndrome** Fukuda K, Straus SE, Hickie I, et al. The CFS: A comprehensive approach to its definition and study. Ann Intern Med 1994; 121(12):953–9.	(Sx 4) Persistent fatigue not relieved with rest	(Sx 12) Impaired memory, concentration or attention Sore throat (Sx 1) Muscle pain Multijoint pain without swelling New headaches Unrefreshing sleep Postexertion malaise Tender lymph nodes	N/A	Must say YES to 2A (Criterion 1) Must say YES to 2J (Criterion 2) To fulfill Criterion 2, subjects should have "concurrent occurrence of at least 4/8 additional symptoms, all of which must have persisted or recurred during ≥6 consecutive months of illness and must not have predated the fatigue." Fukuda criteria: Must say YES to 2A and YES to ≥ 4/8 from 2D–2K
[ ] Yes	[ ] No	2A	**Criterion 1:** Persistent fatigue not relieved with rest (Sx 4) that limits activities		
[ ] Yes	[ ] No	2B	Impaired memory, concentration, or attention (Sx 12) (Difficulty with thinking; confusion)		
[ ] Yes	[ ] No	2C	Sore throat		
[ ] Yes	[ ] No	2D	Muscle pain (Sx 1)		
[ ] Yes	[ ] No	2E	Multijoint pain without swelling		
[ ] Yes	[ ] No	2F	New headaches		
[ ] Yes	[ ] No	2G	Unrefreshing sleep		
[ ] Yes	[ ] No	2H	Postexertion malaise		
[ ] Yes	[ ] No	2I	Tender cervical or axillary lymph nodes		
[ ] Yes	[ ] No	2J	**Criterion 2: YES to ≥4/8 (2B–2I) ≥6 mo**		
[ ] Yes	[ ] No	M:CFS	**Diagnosis: YES to 2A and 2J**		

Module	Diagnosis Criteria Citation	Symptom Question	Supporting Symptoms/ Qualifiers	Physical Exam	Notes
M: IBS	Irritable Bowel Syndrome Drossman AD. Rome III Criteria; 2006.	(Sx 19) Abdominal pain or discomfort	Recurrent abdominal pain or discomfort (at least 3 d/mo during the last 3 mo with symptom onset at least 6 mo prior to diagnosis), that: • Is relieved with bowel movement (at least sometimes) • Has onset associated with a change in stool frequency (at least sometimes) • Has onset associated with a change in stool form or appearance (at least sometimes) Hard or lumpy stools >25% of BM Loose (mushy) or watery stools >25% of BM Abnormal stool frequency (>3/d or <3/wk)	N/A	Abdominal pain or discomfort for at least 3 d/mo during the previous 3 mo. Four bowel patterns may be seen with IBS: (1) IBS with constipation (IBS-C): hard or lumpy stools >25%, and loose (mushy) or watery stools <25% of BM (2) IBS with diarrhea (IBS-D): loose (mushy) or watery stools, and hard or lumpy stool <25% of BM (3) Mixed IBS (IBS-M): hard or lumpy stools >25% and loose (mushy or watery stools >25% of BM (4) Unsubtyped IBS (IBS-U): insufficient abnormality of stool consistency to meet criteria IBS-C, -D or -M

[ ] Yes	[ ] No	3A	Recurrent abdominal pain or discomfort (at least 3 d/mo during the last 3 mo with symptom onset at least 6 mo prior to diagnosis) that:
[ ] Yes	[ ] No	3Aa	Is relieved with bowel movement (at least sometimes)
[ ] Yes	[ ] No	3Ab	Has onset associated with a change in stool frequency (at least sometimes)
[ ] Yes	[ ] No	3Ac	Has onset associated with a change in stool form or appearance (at least sometimes)
[ ] Yes	[ ] No	3B	Hard or lumpy stools >25% of bowel movements
[ ] Yes	[ ] No	3C	Loose (mushy) or watery stools >25% of bowel movements
[ ] Yes	[ ] No	3D	Abnormal stool frequency (>3/d or <3/wk)
[ ] Yes	[ ] No	M:IBS	**Diagnosis: YES to 3A and ≥2/3 of 3Aa, 3Ab, 3Ac. Criterion must be fulfilled for the last 3 mo with symptom onset at least 6 mo to diagnosis.**

Module	Diagnosis Criteria Citation	Symptom Question	Supporting Symptoms/ Qualifiers	Physical Exam	Notes
M: VDYN	**Vulvodynia** McKay M. Vulvodynia: Diagnostic patterns. Dermatologic Clinics 1992;10(2): 423–433. Vulvar vestibulitis and vestibular papillomatosis: Report of the ISSVD Committee on vulvodynia. J Reprod Med 1991;36(6): 413–415. Burning vulva syndrome: Report of the ISSVD Task Force. J Reprod Med 1984; 29:457.	(Sx 40) Constant burning or raw feeling at the opening of the vagina (Sx 41) Itching at the opening of the vagina (absent)	Discomfort relieved by anticandidal therapy (absent) Vaginal or vulvar dermatoses (absent)	N/A	Must respond NO to Sx 41 Diagnosis by exclusion: R/O infection R/O dermatoses As defined by the International Society for the Study of Vulvar Disease: *"chronic vulvar discomfort, especially that characterized by the patient's complaint of burning, stinging, irritation, or rawness."*

[ ] Yes	[ ] No	4A	Constant burning or raw feeling at the opening of the vagina (Sx 40)
[ ] Yes	[ ] No	4B	Tender to touch, or pain with tampon insertion and/or intercourse
[ ] Yes	[ ] No	4C	Itching at the opening of the vagina (Sx 41)
[ ] Yes	[ ] No	4D	Relieved by anticandidal therapy?
[ ] Yes	[ ] No	M:VDYN	**Diagnosis: YES to 4A *and/or* 4B and NO to 4C and 4D**

Module	Diagnosis Criteria Citation	Symptom Question	Supporting Smptoms/ Qualifiers	Physical Exam	Notes
M: MI	**Migraine** Headache Classification Committee of the International Headache Society. Classification and diagnostic criteria for headache disorders, cranial neuralgias and facial pain. Cephalalgia 1988;8 (suppl 7): 1–96.	(Sx 36) Pulsating and/or one-sided headache pain or migraines	**Criterion 1** • Headache attacks last for 4–72 h (untreated or unsuccessfully treated) **Criterion 2** • Unilateral pain • Pulsating quality • Moderate or severe intensity that inhibits or prohibits normal daily activities • Aggravation by walking stairs or similar routine physical activity **Criterion 3** • Nausea and/or vomiting during the headache attack • Photophobia and phonophobia	N/A	Must have <5 attacks that meet the following criteria: **Criterion 1** YES to >2/4 symptoms from Criterion 2 YES to >1/2 symptoms from Criterion 3 that occur during the headache (HA) The following must be ruled out or, the first migraine attack did not occur in close temporal relation to the disorder: • HA associated with head trauma • HA associated with vascular disorders • HA associated with nonvascular intracranial disorder • HA associated with substances or their withdrawal • HA associated with noncephalic infection • HA associated with metabolic disorder • HA or facial pain associated with disorder of the cranium, neck, eyes, ears, nose, sinuses, teeth, mouth, or other facial or cranial structures

[ ] Yes	[ ] No	5A	**Criterion 1** = headache attacks last for 4–72 h (untreated or unsuccessfully treated)
[ ] Yes	[ ] No	5B	Unilateral pain
[ ] Yes	[ ] No	5C	Pulsating quality to the pain
[ ] Yes	[ ] No	5D	Moderate to severe intensity that inhibits or prohibits normal daily activities
[ ] Yes	[ ] No	5E	Aggravation by walking up stairs, or similar routine physical activity
[ ] Yes	[ ] No	5F	**Criterion 2** $\geq$ 2/4 symptoms from 5B–5E
[ ] Yes	[ ] No	5G	Nausea and/or vomiting during the headache attack
[ ] Yes	[ ] No	5H	Photophobia and phonophobia
[ ] Yes	[ ] No	5I	**Criterion 3** $\geq$ 1/2 symptoms from 5G–5H
Rule out: Must answer all NOs to meet the diagnostic criteria for M:MI (migraine headache):			
[ ] Yes	[ ] No	5J	Headache (HA) associated with head trauma
[ ] Yes	[ ] No	5K	HA associated with vascular disorders
[ ] Yes	[ ] No	5L	HA associated with nonvascular intracranial disorders
[ ] Yes	[ ] No	5M	HA associated with substances or withdrawal
[ ] Yes	[ ] No	5N	HA associated with noncephalic infection
[ ] Yes	[ ] No	5O	HA associated with metabolic disorder
[ ] Yes	[ ] No	5P	HA or facial pain associated with disorder of the cranium, neck, eyes, ears, nose, sinuses, teeth, mouth, or other facial or cranial structure
[ ] Yes	[ ] No	5Q	**Criterion 4**: Must answer all NO to 5J–5P
[ ] Yes	[ ] No	M:MI	**Diagnosis: YES to 5A, 5F, 5I and 5Q**

Module	Diagnosis Criteria Citation	Symptom Question	Supporting Symptoms/ Qualifiers	Physical Exam	Notes
M:TMDJ	**Temporomandibular Joint Disorder** Dworkin SF. Research diagnostic criteria for temporomandibular disorders: review, criteria, examinations and specifications, critique. J Craniomandib Disord Facial Oral Pain 1992;6(4): 327–355.	(Sx 31) Jaw and/or face pain (Sx 32) Temple pain (Sx 23) Ear pain	Tight jaw	Tender point exam • ≥ 3 TP to 1 kg of digital pressure • ≥ 1 TP must be ipsolateral to complaint of pain	Must have at least 1/3 symptoms in addition to a positive TP exam; Myofacial TMDJ with limited opening fulfilling above criteria, plus pain-free unassisted mandibular opening of <40 mm, plus maximum assisted opening (passive stretch) of ≥ 5 mm greater than pain-free unassisted opening

[ ] Yes [ ] No	7A	Jaw and/or face pain (Sx 31)	If YES to 7A, 7B, or 7C, perform tender point exam.
[ ] Yes [ ] No	7B	Temple pain (Sx 32)	
[ ] Yes [ ] No	7C	Ear pain (Sx 23)	
[ ] Yes [ ] No	7D	≥ 3 tender points	
[ ] Yes [ ] No	M:TMDJ	**Diagnosis: YES to $\geq 1/3$ 7A–7C and 7D**	
[ ] Yes [ ] No	7E	TMDJ with limited ROM = YES CMSI-TMDJ *and* pain-free unassisted mandibular opening of <40 mm, *plus* maximum assisted opening (passive stretch) of ≥ 5 mm greater than pain-free unassisted opening	
[ ] Yes [ ] No	7F	TMDJ without limited ROM = YES to CMSI-TMDJ	

Pharmacotherapy of Fibromyalgia

Philip J. Mease, MD[a,b,]*, Ernest H. Choy, MD, FRCP[c]

KEYWORDS

- Fibromyalgia • Pharmacotherapy • Pain • Neuromodulation
- Treatment

Historically, clinicians have empirically prescribed pharmacologic therapy for fibromyalgia (FM) based on patterns of specific symptom domains without the imprimatur of formal approval by regulatory agencies or even a clear understanding of the pathophysiology of the condition to guide treatment choice. For example, it has been common to treat musculoskeletal tenderness with medications such as nonsteroidal anti-inflammatory drugs (NSAIDs), muscle relaxants, and narcotic analgesics, sleep disturbance with sedative hypnotics, and mood disturbance with antidepressants. The National Fibromyalgia Association in the United States conducted an Internet survey in 2005 amongst 2596 patients and noted an array of medications being used.[1] The most commonly "ever used" medications were acetaminophen, NSAIDs, tricyclic antidepressants (TCAs), and cyclobenzaprine. The most "helpful" medications were hydrocodone, oxycodone, and codeine preparations, alprazolam, zolpidem, clonazepam, and cyclobenzaprine. None of these medications have been formally approved for the treatment of FM, and only a few have been assessed in controlled treatment trials.

The landscape of pharmacotherapy of FM and its guidance have changed, particularly over the last decade. Since the last time the subject of pharmacotherapy in FM was reviewed by Barkhuizen in an issue of *Rheumatic Disease Clinics of North America*,[2] the field of clinical trial development in FM has matured and the number of medicines tested has increased, but many of the same principles and approaches recommended have remained consistent. To establish efficacy of treatment in FM, it is important to establish the key domains of the condition so that one may assess the impact of treatment on those domains, either singly or in a composite manner. Consortia of FM researchers have established a core set of symptom domains of FM

[a] Seattle Rheumatology Associates, Swedish Medical Center, 1101 Madison Street, Suite 1000, Seattle, WA 98104, USA
[b] University of Washington, Seattle, WA, USA
[c] Sir Alfred Baring Garrod Clinical Trials Unit, Academic Department Rheumatology, King's College London, London, UK
* Corresponding author. Seattle Rheumatology Associates, Swedish Medical Center, 1101 Madison Street, Suite 1000, Seattle, WA 98104.
E-mail address: pmease@nwlink.com (P.J. Mease).

Rheum Dis Clin N Am 35 (2009) 359–372
doi:10.1016/j.rdc.2009.06.007
0889-857X/09/$ – see front matter © 2009 Elsevier Inc. All rights reserved.

rheumatic.theclinics.com

which should be assessed in clinical trials of therapy[3–7] and have recommended outcome measures to assess those symptom domains, which, with variable psychometric quality, have performed reasonably well in distinguishing treatment from placebo arms in clinical trials.[4–8]

The FM working group of the association Outcome Measures in Rheumatology Clinical Trials (OMERACT) has identified three levels of symptom domains in FM that should be assessed in clinical trials because they could potentially be benefited by treatment. The process of the working group, which included an analysis of patient focus groups and physician expert as well as patient Delphi exercises, data mining of controlled clinical trials, and discussions and voting at OMERACT meetings in 2004, 2006, and 2008, are described in the article by Choy in this issue[3] and in a series of other articles.[6–9] The "core" set that should be measured in all clinical trials includes pain, tenderness, fatigue, sleep disturbance, the patient "global" sense of well-being as impacted by FM, and multidimensional function, which includes not only physical but also social and psycho-emotional aspects of function. A second set of symptoms that should be assessed in some trials of a medication include those of depression and "dyscognition" or cognitive dysfunction. The latter domain is not in the core set partly because it has not as yet been fully characterized in FM, nor is it best known how to assess it. A third or "research" set of domains that might be investigated includes "stiffness," which is often described by patients but not well characterized in FM, anxiety, and biomarkers such as cerebrospinal fluid neuropeptides and neuroimaging (**Fig. 1**).[8]

Although these symptoms and signs and possibly often associated conditions such as irritable bowel and bladder syndrome, temporomandibular joint disorder, and headache would ideally be improved by a medication, it is perhaps too much to ask of a single therapy. Indeed, the US Food and Drug Administration (FDA) primarily focuses on efficacy in pain as it considers approval; however, as clinicians, we would like to know that a recommended medicine can have a clinically meaningful effect in multiple FM symptom domains, including patient global well-being as well as function

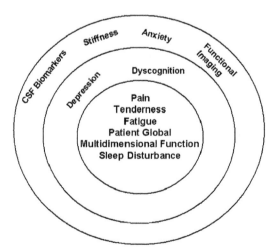

Fig. 1. Domains for fibromyalgia. This concentric circle diagram reflects the hierarchy of domains. Inner circle includes the core set of domains to be assessed in all clinical trials of FM. The second concentric circle includes the outer core set of domains to be assessed in some but not all FM trials. The outermost circle includes the domains on the research agenda that may or may not be included in FM trials. CSF, cerebrospinal fluid.

and not necessarily pain alone. The key outcomes reported in more recent drug trials have been efficacy in pain, patient global well-being, and function, typically as individual variables, although in some trials they have been evaluated in composite measures in which a patient, to be a successful "responder," has to achieve a "clinically meaningful" improvement in at least two if not three of these domains simultaneously and at more enduring time points of at least 3 months if not 6 or longer. Farrar[10] analyzed several different trials of pregabalin in different pain conditions and noted that a "very much improved" and "much improved" response on the Patient Global Impression of Change (PGIC) scale correlated with a 30% improvement in pain Visual Analogue Score (VAS), establishing this as a benchmark of clinically meaningful improvement. In that same study, a response of "very much improved" correlated with a 50% improvement in pain. Demonstration of achievement of these higher hurdles of response, statistically separated from placebo, reinforces the sense that these agents are truly benefiting specific pathophysiologic mechanisms separate from the placebo response that can occur from simply being shown attention in a clinical trial. In most studies, other important domains are being assessed as "secondary" measures, including measures of sleep, fatigue, and cognition.

A variety of outcome measures for all of these domains have been used in clinical trials. Pain measures have included the pain VAS measured on paper or electronically with patient experience diary devices and multiquestion assessments such as the Brief Pain Inventory (BPI). Multidimensional function can be measured with instruments such as the Fibromyalgia Impact Questionnaire (FIQ), an instrument validated in FM, and a more general questionnaire such as the SF-36. Patient global well-being is usually measured on a VAS or Likert scale. A variety of sleep measures, such as the Medical Outcomes Survey, have been used. Fatigue is typically measured by a multidimensional questionnaire such as the Multidimensional Fatigue Inventory (MFI) or Multidimensional Assessment of Fatigue instrument. Cognition has been measured in an exploratory fashion by a self-report instrument, the Multiple Ability Self-report Questionnaire (MASQ); more objective administered measures of cognitive function have not yet been used in large clinical trials. These and other measures used in clinical trials have been reviewed[5] and their psychometric quality of performance evaluated by the OMERACT group.[6-8]

As discussed in several articles in this issue, the pathophysiology of FM is being more clearly elucidated. A complex interplay among genetics, developmental influences, triggering factors, and the neurophysiologic and psycho-emotional substrate of the individual is thought to yield the mix of symptom domains experienced by the patient.

In parallel with this methodologic and basic science work, several large controlled trials with drugs targeting the known neuropathophysiologic pathways of the disease have been completed, generally successfully. As a result of this cumulative work, the FDA and other regulatory agencies have been able to develop a regulatory pathway for approval of FM therapies, resulting in three currently approved therapies (pregabalin, duloxetine, and milnacipran), with more agents with diverse mechanisms likely on the way. A similar process is now occurring in Europe. This work has also raised the level of understanding about the illness, its pathophysiology, and rational treatment approaches among clinicians and the public, leading to greater acceptance of the FM paradigm and an improved likelihood that patients will be steered toward appropriate multimodal (pharmacologic and nonpharmacologic) therapy. The remainder of this article focuses on the evidence for efficacy, tolerability, and safety of a variety of medicines used to treat FM, indicating efficacy in several individual domains of the condition and, where available, efficacy in multiple domains measured in a composite fashion. A methodologic research effort is currently underway by the OMERACT FM group to develop measures of disease state severity and a responder index to take into account the multiple symptom domains of patients in an attempt to provide a more coherent and clinically meaningful approach to measurement of treatment effect in FM.

SEROTONIN AND NOREPINEPHRINE MODULATION IN FIBROMYALGIA

Many would attribute the beginnings of exploration of "rational" therapy for FM to the pioneering sleep studies of Moldofsky and Smythe.[11,12] The demonstration of abnormal sleep physiology in FM patients suggested that the pathology was central and potentially could be improved by the use of central neurotransmitter modulators.

TCAs were initially investigated after identification of alpha-delta nonrapid eye movement sleep disruptions in FM patients caused by abnormalities in central serotonergic neurotransmission.[5,12–18] Tertiary amine tricyclics (TCAs) such as amitriptyline became the initial candidate agents for FM because of their effect as an serotonin-norepinephrine reuptake inhibitor, leading to increased synaptic concentration of these neuropeptides.[5,13,14,17] Three meta-analyses of TCA trials in FM have demonstrated a beneficial effect on sleep quality and a more variable and moderate effect on pain. FM patients demonstrated benefit for pain, sleep, and overall sense of well-being with amitriptyline doses of 25 to 50 mg at bedtime, with cyclobenzaprine (officially classed as a muscle relaxant although a TCA by structure) doses of 10 to 40 mg in short-term studies, and to a lesser extent with other medications classed as TCAs.[14,19,20] Not all controlled trials were able to demonstrate benefit. When Carette studied amitriptyline over a 24-week period, statistically significant separation from placebo was lost, impugning the ability of these agents to provide durable benefit.[14,21] A further drawback to TCA use has been tolerability problems arising from anticholinergic, antiadrenergic, antihistaminergic, and quindine-like effects, including sedation, constipation, and cardiovascular issues which diminish compliance and limit their long-term utility.[13]

Another category of antidepressants evaluated for efficacy in FM is the selective serotonin reuptake inhibitors (SSRIs), such as fluoxetine, citalopram, and paroxetine.[13,14,22] Several controlled trials with these agents in FM have generally shown negative results regarding efficacy in pain, even though these agents are generally better tolerated.[14,22] For example, Wolfe and colleagues[23] found that fluoxetine in a standard fixed dose of 20 mg per day was not superior to placebo. On the other hand, Arnold and colleagues[24] when allowing adjustable dosing found that higher doses yielded greater symptom benefit in FM patients. It is generally agreed that SSRIs have less impact on the pain of FM than do TCAs or the newer serotonin-norepinephrine reuptake inhibitors (SNRIs), even though they may be helpful for clinical domains such as mood disorder or fatigue.[14,22]

Building on the observation of benefit from agents that have dual serotonergic and noradrenergic properties, there have been several large trials of newer SNRIs. These agents have greater neuroreceptor selectivity, are potentially more potent, and are better tolerated than the older TCAs. The first of this newer class of SNRIs, venlafaxine, has been suggested to aid in the management of neuropathic pain and the prevention of migraine and tension headaches;[25] however, venlafaxine shows conflicting results for efficacy in FM, with small open trials suggesting benefit but a larger controlled trial, albeit, with low dose (75 mg), not showing clear benefit over placebo.[25,26]

Two newer SNRIs, duloxetine and milnacipran, have demonstrated more positive benefits for FM patients. Duloxetine is approved in the United States for the treatment of depression, the pain of diabetic peripheral neuropathy, and FM. Its efficacy in FM was demonstrated in two pivotal registry trials.[27–29] The first study assessed both a 60-mg daily and a 60-mg twice daily dose versus placebo in 354 women with FM for 12 weeks. Greater than or equal to a 30% response of the BPI average pain severity score was seen in 55, 54, and 33% of the 60-mg per day, 60-mg twice daily, and placebo groups, respectively, and a 50% or greater response in 41, 41, and 23% of these groups, respectively (each dose group statistically significant relative to placebo). The Patient Global Impression of Improvement (PGII) and total FIQ scores (used as a measure of function and quality of life) were also significantly improved. Patients with a concomitant diagnosis of major depressive disorder (MDD) were allowed to participate; approximately a quarter of the patients had this diagnosis. The response rates in the MDD subgroup were similar to the response rates in the group without MDD. A regression methodology, known as PATH analysis, demonstrated that the majority of the drug's impact on pain was a direct effect and not indirectly mediated through its effect on depression. The idea that the effect of antidepressants on FM symptomatology occurs only because of their effects on psychiatric elements is a common misconception. The most common side effect was nausea, which was generally mild and typically improved with continued use of duloxetine. In general, patients did not gain weight.

A second pivotal study assessed 520 FM patients of both genders for 6 months given placebo controlled versus duloxetine in a similar dosing regimen.[29] Approximately one third of the duloxetine-treated patients had a 50% or greater improvement in the BPI average pain score compared with approximately one fifth of the placebo group, which was statistically significant. Other secondary measures that showed improvement at both the 3- and 6-month assessments in one or both duloxetine dose arms included the PGII, total FIQ, and several components of the fatigue measure MFI. PATH analysis in this study similarly showed that the majority of the pain-relieving effect of duloxetine was direct as opposed to indirect effect through improvement in mood. The adverse event profile in this study was similar; generally, the drug was well tolerated. Measures of sleep in duloxetine trials have shown that it does not specifically help with sleep, nor does it interfere with sleep. Based on the similarity of efficacy of the two different dosages of duloxetine that have been tested in FM, the FDA has approved a dose of 60 mg once a day.

Milnacipran, an SNRI approved for the treatment of depression in parts of Europe and Asia, has now been approved for the management of FM in the United States. The drug displays serotonin and norepinephrine reuptake inhibitor properties and mild N-methyl-D-aspartate inhibitor properties. It has a greater ratio of norepinephrine to serotonin effect than other agents discussed herein, tends to have little in the way of drug-drug adverse interactions, and is dosed twice daily. Studies of milnacipran, in contrast to duloxetine, screened out subjects with depression. The primary outcome measures used in two pivotal trials of milnacipran in FM were "FM responders," defined as patients who fulfilled composite responder indices of 30% improvement in pain VAS, "very much" or "much improved" on the PGIC scale, and six-point improvement of the SF-36 physical component score, and "FM pain responders," defined as patients having a response of pain and patient global measures but not including the SF-36 function component.[30,31]

The first study included 888 FM patients of both genders randomized 1:1:2 to placebo, 50 mg twice daily, and 100 mg twice daily of milnacipran, respectively.[31] At the primary endpoint of 15 weeks, 33% of observed cases achieved FM responder status in both milnacipran dose arms versus 19% of placebo patients. Using a strict baseline observation carried forward (BOCF) analysis, approximately 19% of treated patients versus 12% of placebo patients did so. Both analyses showed a statistically significant separation of milnacipran treatment from placebo. FM pain responder status was achieved by 45% of milnacipran-treated versus 27% of placebo-treated patients using an observed cases analysis and by 27% versus 19% of patients using a BOCF analysis. Secondary measures that showed statistically significant improvement included fatigue as measured by the MFI and a self-reported measure of cognition as measured by the MASQ. Efficacy was generally maintained through the second timepoint of assessment, 27 weeks. The most prominent side effects were mild-to-moderate nausea and headache, which resolved with continued use of the medication. The patients did not gain weight, not unlike the experience with duloxetine. A 12-month treatment group showed that long-term treatment with milnacipran maintains positive effects and is safe.[32]

A second pivotal trial of milnacipran in FM assessed 1196 patients randomized 1:1:1 to placebo, 50 mg twice daily, and 100 mg twice daily of milnacipran for 15 weeks.[30] The same measures of response were used and the results were similar, showing statistically significant separation of response of both dose arms in comparison with placebo in FM responder and FM pain responder rates per BOCF and observed cases methods of analysis. Key secondary measures that showed statistically significant improvement included the PGIC, function (SF-36), and fatigue (MFI) assessments. The adverse event profile was similar to that of the first study. With this agent as well as with duloxetine, patients tended to accommodate better to the drug when a gradual initial dose titration was employed. Also similar to duloxetine, milnacipran neither helped nor hindered sleep quality. Based on the data from these trials, the FDA has approved milnacipran for the management of FM in both the 50-mg twice daily and 100-mg twice daily dosage.

Antiepileptic Drugs

It has long been known that certain drugs originally developed for the treatment of epilepsy can have pain-relieving effects. The most clear evidence for this has been with pregabalin and gabapentin. Pregabalin, approved for the treatment of diabetic peripheral neuropathy, postherpetic neuralgia, as well as adjunctive therapy in partial onset seizures, was the first pharmaceutical approved by the FDA for FM treatment. It binds to the $\alpha_2\delta$ auxiliary protein associated with voltage-gated calcium channels and modulates neuronal calcium influx. The result is a reduction of release of several pain pathway neurotransmitters which have a role in pain processing, such as glutamate and substance P. Efficacy in FM was first established in an 8-week trial in 529 FM patients using dosages of 150, 300, and 450 mg in a total daily dose (divided three times daily) versus placebo. The two higher dose arms showed statistically significant improvements in pain, patient global impression of improvement with therapy, sleep disturbance, fatigue, and health-related quality of life in FM patients.[33] Statistically significant responder rates using the pain VAS showed a 50% or greater response in 29% of the 450-mg group versus 13% of the placebo group and a 30% or greater response in 48% and 27% of the 450-mg and placebo groups, respectively. The 300-mg and 150-mg groups did not separate from placebo statistically. Phase three trials of pregabalin confirmed these observations, including efficacy in the three key domains of pain, patient global improvement, and function, and supported longer term durability of effect out to 6 months.[34–36] An important secondary domain that demonstrated improvement was sleep. Adverse effects experienced by some patients included dizziness and sedation, which tended to improve and resolve during the initial period of use, as well as weight gain in a small percentage of patients. Based on these results, the FDA granted approval for the use of pregabalin for the management of FM in dosages of 300 to 450 mg. Further study of pregabalin continues to confirm the safety and efficacy of long-term use.[37–39] As with the SNRIs, gradual dose titration improves initial tolerability with this agent.

A single controlled trial with the agent gabapentin showed efficacy in multiple FM symptom domains, including pain, PGIC, function, and sleep.[40] The median dose used by 150 patients randomized to gabapentin versus placebo was 1800 mg in divided doses per day (range, 1200–2400 mg allowed and titrated to tolerance). The side effect profile was similar to that of pregabalin. Although mechanistically similar to pregabalin, the pharmacokinetic and pharmacodynamic profile of gabapentin is not as favorable as that of pregabalin.

Sedative Hypnotics

Sedative hypnotics may aid in restoring disrupted or nonrestorative sleep in FM patients. Improved sleep contributes to diminishing other symptoms including fatigue and dyscognition. Sodium oxybate, approved for the treatment of narcolepsy, is the sodium salt of gamma hydroxybutyrate, which, in turn, is a precursor of gamma aminobutyric acid, which has sedating properties. An 8-week phase 2 study of this agent in 88 FM patients evaluated a dosage of 4.5 and 6 g versus placebo taken in two divided doses at bedtime and 2.5 to 4 hours later. Statistically significant improvements in pain, patient global improvement, function (FIQ), fatigue, and sleep quality changes were demonstrated.[41] These results have been confirmed in a larger 12-week study.[42] The most common side effects were nausea and dizziness, but overall the drug was well tolerated. A practical point regarding this agent is that its use is highly regulated because of recreational abuse potential. Other sedative hypnotics studied in FM patients are zolpidem and zopiclone, short-acting non-benzodiazeprine sedatives.[13,43–45] These drugs improved sleep but not pain in patients, rendering them potentially useful adjunctive treatment medications.

Analgesics

Analgesics have been employed in an attempt to mitigate the primary symptom of pain in FM patients. A clinic survey found that about 14% of FM patients are treated with opiates[46]; however, a double-blind, placebo-controlled study of intravenous morphine did not show reduction in pain.[47] One could argue that the stronger opioid agents have not been adequately tested in FM; however, a cautionary point about their routine use in FM is their addictive potential, side effect profile, and theoretical potential to cause opioid-induced hyperalgesia.[48] Tramadol, which is a mild opioid that also has mild SSRI properties, has been assessed in two controlled trials in FM patients and has demonstrated efficacy in pain as well as several subscales of the FIQ and SF-36 function measures.[49,50] Tramadol may be considered as an adjunctive measure for the treatment of pain in FM.

NSAIDs appear to have no effect when used alone in FM but may be modestly helpful when combined with a TCA.[51] NSAIDs may be beneficial in ameliorating peripheral pain generators, such as the pain of osteoarthritis, which may be partly responsible for some of the symptom burden of patients who have such a condition concomitant with FM. This same concept holds for other comorbid painful conditions such as rheumatoid arthritis and lupus, that is, effective treatment of the comorbid condition with appropriately targeted medications may reduce the overall symptom burden of the patient, which may indirectly benefit their experience of FM.

Other Pharmacologic Approaches

Other pharmacologic approaches have been or are in the process of being tried in FM. As discussed in other articles in this issue, there is some evidence that there may be functional or quantitative deficiency of dopamine in FM. Holman has assessed this class of medication in FM patients. The promising results of a non-monotherapy trial in FM with the dopamine agonist agent pramipexole are discussed herein in the section on combination pharmacotherapy.[52] A monotherapy trial needs to be performed with this class of agent to ascertain its effect size in various symptom domains of FM. In patients with concomitant restless leg syndrome, this class of agent would be a useful adjunct.

Tropisetron, an intravenous $5\text{-}HT_3$ antagonist with analgesic effects, has shown efficacy in small trials of FM patients in a bell-shaped curve dose effect.[53] These results may be due in part to the fact that there are receptors for this neurotransmitter on both ascending pain fibers that transmit nociceptive information as well as inhibitory dorsal horn neurons, potentially leading to contradictory effects depending on the dosage used.

When corticosteroids have been assessed in FM, they have not been shown to have a beneficial effect on FM itself,[54] although as is true for NSAIDs, they may have adjunctive utility in reducing inflammation-induced pain from comorbid inflammatory conditions such as rheumatoid arthritis or lupus.

Several other exploratory trials of drugs whose mechanisms have the potential to demonstrate antinociceptive neuromodulation through one or more of the postulated mechanisms of FM are currently underway or are in development and can be tracked through the FDA Web site.

Devices

Although this article is focused on pharmacotherapy for FM, it seems appropriate to acknowledge that several device strategies are in development for the treatment of FM and other chronic pain conditions. Three electromagnetic wave devices show efficacy for treating FM symptoms: transcranial direct current stimulation (tDCS), repetitive transcranial magnetic stimulation (rTMS), and complex neural pulse stimulation (CNP).[55–57] The presumed mechanism of these devices is to modulate neural pain signaling by means of transcranial electromagnetic impulses. The tDCS device modifies brain activity by applying a weak DC current for 20 minutes into the brain via electrodes placed on the cranium by a technician. Daily use of the tDCS device improved pain and physical function in FM patients.[55] The rTMS device applies magnetic waves to the cranium and is also administered by a technician. When used everyday for 30 minutes, the device improved pain in FM.[56] The CNP device uses a lower power magnetic pulse applied to the cranium through a headset used by the patient everyday for 40 minutes. Because it is self-administered, this approach is more convenient for the patient. Preliminary studies of the CNP device indicate improvement in the chronic pain associated with FM,[57] but more definitive controlled trials are needed to know if this approach can be effective. In the future, other medical devices used to treat related pain conditions may show efficacy for treating FM symptoms.

COMBINATION PHARMACOTHERAPY

As indicated previously, patients with FM experience multiple symptoms that may benefit from several different medications that have different mechanisms of action and may preferentially benefit one symptom domain over another. As indicated in the National Fibromyalgia Association survey,[1] multiple medications are commonly used, often in combination. For example, if a medicine has a significant impact on pain yet little benefit on sleep, it would be reasonable to use it along with a medicine that particularly improves sleep, as long as there is not a pharmacologic or adverse event issue that is a contraindication to use the two together. If two medicines that have a significant impact on pain are used and one also benefits fatigue and the other has drowsiness as a side effect, it would be sensible to use the former during the day and the latter at bedtime. It is important to have knowledge about potential adverse drug interactions and to work closely with a pharmacist to ensure safe combination therapy. For example, the concomitant use of SSRIs and SNRIs or two SNRIs can result in serotonin syndrome which can be difficult to detect and toxic.[58] Considering our growing understanding about the pathophysiology of FM, rational combination therapy would target the inhibition of nociceptive signaling in ascending pain fibers, such as with the agent pregabalin, along with an agent that augments norepinephrine and serotonin signaling in descending neurons that have a pain modulation role, such as one of the SNRIs such as duloxetine or milnacipran. If a patient prefers to keep their medication use to a minimum, it would make sense to choose one or two medicines that can impact several symptom domains effectively rather than just one. Use of an SNRI that can benefit pain and mood or a medicine such as pregabalin that can improve pain and sleep rather than a pure analgesic that only benefits pain would be examples.

Do we have definitive data that such rational combinations are truly additive or synergistic in their effect and yield greater effectiveness in multiple symptom domains than monotherapy? Now that several drugs are being approved for FM based on monotherapy data, trials are being developed to test this question as well as assess the safety and tolerability of combinations. An example of an ideal design for such a trial would be four treatment arms: (1) placebo versus (2) drug A versus (3) drug B versus (4) drug A plus B. If the fourth arm of this study yielded significantly greater benefit in several symptom domains, such as pain, fatigue, and sleep, and did not have significantly more side effects than the second or third arms, combination therapy would be supported. An ideal goal would be to address as many of the slices of the pie diagram in **Fig. 2** as is feasible.

Often when combinations of medicines are used, they are best introduced sequentially so that a patient can gain a sense of the effectiveness of one medicine and adjust to adverse effects that may be more prominent initially and then diminish or resolve before introducing a second medicine. The prominence of one symptom domain over another may impact the sequential choice of medicines. A corollary point is that, when first seen, a patient may portray a symptom such as pain as the most prominent symptom to address. With effective treatment of pain, other symptoms may become more prominent, such as sleep disturbance or dyscognition, which will dictate the next steps in sequential medicine choice.

Some clinical trials have not required washout of all drugs that can treat FM, allowing demonstration of the effect of a tested drug when added to background therapy. This method gives a sense of the safety and tolerability of combinations of drugs but does not allow a true quantization of additive effect. A trial of tramadol and acetaminophen allowed background low dose SSRI, zolpidem, and flurazepam but excluded a TENs device, other antidepressants, or antiepileptic drugs.[49] The primary endpoint of this study, the difference in the dropout rate over time in the treatment and placebo groups, achieved statistical significance. A trial with pramipexole allowed concomitant treatment with antiepileptic, anti-inflammatory, antidepressant, or analgesic agents (including opioids).[52] This trial suggested that pramipexole with other treatments

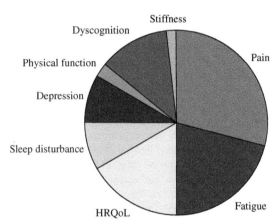

Fig. 2. Hypothetical mix of symptom domains in an FM patient: constructs for the customization of treatment. A pie diagram demonstrating hypothetical mix of symptom domains in a patient with FM characterizing the multiplicity of symptoms and illustrating that the amount of symptom involvement can vary from patient to patient. HRQoL, health-related quality of life.

improved pain, fatigue, function, and global status and was adequately tolerated. A controlled monotherapy trial with this agent is needed to more clearly determine its efficacy in FM.

Although this article is focused on pharmacotherapy of FM, it is important to keep in mind that the multiple symptoms typically occurring in FM are commonly associated with several comorbid conditions, such as irritable bowel and bladder syndrome, headache, restless leg syndrome, and so forth. Each of these conditions may have its own set of approved therapies as well as therapies that overlap with those approved for FM. Keeping in mind drug-drug interactions, this is another area in which combination pharmacotherapy occurs. Furthermore, these therapies may be initiated and managed by other clinicians such as gastroenterologists, urologists, neurologists, or primary care physicians. Open lines of communication must be maintained with this team to keep track of all the medications the patient is taking to avoid problematic drug interactions.

EVIDENCE-BASED TREATMENT RECOMMENDATIONS

As an increasing number of controlled trials of pharmacologic and nonpharmacologic treatments for FM emerge, it is important to note the efforts of researchers to perform methodologically sound meta-analyses of these trials to help guide clinicians regarding treatment choices. These are not guidelines with inherently more codified approaches but rather recommendations, which more flexibly take into account the many individual nuances which determine optimal care. Several of these recommendations have already been referenced in this article, including meta-analyses of the antidepressant class of medicines[14,19,20] and the management recommendations by Goldenberg and colleagues.[15] Rossy and colleagues[22] published in 1999 a meta-analysis of both pharmacologic and nonpharmacologic treatment approaches in FM. The most recent overall meta-analysis of FM treatments was conducted by Carville and colleagues[59] on behalf of the European League Against Rheumatism consortium led by Choy. Based on the evidence from peer-reviewed journal articles and certain abstracts published through 2005 on FM treatment, a series of recommendations was rendered based on the quality of evidence and consensus among consortium members. In concert with several other previously made observations, this group suggested evidence for the effectiveness of medicines of the antidepressant class, especially SNRIs, pregabalin, tramadol, tropisetron, and possibly pramipexole and simple analgesics.

SUMMARY

As understanding of the pathophysiology of FM has become clearer, the ability to treat the condition has also improved. Neuromodulatory agents of a variety of classes (eg, drugs that help to restore toward normal key noradrenergic- and serotonergic-mediated inhibitory pain pathways, that diminish nociceptive signaling in ascending pain pathways, and that beneficially impact symptom domains beyond pain, such as disturbed sleep and cognition as well as fatigue) have been shown in well-designed controlled trials to improve the key symptom domains of FM. Because improved methods of measuring disease severity and the impact of therapy are being used in these trials, we can be more confident that the improvements are real and meaningful. Currently approved treatments do not benefit all patients either because of inadequate efficacy or a lack of tolerability. Nevertheless, the results are better than what has been shown with older, less efficacious, or poorly tolerated medicines. Several new treatment approaches are in development now that the pathophysiology is better understood and the approach to clinical trial conduct and regulatory approval is clearer. It is hoped this will provide more effective tools for treatment, either in monotherapy or combination therapy format, to be used in conjunction with nonpharmacologic approaches.

REFERENCES

1. Bennett RM, Jones J, Turk DC, et al. An internet survey of 2596 people with fibromyalgia. BMC Musculoskelet Disord 2007;9:27–38.
2. Barkhuizen A. Rational and targeted pharmacologic treatment of fibromyalgia. Rheum Dis Clin North Am 2002;28:261–90.
3. Choy EH. Key symptom domains to be assessed in FM. Rheum Dis Clin North Am, in progress.
4. Choy EH, Arnold LM, Clauw D, et al. Content and criterion validity of the preliminary core dataset for clinical trials in fibromyalgia syndrome. J Rheumatol, in press.
5. Mease P. Fibromyalgia syndrome: review of clinical presentation, pathogenesis, outcome measures, and treatment. J Rheumatol 2005;32:6–21.
6. Mease P, Arnold LM, Bennett R, et al. Fibromyalgia syndrome. J Rheumatol 2007; 34:1415–25.
7. Mease PJ, Clauw DJ, Arnold LM, et al. Fibromyalgia syndrome. J Rheumatol 2005;32:2270.
8. Mease P, Arnold LM, Choy EH, et al. Fibromyalgia syndrome. J Rheumatol, in press.
9. Mease PJ, Arnold LM, Crofford LJ, et al. Identifying the clinical domains of fibromyalgia: contributions from clinical and patients Delphi exercises. Arthritis Care Res 2008;59:952–60.
10. Farrar JT, Young JP Jr, LaMoreaux L, et al. Clinical importance of changes in chronic pain intensity measured on an 11-point numerical pain rating scale. Pain 2001;94:149–58.

11. Moldofsky H. Sleep and FM. Rheum Dis Clin North Am, in progress.
12. Moldofsky H, Scarisbrick P, England R, et al. Musculoskeletal symptoms and non-REM sleep disturbance in patients with "fibrositis syndrome" and healthy subjects. Psychosom Med 1975;37:341–5.
13. Arnold LM. New therapies in fibromyalgia. Arthritis Res Ther 2006;8:212–32.
14. Arnold LM, Keck PE Jr, Welge JA. Antidepressant treatment of fibromyalgia: a meta-analysis and review. Psychosomatics 2000;41:104–13.
15. Goldenberg D, Burckhardt C, Crofford L. Management of fibromyalgia syndrome. JAMA 2004;292:2388–95.
16. Mease PJ, Seymour K. Fibromyalgia syndrome update: emerging pharmacologic treatments. J Musculoskel Med 2007;24:436–45.
17. Mease PJ, Seymour K. Fibromyalgia: should the treatment paradigm be monotherapy or combination pharmacotherapy? Curr Pain Headache Rep 2008;12:399–405.
18. Moldofsky H, Scarisbrick P. Induction of neurasthenic musculoskeletal pain syndrome by selective sleep stage deprivation. Psychosom Med 1975;38:35–44.
19. O'Malley PG, Balden E, Tomkins G, et al. Treatment of fibromyalgia with antidepressants: a meta-analysis. J Gen Intern Med 2000;15:659–66.
20. Tofferi JK, Jackson JL, O'Malley PG. Treatment of fibromyalgia with cyclobenzaprine: a meta-analysis. Arthritis Rheum 2004;51:9–13.
21. Carette S, Bell MJ, Reynolds WJ, et al. Comparison of amitriptyline, cyclobenzaprine, and placebo in the treatment of fibromyalgia: a randomised, double blind clinical trial. Arthritis Rheum 1994;37:32–40.
22. Rossy LA, Buckelew SP, Dorr N, et al. A meta-analysis of fibromyalgia treatment interventions. Ann Behav Med 1999;21:180–91.
23. Wolfe F, Cathey MA, Hawley DJ. A double-blind placebo controlled trial of fluoxetine in fibromyalgia. Scand J Rheumatol 1994;23:255–9.
24. Arnold LM, Hess EV, Hudson JI, et al. A randomized, placebo-controlled, double-blind, flexible-dose study of fluoxetine in the treatment of women with fibromyalgia. Am J Med 2002;112:191–7.
25. Sayar K, Aksu G, Ak I, et al. Venlafaxine treatment of fibromyalgia. Ann Pharmacother 2003;37:1561–5.
26. Zijsltra TR, Barendregt PJ, van de Laar MA. Venlafaxine in fibromyalgia: results of a randomized, placebo-controlled, double-blind trial. Arthritis Rheum 2002;46:S105.
27. Arnold LM, Rosen A, Pritchett YL, et al. Duloxetine in the treatment of fibromyalgia in women: results from two clinical trials. Pain 2005;119:5–15.
28. Mease PJ, Russell IJ, Kajdasz DK, et al. Long-term safety, tolerability, and efficacy of duloxetine in the treatment of fibromyalgia. [Epub ahead of print]. Semin Arthritis Rheum 2009.
29. Russell IJ, Mease PJ, Smith TR, et al. Efficacy and safety of duloxetine for treatment of fibromyalgia in patients with or without major depressive disorder: results from a 6-month, randomized, double-blind, placebo-controlled, fixed-dose trial. Pain 2008;136:432–44.
30. Clauw DJ, Mease P, Palmer RH, et al. Milnacipran for the treatment of fibromyalgia in adults: a 15-week, multicenter, randomized, double-blind, placebo-controlled, multiple-dose clinical trial. Clin Ther 2008;30:1988–2004.
31. Mease PJ, Clauw DJ, Gendreau RM, et al. The efficacy and safety of milnacipran for treatment of fibromyalgia: a randomized, double-blind, placebo-controlled trial. J Rheumatol 2009;36:398–409.

32. Goldenberg D, Clauw DJ, Palmer RH, et al. One-year durability of response to milnacipran treatment for fibromyalgia [abstract]. Arthritis Rheum 2007;S603.
33. Crofford L, Rowbotham M, Mease P, et al. Pregabalin for the treatment of fibromyalgia syndrome: results of a randomized, double-blind, placebo-controlled trial. Arthritis Rheum 2005;52:1264–73.
34. Arnold LM, Russell IJ, Diri EW, et al. A 14-week, randomized, double-blind, placebo-controlled, durability of effect study of pregabalin for pain associated with fibromyalgia. J Pain 2008;9:792–805.
35. Crofford LJ, Mease PJ, Simpson SL, et al. Fibromyalgia relapse evaluation and efficacy for durability of meaningful relief (FREEDOM): a 6-month, double-blind, placebo-controlled trial with pregabalin. Pain 2008;136:419–31.
36. Mease PJ, Russell IJ, Arnold LM, et al. A randomized, double-blind, placebo-controlled, phase III trial of pregabalin in the treatment of patients with fibromyalgia. J Rheumatol 2008;35:502–14.
37. Duan WR, Florian H, Young JP, et al. Pregabalin monotherapy for management of fibromyalgia: analysis of two double-blind, randomized, placebo-controlled trials. Arthritis Rheum 2007;56:S602.
38. Florian H, Young JP, Haig G, et al. Efficacy and safety of pregabalin as long-term treatment of pain associated with fibromyalgia: a 1-year, open-label study [abstract]. Arthritis Rheum 2007;S602.
39. Simpson SL, Young JP, Haig G, et al. Pregabalin therapy for durability of meaningful relief of fibromyalgia. In: Program and abstracts of the American College of Rheumatology 2007 Annual Scientific Meeting. Boston, November 6–11, 2007.
40. Arnold LM, Goldenberg D, Stratford SB, et al. Gabapentin in the treatment of fibromyalgia. Arthritis Rheum 2006;54:S827.
41. Russell IJ, Perkins AT, Michalek JE, et al. Sodium oxybate relieves pain and improves function in fibromyalgia syndrome: a randomized, double-blind, placebo-controlled, multicenter clinical trial. Arthritis Rheum 2009;60:299–309.
42. Swick TJ, Alvarez-Horine S, Zheng Y, et al. Sodium oxybate improved pain, fatigue, and sleep in patients with fibromyalgia: results from a 14-week randomized, double-blind, placebo-controlled trial. Sleep 2009;32:A321.
43. Drewes AM, Andreasen A, Jennum P, et al. Zopiclone in the treatment of sleep abnormalities in fibromyalgia. Scand J Rheumatol 1991;20:288–93.
44. Gronblad M, Nykanen J, Konttinen Y, et al. Effect of zopiclone on sleep quality, morning stiffness, widespread tenderness and pain and general discomfort in primary fibromyalgia patients: a double-blind randomized trial. Clin Rheumatol 1993;12:186–91.
45. Moldofsky H, Lue FA, Mously C, et al. The effect of zolpidem in patients with fibromyalgia: a dose ranging, double-blind, placebo controlled, modified crossover study. J Rheumatol 1996;23:529–33.
46. Wolfe F, Anderson J, Harkness D, et al. A prospective, longitudinal, multicenter study of service utilization and costs in fibromyalgia. Arthritis Rheum 1997;40:1560–70.
47. Sorensen J, Bengtsson A, Backman E, et al. Pain analysis in patients with fibromyalgia: effects of intravenous morphine, lidocaine, and ketamine. Scand J Rheumatol 1995;24:360–5.
48. Chu LF, Clark DJ, Angst MS. Opioid tolerance and hyperalgesia in chronic pain patients after one month of oral morphine therapy: a preliminary prospective study. J Pain 2006;7:43–8.

49. Bennett RM, Kamin M, Karim R, et al. Tramadol and acetaminophen combination tablets in the treatment of fibromyalgia pain: a double-blind, randomized, placebo-controlled study. Am J Med 2003;114:537–45.
50. Russell I, Kamin M, Bennett RM, et al. Efficacy of tramadol in treatment of pain in fibromyalgia. J Clin Rheumatol 2000;6:250–7.
51. Goldenberg DL, Felson DT, Dinerman H. A randomized, controlled trial of amitriptyline and naproxen in the treatment of patients with fibromyalgia. Arthritis Rheum 1986;29:1371–7.
52. Holman AJ, Myers RR. A randomized, double-blind, placebo-controlled trial of pramipexole, a dopamine agonist, in patients with fibromyalgia receiving concomitant medications. Arthritis Rheum 2005;52:2495–505.
53. Spath M, Stratz T, Neeck G, et al. Efficacy and tolerability of intravenous tropisetron in the treatment of fibromyalgia. Scand J Rheumatol 2004;33:267–76.
54. Clark S, Tindall E, Bennett RM. A double blind crossover trial of prednisone versus placebo in the treatment of fibrositis. J Rheumatol 1985;12:980–3.
55. Fregni F, Gimenes R, Valle AC, et al. A randomized, sham-controlled, proof of principle study of transcranial direct current stimulation for the treatment of pain in fibromyalgia. Arthritis Rheum 2006;54:3988–98.
56. Sampson SM, Rome JD, Rummans TA. Slow-frequency rTMS reduced fibromyalgia pain. Pain Med 2006;7:115–8.
57. Thomas AW, Graham K, Prato FS, et al. A randomized, double-blind, placebo-controlled clinical trial using a low-frequency magnetic field in the treatment of musculoskeletal chronic pain. Pain Res Manag 2007;12:249–58.
58. Boyer EW, Shannon M. The serotonin syndrome. N Engl J Med 2005;352:112–20.
59. Carville SF, Arendt-Nielsen S, Bliddal H, et al. EULAR evidence-based recommendations for the management of fibromyalgia syndrome. Ann Rheum Dis 2008;67:536–41.

Exercise Interventions in Fibromyalgia: Clinical Applications from the Evidence

Kim D. Jones, PhD, RN, FNP[a],*, Ginevra L. Liptan, MD[b,c]

KEYWORDS

- Fibromyalgia • Exercise interventions • Exercise prescription
- Eccentric contraction • Self-efficacy

Most clinicians are aware of the benefits of exercise for patients who have fibromyalgia (FM). Many express frustration, however, with poor patient compliance with exercise recommendations. Viewed from a broader context, regular exercise eludes at least 70% of Americans.[1] It is thus not surprising that patients with the pain, fatigue, and disrupted sleep of FM would face additional challenges in adopting and maintaining an exercise program. In fact, 83% of patients who have FM do not engage in aerobic exercise, and most of those tested have below-average fitness levels. In physical self-report or functional testing, the average 40-year-old patient who has FM was found to be as physically unfit as an 80-year-old person who does not have FM.[2,3]

This article summarizes physiologic obstacles to exercise and reviews exercise interventions in FM. In addition, the authors describe the top 10 principles for successfully prescribing exercise in the comprehensive treatment of FM and provide a practical exercise resource table to share with patients.

POTENTIAL "PHYSIOLOGIC" OBSTACLES TO ADEQUATE EXERCISE IN PATIENTS WHO HAVE FIBROMYALGIA

The common complaint of many patients who have FM is that they hurt and feel more fatigued after exercise. There are a few observations worthy of note that may be

This work was supported by National Institutes of Health (NIH)/National Institute of Arthritis & Musculoskeletal Health & Skin Disease grant SR21AR05359, NIH/National Institute of Diabetes and Digestive and Kidney Diseases grant RH133G070214, NIH/National Institute of Mental Health grant R01 MH0709818-0, and the Fibromyalgia Information Foundation.
[a] Office of Research and Development, School of Nursing, Oregon Health & Science University, 3455 SW US Veterans Hospital Road, SN-ORD, Portland, OR 97239–2941, USA
[b] Division of Arthritis and Rheumatic Diseases, Oregon Health & Science University, 3181 SW Sam Jackson Park Road OP-09, Portland, OR 97239, USA
[c] Legacy Good Samaritan Pain Management Center, 1130 NW 22nd Avenue, Suite 345, Portland, OR 97210, USA
* Corresponding author.
E-mail address: joneskim@ohsu.edu (K.D. Jones).

relevant to postexertional pain and fatigue in patients who have FM. Kosek's group[4,5] has reported that patients who have FM have reduced muscle blood flow to the infraspinatus muscle during dynamic and static exercise and that such exercise is more painful than in healthy controls. Reduced muscle blood flow in FM was originally reported in 1982 by Klemp and colleagues[6] and then by Bennett[7] and McIver and colleagues.[8] It has been hypothesized that exertional pain in FM may partially be a result of muscle ischemia. Exercise is generally considered to evoke an inhibitory effect on pain by the production of endorphins[9,10] and activation of the descending inhibitory pathways. The hypothalamic pituitary adrenergic response to exercise is blunted in patients who have FM,[11] and a concomitant reduction in the release of endorphins would be expected;[12] however, this has not so far been tested in patients who have FM. Furthermore, patients who have FM have been reported to have reduced μ-opioid receptor binding in several brain regions involved in pain modulation.[13] These findings indicate that the μ-opioid receptors are nearly saturated in patients who have FM, making them less responsive to the secretion of endogenous opioids. The descending bulbospinal pathways are critical in reducing the perception of ongoing painful stimuli.[14] Staud and colleagues[15] have reported that sustained muscular contraction induced widespread inhibition of pain perception in healthy individuals but not in patients who had FM; on the contrary, sustained muscle contraction induced an increase in the hyperalgesia of patients who had FM. The authors hypothesize that the inability of patients who have FM to develop postexercise hypoalgesia may be the result of an impaired response of the inhibitory bulbospinal pathways.

The stress response system is abnormal in FM, with perturbations in the autonomic nervous system that may be manifested as postural orthostatic tachycardia syndrome, neurally mediated hypotension, and fatigue.[11,16,17] These autonomic perturbations can contribute to poor exercise tolerance in patients who have FM. The endocrine arm of the stress system has also been reported to be dysfunctional, with cortisol and growth hormone (GH) imbalances.[18,19] Jones and colleagues[20] have reported a defective GH response to exercise in more than 90% of patients who have FM. GH is important in muscle growth and repair, and it is hypothesized that defective GH production impairs the resolution of exercise-induced muscle microtrauma.[21] Finally, levels of exercise that are excessive for a given individual result in the production of proinflammatory cytokines,[22] which results in feeling increased fatigue as a consequence of the cytokine-associated "sickness syndrome".[23] Whether these problems are a result of being deconditioned, and hence improve with gradual escalation of exercise intensity, or whether they represent a "physiologic" block resulting from having FM is not fully understood at this time. It is probable that both notions have some degree of truth and underline the necessity for a strictly graduated approach to exercise therapy in patients who have FM.

REVIEW OF FIBROMYALGIA EXERCISE INTERVENTIONS: TWO DECADES OF PROGRESS

The first consideration of exercise as a possible therapeutic intervention in FM arose from a sleep laboratory in the 1970s. Researchers repeatedly startled healthy college students awake during deep sleep. This manipulation caused muscle pain and tender points in most subjects, although, surprisingly, sparing those who were elite runners.[24] Since that time, 70 exercise interventions in FM have been published. From 1988 through 2008, a total of 4385 subjects completed those studies. Of those studies, 56 were randomized controlled trials. Modalities of exercises studied included aerobics (land and water), strength, flexibility, and various combinations of these. More recently, "movement therapies," such as Qi Gong, T'ai Chi, and yoga, have been tested, with positive results. Outcomes, including heart rate variability and cognition, have been newly published, as has an intervention in juvenile FM (**Fig. 1**).

Multiple exercise reviews, position papers, and clinical guidelines have been published. **Table 1** outlines the major findings of four recent reviews.

High attrition rates have plagued many studies on exercise in FM. The average attrition rate for studies included in the Cochrane Review was 27%. Some early strength training studies had dropout rates as high as 47%.[30] Likewise, programs testing running, calisthenics, and fast dancing have reported up to 67% attrition.[31] Similarly, high-intensity exercise has also been shown to provoke pain compared with low-intensity exercise.[32] Exercise interventions that were lower in intensity and allowed for some individualization in the protocol have yielded attrition rates less than 10%.[33]

Since the publication of the review articles detailed previously, 18 original exercise clinical trials have been published.[34–51] Most were high-quality studies confirming that individualized low-intensity exercise of varying dose and modality was effective at improving function and reducing symptoms. There were some novel contributions in the past year, however. Munguia-Izquierdo and Legaz-Arrese[46] found improvements in cognitive function (paced auditory serial addition, reversal of digits, trail-making tests, controlled oral word association, and Rey auditory verbal learning test) in 35 subjects who had FM compared with 25 controls who had FM after mixed-type water exercise three times weekly for 16 weeks. This finding was not supported by Jones and colleagues[42] and Glass and colleagues,[52] who randomized 165 FM subjects to mixed-type land-based exercise, with or without pyridostigmine, three times weekly for 6 months. Subjects demonstrated significant improvements in GH release, sleep, anxiety, and fatigue but did not experience between-group improvements in cognition as measured by five standardized neurocognitive tasks. Exercise as a treatment for dyscognition in FM is deserving of further study because cognitive dysfunction is rated by many patients as their most distressing symptom.[3]

Stephens and colleagues[48] published the first exercise intervention in children in 2008. Thirty children, ranging in age from 8 to 18 years, who had FM entered (24 completed) the study and were randomly assigned to Qi Gong or aerobics. Overall,

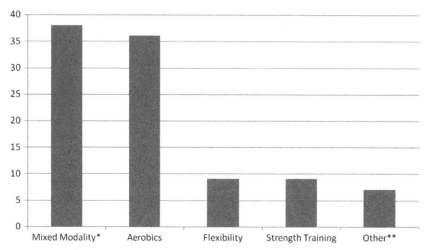

Fig. 1. Percent of exercise modalities studied. Mixed modality includes interventions that combined aerobic, strength, and flexibility training (*). Other includes Qi Gong, T'ai Chi, and lifestyle activity (**). Yoga is included in the flexibility group.

Table 1
Selected fibromyalgia exercise review articles

Review Article	No. Trials	Type of Trial	Exclusion Criteria
Jones et al, 2006[25]	46 trials reviewed from 1988–2005	16 aerobic 5 strength 3 flexibility 4 movement based (T'ai Chi, yoga) 18 mixed-exercise type	Excluded if not an exercise intervention or if the subjects who had FM were analyzed as part of a larger mixed chronic pain cohort
Conclusion: strongest evidence in support of aerobic exercise. Better results were seen with lower intensity exercise programs that were individualized to patient needs.			
Cochrane Database review, 2007[26]	34 trials reviewed from 1988–2005	15 aerobic 3 strength 3 flexibility 11 mixed-exercise type	Excluded if not RCT or inadequate description of exercise
Conclusion: "gold" level evidence for aerobic exercise on physical capacity and FM symptoms. Strength and flexibility may have benefit, but there is inadequate evidence at this point.			
Ottawa Panel evidence-based guidelines, 2008[27,28]	21 trials reviewed from 1988–2006	16 aerobic 5 strength	Excluded if not RCT, attrition greater than 20%, sample size smaller than 5, or not published in English or French
Conclusion: aerobic exercise provides clinically and statistically significant benefits in FM. It was also concluded that strengthening exercises are beneficial for the overall management of FM.			
Gowans et al, 2007[29]	8 trials reviewed from 1999–2006	All pool-based aerobic exercise	Excluded if not pool-based exercise
Conclusion: aerobic exercise in warm pools seems to be as beneficial as land-based aerobic exercise, with additional benefits seen in mood and sleep duration.			

Abbreviation: RCT, randomized clinical trial.

the aerobics group demonstrated a greater number of improvements compared with the Qi Gong group, but both groups had significant and similar improvements in pain, anaerobic function, tender point count, and symptom severity. FM in children is increasingly recognized, and clinicians are often called on to write recommendation letters to their young patients' physical education instructors. Further study of exercise in juvenile FM is needed.

A final novel contribution of 2008 was from Figueroa and colleagues,[38] who studied 10 female subjects who had FM compared with nine healthy controls. The subjects who had FM only undertook twice-weekly strength training with resistance machines for 16 weeks. As expected, the subjects who had FM demonstrated perturbed heart rate variability compared with healthy controls. After the intervention, the subjects who had FM and exercised, compared with FM sedentary controls, demonstrated improvement in total power, cardiac parasympathetic tone, pain, and muscle strength. Exercise as a treatment for autonomic deraignment deserves further evaluation.

In summary, the recent reviews, coupled with 69 exercise interventions in FM, are generally positive, with benefits seen in FM symptoms and physical functioning. Key to compliance with the interventions was the use of low-intensity low-impact programs and maintenance of the ability to individualize the protocol. Evidence for mixed-type or aerobic exercise is strongest, with mounting evidence for beneficial effects from strength training.[30,33,38,43,51,53–57] Some position statements incorporate the fact that there is "no or poor" evidence for adding flexibility training to the exercise prescription in FM.[58] This is primarily attributable to the small number of trials that have isolated tested flexibility training alone. The results of flexibility training, including yoga studies, are positive, but there is not yet a preponderance of evidence that supports the use of flexibility training as a single modality in FM.[33,35,45,59–62] More research needs to be done to evaluate the effectiveness of movement-based therapies in FM, such as Qi Gong and T'ai Chi, because emerging evidence in these modalities is positive.[41,48,63–66]

STRATEGIES TO OPTIMIZE YOUR PATIENTS' EXERCISE SUCCESS

Given the high attrition rates in many exercise studies and altered physiology of FM, successful prescribing of exercise in clinical practice requires finesse. Among clinicians treating FM, there was once an attitude of "Until a FM patient helps himself or herself by exercising, there is nothing I can do for him or her." Providers are increasingly realizing that the opposite approach is much more effective. Once a patient's poor sleep, mood, and peripheral pain generators are addressed with appropriate medical therapy, he or she is then more likely to be compliant with an exercise program and to gain its full benefits.

The following approach is recommended to incorporate exercise into a comprehensive treatment strategy of FM:[67]

Confirm the diagnosis of FM on the first visit, and take a focused medical history, with particular emphasis on pain, sleep, fatigue, stiffness, mood disorders, and cognition. Use of a body pain diagram can help to identify peripheral pain generators.

Begin medications depending on which symptoms are most severe or distressing.

As symptoms begin to improve, provide education about FM and exercise techniques, mostly through books and Web resources (**Table 2**).

During the next few visits, optimize medical management and refer patients for further treatment as needed (eg, refer to psychiatry for severe mood disorder or for a sleep study to evaluate for obstructive sleep apnea).

Table 2
Selected patient resources for exercise with fibromyalgia

Books

Crotzer SL. Yoga for fibromyalgia: move, breathe, and relax to improve your quality of life. Yoga Shorts. Berkely (CA): Rodmell Press; 2008.	Gentle movements tailored for FM; moves avoid overstretching and use towels and chairs to modify poses
Bigelow SL. Fibromyalgia: simple relief through movement. New York: Wiley; 2000.	Excellent, practical, easy-to-read book written by a person who has FM
Rose DJ. Fallproof!: a comprehensive balance and mobility training program. Danvers (MA): Human Kinetics Publishers; 2003.	Picture-guided tour of exercises and postures to reduce the risks for falling and improve balance confidence; written by a leading balance researcher and an exercise physiologist who has FM
Turk DC. The pain survival guide: how to reclaim your life. Washington, DC: APA Lifetools; 2005.	A practical guide for people who have FM written by a leading FM researcher and psychologist; focus on sections regarding balance rest and activity; one paragraph diminishes the role of pharmacologic agents, a tenet that is not necessarily endorsed by other FM researchers and clinicians
Matallana L. The complete idiot's guide to fibromyalgia. New York: Alpha; 2009.	Second edition of a practical guide to understanding and treating FM; written by a patient who has FM and is also the president and founder of the National Fibromyalgia Association
Bond M. The new rules of posture: how to sit, stand, and move in the modern world. Montpelier (VT): Healing Arts Press; 2007.	An illustrated book of posture poses to use as exercise and to decrease pain; not written specifically for FM but translates safely to the special needs of people who have FM
Silver JK, editor. Understanding fitness how exercise fuels health and fights disease. Westport (CT): Praeger Publishers.	Exercise chapter on FM written by Janice Hoffman and Dr. Kim Dupree Jones, FM exercise specialists
Blahnik J. Full-body flexibility for optimal mobility and strength. Champaign (IL): Human Kinetics; 2004.	Offers gentle moves adapted from yoga, Pilates, and martial arts to focus on equalized strength and flexibility in opposing muscle groups; not written specifically for FM but translates safely to the special needs of people who have FM
Andes K. A woman's book of strength. New York: Penguin Putnam, The Berkley Publishing Group; 1995.	Do not be intimidated by the unrealistic picture on the cover. This book provides physical and spiritual strength to maximize relaxation and promote strength through "circular feminine movement patterns"; not written specifically for FM but translates safely to the special needs of people who have FM.

Austin A. Beginner's guide to T'ai Chi. London: Axis Publishing; 2004.	Unlike yoga, T'ai Chi emphasizes body motions rather than positions. This color photograph manual offers instruction and advice on creating an individually tailored T'ai Chi program, based on a 24-step Beijing short form; not written specifically for FM but translates safely to the special needs of people who have FM.
Otis J. Managing chronic pain: A CBT approach. New York: Oxford University Press; 2007.	This book provides education on chronic pain, theories of pain and diaphragmatic breathing, progressive muscle relaxation and visual imagery, automatic thoughts and pain, cognitive restructuring, stress management, time-based pacing, pleasant activity scheduling, anger management, sleep hygiene, and relapse prevention. Using these techniques helps people who have FM to regain a sense of control and improve their quality of life.

Videotape/digital versatile disc

Balance and strength, exercise training in fibromyalgia. Available at: www.myalgia.com	Created by the Fibromyalgia Information Foundation, this digital versatile disc (DVD) features Dr. Kim Dupree Jones demonstrating body alignment and balance testing. Janice Hoffman, a certified exercise specialist, leads a group of people who have FM and are exercising at various levels depending on their FM severity and fitness level. Cinda Hugos, a physical therapist, discusses balance aids, footwear, and strategies for navigating in crowded public locations. Dr. Robert Bennett presents the essential elements of comprehensive FM management.
Stretching and relaxation tape for patients who have fibromyalgia. Available at: www.myalgia.com	Created by the Fibromyalgia Information Foundation, this DVD features people who have FM and are led in gentle stretching of all muscle groups. Janice Hoffman also provides a relaxation session to soothing music. Dr. Robert Bennett discusses the importance of identifying and treating pain generators through range of motion and with an actual demonstration of myofascial trigger point injection on a patient who has FM.
Aerobic exercise for patients who have fibromyalgia. Available at: www.myalgia.com	Created by the Fibromyalgia Information Foundation, this DVD provides a gentle realistic aerobic workout routine featuring four people who have FM and two exercise specialists, including Dr. Sharon Clark. Dr. Robert Bennett explains why people with FM experience widespread pain and should consider a comprehensive treatment program, including exercise.

(continued on next page)

Table 2
(continued)

Get your motor running. Available at: www.fmaware.org	Three-level exercise program developed specifically for people who have FM by Dr. Jessie Jones, an exercise physiologist and patient who has FM
Yee R. Back care yoga for beginners. Available at: www.gaiam.com	20-minute gentle yoga workout using a chair and gentle poses; not developed specifically for people who have FM but works well for fibromyalgia back pain
Web resources	
Clark SR. A fibromyalgia patient's guide to exercise. Available at: www.myalgia.com/exercise	This printout describes the how and why of modifying exercise in FM. Furthermore, it includes advice on how to tailor activities of daily living to minimize eccentric muscle work, modify your posture, and monitor your breathing.
Hoffman JH. Everyday flexibility moves. Available at: www.myalgia.com/exercise	Great to take to personal trainers or to use at home, this PDF printout with line drawings and simple explanations was designed by a FM exercise expert.
Jones K, Hoffman J. Functional fitness. Available at: www.myalgia.com/excercise	This publication provides exercise and other treatments for FM. It highlights how to modify posture, strength training, and balance and aerobic activities while featuring color pictures of people who have FM performing exercises.
FMaware.org. Available at: www.fmaware.org (type exercise in the search engine)	The National Fibromyalgia Association provides 261 "hits" for exercise when entered in the search engine. Many are from their magazine, FMAware, and are written for lay persons rather than clinicians or scientists.
FMnetnews.com. Available at: www.fmnetnews.com/resources-daily-exercise	A practical two-page guide to diet and exercise in FM, with scientifically sound exercise bullet points that focus on maintaining functionality
Egoscue P. Pain free radio. Available at: http://talkradio1370am.com/ Pain-Free-Radio-with-Pete-Egoscue/298,761	This weekly radio program can be heard live on the link provided or downloaded to an I-Pod or MP3 player to enjoy while resting or exercising. Pete Egoscue fields live calls and provides practical low-technology solutions to pain based on posture and body alignment. Occasionally, he takes a negative stand on surgery or medication, which needs to be individualized to each patient by a health care provider who can examine the patient in person.

At this point in the patient-provider relationship, patients generally trust the provider enough to attempt exercise and be given a formal exercise prescription.

All modes of exercise can be successfully modified for FM. For a sedentary person who has moderate to severe FM, the authors recommend the following progression: (1) breath, posture, and relaxation training; (2) flexibility; (3) strength and balance; and (4) aerobics.[68]

TOP 10 PRINCIPLES FOR PRESCRIBING EXERCISE IN FIBROMYALGIA
Treat Peripheral Pain Generators to Minimize Central Sensitization

People who have FM have an enhanced awareness of pain arising from skin, muscle, and joint structures attributable to central sensitization, which has been found to be an important component in the pathophysiology of FM.[69] It is critical to identify peripheral pain generators, such as osteoarthritis, spine pathologic conditions, bursitis, tendonitis, plantar fasciitis, and myofascial trigger points. Treatments of peripheral pain generators with medications, injections, manual therapies, and lidocaine or capsaicin patches, as appropriate, can increase the likelihood of exercise success.

Exercise should also be modified to minimize aggravation of the peripheral pain generators. It is important to choose a type of exercise that does not exacerbate these peripheral pain generators. For example, patients who have significant knee osteoarthritis and stiffness may do better with water-based aerobics than land-based aerobics. A patient with significant gluteal and trochanteric trigger points has less aggravation of his or her tender points if using an elliptic trainer rather than a stationary bike. If joints are hypermobile, patients should be referred to a physical therapist who can teach them to rest and exercise with their joints within the normal joint line, thereby reducing another source of peripheral pain generation.

Posture and body alignment work decreases peripheral pain generators. Posture prescriptions are generally focused on stretching or strength training without added weights (eg, isometric muscle contractions). Pain-perpetuating postures are common in FM and include shortening of the neck and upper back muscles as the patient assumes a head-forward, shoulders-raised, back-rounded posture. Lower body changes, often present as hip flexion or rotation, may occur in response to pain. Providers can do a cursory evaluation of posture as described in **Box 1**. Simple postural adjustments reduce spine pain, a symptom endured by all patients who have FM.

Stretching can also aid in the release of peripheral pain generators, especially trigger points. Specifically, tightened muscle bands and contraction knots within muscle are lessened as the Golgi tendon apparatus signals the muscle fibers to relax. The dose of stretching is key—patients cannot stretch too often, but they can stretch too far. Stretches should not produce immediate muscle burning and should be static rather than ballistic (avoid bouncing). Patients who experience too much pain to stretch may find relief with fluorometholone spray and stretch techniques. This technique requires a prescription spray from the provider, usually given in concert with a referral to a physical therapist, who teaches the patient how to use the spray and how to stretch at home. Alternatively, patients can stretch in a warm bath or shower.

Minimize Eccentric Muscle Work

To avoid causing unnecessary strain on the muscles of patients who have FM, it is important to minimize eccentric muscle use. Eccentric muscle use is muscle lengthening against resistance.[42,70] Exercise tailoring to minimize muscle work can be

---

Box 1
Office evaluation of posture in fibromyalgia

- Ask the patient to stand, without looking at his or her feet, and place the feet parallel under the hips.

- Ask the patient where he or she feels the weight. It should be equal between the feet, with roughly 50% on the heels and 50% on the balls of the feet, and equal bilaterally.

- Ask the patient to look down and help him or her to realign the feet so that the feet are hip distance over knees and ankles. Often, feet are everted (toes pointing out) and not symmetric. This may stem from pelvic rotation or unnatural pelvic flexion or extension (loss of the natural S-shaped curve in the spine).

- Help the patient to align his or her feet. This may feel "pigeon toed" to many patients. Then ask the patient to adjust his or her weight as described previously.

- Observe the patient's hand position while standing, arms straight, resting at his or her sides. The thumbs should be pointed forward. If the backs of the hands are facing forward, the shoulders are often rounded forward.

---

done in classes, with gym equipment, or even in activities of daily living (ADLs). For example, while walking downhill, load is placed on elongated muscles, creating greater eccentric muscle work. Patients who prefer treadmill walking should walk at a flat, rather than downward, sloping grade to minimize eccentric muscle use. Use small steps and limited arm extension when walking, mopping, or vacuuming to minimize eccentric work in the hips and thighs. Also keep movements near the midline of the body and minimize overhead work and repetitive motion, particularly of small muscle groups. Most gym equipment for aerobic training relies on repetitive movements. To minimize eccentric muscle work on machines, such as elliptic trainers, stair steppers, and Nordic tracks, use the lowest hand grip available or let the arms rest on the support bars. A better approach to these types of equipment is to switch machines every 10 minutes or less, based on fitness level. Care should be taken with recumbent bikes to avoid knee hyperextension. When using machine or free weights, spend more time in concentric contraction compared with eccentric contraction. For example, bicep contraction could be up 1-2-3-4-5-6, down 1-2-3, and rest 1-2-3 to allow the muscle to return to full baseline resting state.[71] Strength training movements should be kept on a parallel plane and near the midline of the body when possible.

Consider using lighter weight than age-predicted norms, often less than 50% of the one-repetition maximum recommended. Training should begin with single sets of six repetitions, increasing slowly. Soft elastic bands have the advantage of providing resistance without requiring heavy lifting, a tight grip, or sustained contraction. These are helpful in patients who have wrist pain or carpal tunnel syndrome. For those who wish to use free weights, consider employing a personal trainer to ensure proper positioning. Trainers can also aid in counting repetitions and limiting time spent in eccentric contraction. A clinician can write a prescription for exercise, as can a personal trainer, and the cost may often be reimbursed through an employer-sponsored health care flexible spending account.

Program Low-intensity Nonrepetitive Exercise

Early exercise interventions in FM offered trials that were more similar in dose to those recommended by the American College of Sports Medicine, whose original audience was elite athletes. Patients who had FM and could tolerate the interventions demonstrated improvements in physical fitness, but results were mixed in terms of symptom reduction. One way to conceptualize the dose of exercise needed in FM is to realize that the therapeutic window is narrow: too much exercise results in symptom exacerbation, and too little exercise is inadequate to obtain results. Aerobic activity in FM is best accomplished by moving the large muscle groups of the legs and hips, with lesser involvement of the upper extremities. The program should avoid repetitive movements by alternating limbs, building in rest periods that are individualized by the participant, and changing movement patterns frequently. These recommendations are difficult for instructors who use "add-on" routines in which patients learn eight-count dance-type moves, adding more complexity and a greater number of patterns. People who have FM often report difficulty in remembering complex movement patterns, which is perhaps partially attributable to documented cognitive difficulties. Effective exercise can be done on land or in the water individually or in a group. The type of exercise is largely determined by patient preference and access to group classes and warm-water pools. Pool exercise classes should not be confused with swimming. Swimming may induce a flare if done too aggressively because it is an intense upper body exercise that relies heavily on eccentric strokes.

Walking is well supported in the aerobic literature and in the FM literature. It is touted as having the greatest chance of becoming a maintained exercise program.[72–74] In addition to aerobic fitness, walking promotes core strength, and thereby may reduce back pain. When walking, encourage small steps on flat even surfaces, minimize eccentric muscle work, and reduce the risks for falling. Adding ankle or wrist weights to a walking routine is not recommended in FM because aerobic gains are made largely by maximizing the use of large muscles, such as the hips and thighs. Additionally, ankle weights may contribute to falls.

Recognize the Importance of Restorative Sleep

It is important to evaluate and treat patients for obstructive sleep apnea and restless legs syndrome, which are more common in FM.[75,76] People who have FM generally report sleep problems (difficulty in falling asleep, difficulty in staying asleep, or nonrefreshing sleep). Minimal time in stage 3 and 4 sleep, alpha intrusion into delta sleep, and reduced sleep efficiency are well documented in sleep studies of patients who have FM.[77,78] In fact, minimal time in stage 3 and 4 sleep may be responsible, in part, for a disordered hypothalamic pituitary GH axis because 80% of GH is made during deep sleep. This dysfunction manifests itself as low insulin-like GH levels in at least 30% of persons who have FM and low GH secretion in response to acute exercise in 90% of persons who have FM.[79] GH in adults has the critical function in adulthood of repairing muscle microtrauma after activity. A combination of medications and sleep hygiene generally improves sleep quality, fatigue, and ability to exercise. A provider who finds it uncomfortable to prescribe long-term sleep medications may find it beneficial to refer sleep management to a sleep specialist, psychiatrist, or psychiatric mental health nurse practitioner.

The exercise modification may be to choose a class that takes place during the patient's optimal hours of function (often 10:00 AM to 3:00 PM) rather than at the end of the day. Additionally, many patients report an increased ability to tolerate exercise after a short nap. Dysfunctional breathing patterns are common in persons with chronic sleep deprivation and pain postures. In appreciation of this, the instructor should spend ample time in warm-up and cool-down and in breathing practices at the beginning and end of class. Common unhealthy breathing practices include reverse breathing, chest breathing, collapsed breathing, or frozen or shallow breathing. Correcting these patterns in class provides patients with a skill set they can apply throughout their day.

Screen for and Treat Autonomic Dysfunction

Autonomic dysfunction is widely recognized as another component of FM. In particular, this can manifest as severe fatigue, near-syncopal episodes, orthostatic hypotension, and chronic low blood pressure.[80] The clinician can screen for neurally mediated hypotension and postural orthostatic tachycardia syndrome, ordering a tilt table test when appropriate. If persistent low blood pressure is an issue, consider suggesting that patients drink dilute salt water (1 tsp/gal) and wear compression stockings. In severe cases, prescription of fludrocortisone may be necessary to allow patients to tolerate exercise.[81] The exercise instructor should know if patients are taking medications that may worsen orthostatic hypotension or be associated with dizziness. In FM, these medications may include most antihypertensives, tricyclic antidepressants, dopamine agonists, and trazodone.

The exercise modification for autonomic dysfunction includes avoiding prolonged motionless standing. Many patients prefer to exercise from a chair. Transitions from lying to standing positions during exercise should be slow, often taking up to 60 seconds. Finally, instructors should avoid movements that require pivots or fast turns. Temperature dysregulation associated with dysautonomia may be bypassed by dressing in layers for exercise.

Evaluate for Poor Balance and Risks for Falling

People who have FM often have poor balance and are more prone to falls and accidents.[82] Balance has been shown to improve with exercise training in FM.[42,82] Referral to a physical therapist may be beneficial in patients with poor balance. These professionals can teach patients to use lightweight aluminum canes, even during exercise. The canes can be adjusted up or down a notch each day. The patient should also learn to alternate arms when using a cane. Both of these techniques reduce shoulder girdle stress and resultant regional pain.

The exercise instructor can design routines with movements near a wall or with a partner to promote stabilization. Multitasking during exercise and rapid turning should be reduced to decrease the risks for falling. Gentle exercises in bare feet may increase kinesthetic awareness, thereby promoting balance. With regard to exercise equipment for which wearing supportive shoes is a must, a larger treadmill with a color difference between the moving treadmill and the side bar may minimize falls.

Modify Exercise for Common Comorbidities (Central Sensitivity Syndromes)

The provider should look for common comorbidities, such as irritable bowel syndrome, overactive bladder, chronic headaches, and pelvic pain syndromes, that accompany FM.[83] Along with maximizing medical management of these conditions, exercise can be modified for common comorbidities. For irritable bowel or bladder, choose an exercise room within easy access of a restroom. If exercising at home, consider walking around the block several times rather than walking a mile away from the house and a mile back to maintain proximity to a bathroom. For pelvic pain syndromes, such as endometriosis, vulvodynia, and vulvar vestibulitis, patients should avoid jarring or pounding standing exercises, such as jumping jacks. They can use a reclined exercise bike rather than an upright exercise bike and can use a pillow or donut during seated exercises. For chronic headaches, the instructor can institute the exercise studio as a "fragrance-free zone," use a lower volume setting for music, and avoid glaring or flashing lighting. Patients can also wear silicone ear plugs if they find that noise precipitates a headache.

Address Obesity and Deconditioning

The FM patient population is experiencing a steep increase in body mass index, much like the general US population. Obese patients who have FM may face additional challenges when trying to maintain therapeutic exercise and can feel self-conscious about participating in group exercise classes. Provider discussions about obesity should focus on functional improvements rather than body image. It can be helpful to refer a patient to a dietician. If insurance does not cover a visit to a registered dietician, the provider can write a prescription for dietary counseling for obesity and FM, which may be reimbursable through a flexible health care spending account. To ease obese patient concerns about group exercise classes, avoid body image discussion during exercise. Mirrors can be covered, or classes can be oriented away from mirrors. When teaching positions, the instructor should allow for added abdominal girth, instructing patients to separate their knees during seated positions or selected resting positions (eg, child's pose in yoga).

Aerobic and muscular deconditioning is common in FM regardless of body mass index. Both are essential to maintaining functional independence. Furthermore, muscle function in FM is retrainable. Multiple studies have demonstrated strength gains in people who have FM that mirror strength gains seen in healthy controls.[54,56,57] Maintaining strength and aerobic conditioning is thus an essential and realistic component of the exercise prescription. The critical element is understanding the limits of traditional aerobic and strength training, given demonstrated deconditioning and the flare-inducing potential of muscle microtrauma. Patients should be encouraged to increase the exercise intensity by approximately 10% only after the subject feels comfortable for 2 or more weeks at the previous level.

Conserve Energy in Daily Life to Exercise

Unlike the standard exercise recommendations from the surgeon general to increase lifestyle activity (eg, take the stairs instead of the elevator, use manual garage door openers, park farther away), this type of activity has not been shown to be effective in FM. Fontaine and Haaz[39] tested increasing lifestyle activity, such as walking, housework, and yard work by 70%, as assessed by a pedometer, and found that it did not demonstrate statistical significance in FM symptoms and 6-minute walk times compared with an FM education control group. Nevertheless, patients who have FM and are more fit may be able to increase ADLs as recommended by other FM exercise experts.[84] For patients who have been sedentary for longer than 3 months, the authors recommend a fatigue reduction program that allows patients to save their energy for an actual exercise session. For example, in daily life, patients can conserve energy in nonexercise activities (eg, sit in the shower; consider a hairstyle that does not require a morning shower, overhead blow drying, or styling). The ultimate goal of exercise in FM is not elite athletic fitness but a gradual move toward functional independence and fitness. A more fit body allows patients to move through their ADLs without inducing a symptom flare. As aerobic conditioning improves, multiple physiologic adaptations occur that allow the body to work more efficiently without fatiguing. As strength and flexibility return, taut muscle bands are released, creating longer and more supple muscles that are less likely to pull the body into "pain postures" and dysfunctional breathing patterns.[85] Physical therapists, occupational therapists, social workers, psychiatric mental health nurse practitioners, and psychologists are excellent resources in helping patients learn to balance rest with exercise.

Promote Self-efficacy

The final principle, self-efficacy, can be applied in each of the previous nine principles. Self-efficacy involves having, or gaining, the confidence that one can complete a task, such as regular participation in exercise (efficacy expectation). The second critical component is believing that completing a task results in a desired effect, such as fitness or symptom control (efficacy outcome). There are four major ways to promote self-efficacy.[86]

Mastery

Design an exercise program that is realistic and achievable for people who have FM. Most patients who have FM have had the experience of exercising too aggressively and ending up with a symptom flare. Mastery is enhanced by a "start low, go slow" exercise philosophy that is progressive and encourages people to recognize and celebrate their success.

Modeling

Encourage group exercise. Supervised group-based exercise has better adherence in the literature than home-based programs. Invite patients to watch exercise class even if they have no intention of exercising. Often, after weeks of seeing others who have FM being successful, they may be willing to try exercise as well.

Verbal persuasion

Tell your patients that you are confident they are going to be successful in their attempt to exercise. A technique to enhance verbal persuasion is to ask the patient about a time in his or her life when he or she felt successful. Patients may volunteer benchmarks, such as graduation, landing a dream job, marriage, or parenting. The clinician can take this opportunity to suggest to the patient that because past success is a potent predictor of future success, he or she is confident that the patient is going to be successful in his or her exercise attempts. Another verbal persuasion technique is to provide assurance that exercise, appropriately tailored to FM, does not result in permanent muscle or joint damage.[87]

Symptom reduction

Patients may say "I've tried all types of exercise, but always end up in a flare. I just can't do it." It is also understandable that the body's natural response to pain is to be still and guard painful areas. In fact, bed rest was once the treatment for chronic pain. A patient may need to be coached to exercise in a gradually progressive manner. He or she may enhance self-efficacy by noting an improvement in symptoms, particularly stiffness, mood, fatigue, sleep, and physical functioning. Ultimately, improvements in all these areas translate to an overall improvement in quality of life.

SUMMARY

In summary, the FM literature supports the notion that tailored exercise reduces symptoms and improves fitness. A therapeutic alliance between the provider and patient is enhanced if both understand the potential physiologic obstacles to exercise and the top 10 principles for prescribing exercise in FM. Such an alliance increases the likelihood of the patient successfully integrating life-long exercise into his or her comprehensive FM treatment plan.

ACKNOWLEDGMENTS

The authors thank Dr. Robert M. Bennett for his thoughtful critique of this manuscript.

REFERENCES

1. Pratt M, Macera CA, Blanton C. Levels of physical activity and inactivity in children and adults in the US: roundtable consensus statement. Medicine & Science in Sports and Exercise 1999;31(11):S526.
2. Rutledge DN, Jones K, Jones CJ. Predicting high physical function in people with fibromyalgia. J Nurs Scholarsh 2007;39(4):319–24.
3. Shillam CR, Jones KD, Miller L, et al. Physical function in fibromyalgia patients over 50 years of age: influence of symptoms, age and comorbidities. Arthritis Rheum 2009;58(Suppl 9):1408.
4. Kadetoff D, Kosek E. The effects of static muscular contraction on blood pressure, heart rate, pain ratings and pressure pain thresholds in healthy individuals and patients with fibromyalgia. Eur J Pain 2006;11(1):39–47.
5. Elvin A, Siosteen AK, Nilsson A, et al. Decreased muscle blood flow in fibromyalgia patients during standardised muscle exercise: a contrast media enhanced colour Doppler study. Eur J Pain 2006;10(2):137–44.
6. Klemp P, Nielsen HV, Korsgard J, et al. Blood-flow in fibromyotic muscles. Scand J Rehabil Med 1982;14(2):81–2.
7. Bennett RM. Muscle physiology and cold reactivity in the fibromyalgia syndrome. Rheum Dis Clin North Am 1989;15(1):135–47.
8. McIver KL, Evans C, Kraus RM, et al. NO-mediated alterations in skeletal muscle nutritive blood flow and lactate metabolism in fibromyalgia. Pain 2006;120(1–2):161–9.
9. Goldfarb AH, Jamurtas AZ. Beta-endorphin response to exercise. An update. Sports Med 1997;24(1):8–16.
10. Carrasco L, Villaverde C, Oltras CM. Endorphin responses to stress induced by competitive swimming event. J Sports Med Phys Fitness 2007;47(2):239–45.
11. Giske L, Vollestad NK, Mengshoel AM, et al. Attenuated adrenergic responses to exercise in women with fibromyalgia—a controlled study. Eur J Pain 2008;12(3):351–60.
12. Charmandari E, Tsigos C, Chrousos G. Endocrinology of the stress response. Annu Rev Physiol 2005;67:259–84.
13. Harris RE, Clauw DJ, Scott DJ, et al. Decreased central mu-opioid receptor availability in fibromyalgia. J Neurosci 2007;27(37):10000–6.
14. Mense S. Neurobiological concepts of fibromyalgia—the possible role of descending spinal tracts. Scand J Rheumatol Suppl 2000;113:24–9.
15. Staud R, Robinson ME, Price DD. Isometric exercise has opposite effects on central pain mechanisms in fibromyalgia patients compared to normal controls. Pain 2005;118(1–2):176–84.
16. Jones KD, Hugos C, Bhat SS, et al. Can clinicians predict neurally mediated hypotension and postural orthostatic tachycardia syndrome in fibromyalgia patients [abstract]. Arthritis Rheum 2007;56(Suppl 9):125.
17. Staud R. Autonomic dysfunction in fibromyalgia syndrome: postural orthostatic tachycardia. Curr Rheumatol Rep 2008;10(6):463–6.
18. Crofford LJ, Young EA, Engleberg NC, et al. Basal circadian and pulsatile ACTH and cortisol secretion in patients with fibromyalgia and/or chronic fatigue syndrome. Brain Behav Immun 2004;18(4):314–25.
19. Ross R, Jones KD, Wood L, et al. Cytokine perturbations correlate with absent growth hormone response in exercising fibromyalgia subjects [abstract]. Arthritis Rheum 2009;58(Suppl 9).
20. Jones KD, Deodhar AA, Burckhardt CS, et al. A combination of 6 months of treatment with pyridostigmine and triweekly exercise fails to improve insulin-like

growth factor-I levels in fibromyalgia, despite improvement in the acute growth hormone response to exercise. J Rheumatol 2007;34(5):1103–11.

21. Bennett R. Growth hormone in musculoskeletal pain states. Curr Rheumatol Rep 2004;6(4):266–73.

22. Suzuki K, Nakaji S, Yamada M, et al. Systemic inflammatory response to exhaustive exercise. Cytokine kinetics. Exerc Immunol Rev 2002;8:6–48.

23. Dantzer R, Kelley KW. Twenty years of research on cytokine-induced sickness behavior. Brain Behav Immun 2007;21(2):153–60.

24. Moldofsky H, Scarisbrick P. Induction of neurasthenic musculoskeletal pain syndrome by selective sleep stage deprivation. Psychosom Med 1976;38(1): 35–44.

25. Jones KD, Adams D, Winters-Stone K, et al. A comprehensive review of 46 exercise treatment studies in fibromyalgia (1988–2005) [abstract]. Health Qual Life Outcomes 2006;4:67.

26. Busch AJ, Barber KA, Overend TJ, et al. Exercise for treating fibromyalgia syndrome. Cochrane Database Syst Rev 2007;(4):CD003786.

27. Brosseau L, Wells GA, Tugwell P, et al. Ottawa Panel evidence-based clinical practice guidelines for aerobic fitness exercises in the management of fibromyalgia: part 1. Phys Ther 2008;88(7):857–71.

28. Brosseau L, Wells GA, Tugwell P, et al. Ottawa Panel evidence-based clinical practice guidelines for strengthening exercises in the management of fibromyalgia: part 2. Phys Ther 2008;88(7):873–86.

29. Gowans SE, deHueck A. Pool exercise for individuals with fibromyalgia. Curr Opin Rheumatol 2007;19(2):168–73.

30. Kingsley JD, Panton LB, Toole T, et al. The effects of a 12-week strength-training program on strength and functionality in women with fibromyalgia. Arch Phys Med Rehabil 2005;86(9):1713–21.

31. Nørregaard J, Lykkegaard J, Mehlsen J, et al. Exercise training in treatment of fibromyalgia. J Muscoskel Pain 1997;5(1):71–9.

32. van Santen M, Bolwijn P, Landewe R, et al. High or low intensity aerobic fitness training in fibromyalgia: does it matter? J Rheumatol 2002;29(3):582–7.

33. Jones KD, Burckhardt CS, Clark SR, et al. A randomized controlled trial of muscle strengthening versus flexibility training in fibromyalgia. J Rheumatol 2002;29(5): 1041–8.

34. Alentorn-Geli E, Padilla J, Moras G, et al. Six weeks of whole-body vibration exercise improves pain and fatigue in women with fibromyalgia. J Altern Complement Med 2008;14(8):975–81.

35. da Silva GD, Lorenzi-Filho G, Lage LV. Effects of yoga and the addition of Tui Na in patients with fibromyalgia. J Altern Complement Med 2007;13(10):1107–13.

36. de Andrade SC, de Carvalho RF, Soares AS, et al. Thalassotherapy for fibromyalgia: a randomized controlled trial comparing aquatic exercises in sea water and water pool. Rheumatol Int 2008;29(2):147–52.

37. Evcik D, Yigit I, Pusak H, et al. Effectiveness of aquatic therapy in the treatment of fibromyalgia syndrome: a randomized controlled open study. Rheumatol Int 2008; 28(9):885–90.

38. Figueroa A, Kingsley JD, McMillan V, et al. Resistance exercise training improves heart rate variability in women with fibromyalgia. Clin Physiol Funct Imaging 2008; 28(1):49–54.

39. Fontaine K, Haaz S. Effects of lifestyle physical activity on health status, pain, and function in adults with fibromyalgia syndrome. J Muscoskel Pain 2007; 15(1):3–9.

40. Gusi N, Tomas-Carus P. Cost-utility of an 8-month aquatic training for women with fibromyalgia: a randomized controlled trial [abstract]. Arthritis Res Ther 2008; 10(1):R24.
41. Haak T, Scott B. The effect of Qigong on fibromyalgia (FMS): a controlled randomized study. Disabil Rehabil 2008;30(8):625–33.
42. Jones KD, Burckhardt CS, Deodhar AA, et al. A six-month randomized controlled trial of exercise and pyridostigmine in the treatment of fibromyalgia. Arthritis Rheum 2008;58(2):612–22.
43. Kayo A, Sanches C, Montegro-Rodrigues R, et al. Effectiveness of physical exercise on decrease of pain in patients with fibromyalgia [abstract]. Arthritis Rheum 2007;56(9S):532.
44. Mannerkorpi K, Nordeman L, Ericsson A, et al. Pool exercise produces therapeutic effects in patients with fibromyalgia or chronic widespread pain. J Rehabil Med, in press.
45. Matsutani LA, Marques AP, Ferreira EA, et al. Effectiveness of muscle stretching exercises with and without laser therapy at tender points for patients with fibromyalgia. Clin Exp Rheumatol 2007;25(3):410–5.
46. Munguia-Izquierdo D, Legaz-Arrese A. Assessment of the effects of aquatic therapy on global symptomatology in patients with fibromyalgia syndrome: a randomized controlled trial. Arch Phys Med Rehabil 2008;89(12):2250–7.
47. Rooks DS, Gautam S, Romeling M, et al. Group exercise, education, and combination self-management in women with fibromyalgia: a randomized trial. Arch Intern Med 2007;167(20):2192–200.
48. Stephens S, Feldman BM, Bradley N, et al. Feasibility and effectiveness of an aerobic exercise program in children with fibromyalgia: results of a randomized controlled pilot trial. Arthritis Rheum 2008;59(10):1399–406.
49. Tomas-Carus P, Hakkinen A, Gusi N, et al. Aquatic training and detraining on fitness and quality of life in fibromyalgia. Med Sci Sports Exerc 2007;39(7): 1044–50.
50. Tomas-Carus P, Gusi N, Hakkinen A, et al. Eight months of physical training in warm water improves physical and mental health in women with fibromyalgia: a randomized controlled trial. J Rehabil Med 2008;40(4):248–52.
51. Valkeinen H, Alen M, Hakkinen A, et al. Effects of concurrent strength and endurance training on physical fitness and symptoms in postmenopausal women with fibromyalgia: a randomized controlled trial. Arch Phys Med Rehabil 2008;89(9): 1660–6.
52. Glass J, Jones KD, Bennett RM. Cognitive function in fibromyalgia patients correlates with mood and physical symptoms but is not improved by exercise or pyridostigmine. Arthritis Rheum 2006;54(Suppl 9):829.
53. Bircan C, Karasel SA, Akgun B, et al. Effects of muscle strengthening versus aerobic exercise program in fibromyalgia. Rheumatol Int 2008;28(6):527–32.
54. Hakkinen K, Pakarinen A, Hannonen P, et al. Effects of strength training on muscle strength, cross-sectional area, maximal electromyographic activity, and serum hormones in premenopausal women with fibromyalgia. J Rheumatol 2002;29(6):1287–95.
55. Hannonen P, Rahkita P, Kallinen M, et al. Effects of prolonged vs muscle strengthen programs on fibromyalgia [abstract]. J Muscoskel Pain 1995; 70((Suppl 1):34.
56. Valkeinen H, Hakkinen K, Pakarinen A, et al. Muscle hypertrophy, strength development, and serum hormones during strength training in elderly women with fibromyalgia. Scand J Rheumatol 2005;34(4):309–14.

57. Valkeinen H, Hakkinen A, Hannonen P, et al. Acute heavy-resistance exercise-induced pain and neuromuscular fatigue in elderly women with fibromyalgia and in healthy controls: effects of strength training. Arthritis Rheum 2006;54(4): 1334–9.

58. Goldenberg DL, Burckhardt C, Crofford L. Management of fibromyalgia syndrome. JAMA 2004;292(19):2388–95.

59. Martin L, Nutting A, MacIntosh BR, et al. An exercise program in the treatment of fibromyalgia. J Rheumatol 1996;23(6):1050–3.

60. McCain GA, Bell DA, Mai FM, et al. A controlled study of the effects of a supervised cardiovascular fitness training program on the manifestations of primary fibromyalgia. Arthritis Rheum 1988;31(9):1135–41.

61. Richards SC, Scott DL. Prescribed exercise in people with fibromyalgia: parallel group randomised controlled trial. BMJ 2002;325(7357):185.

62. Valim V, Oliveira L, Suda A, et al. Aerobic fitness effects in fibromyalgia. J Rheumatol 2003;30(5):1060–9.

63. Astin JA, Berman BM, Bausell B, et al. The efficacy of mindfulness meditation plus Qigong movement therapy in the treatment of fibromyalgia: a randomized controlled trial. J Rheumatol 2003;30(10):2257–62.

64. Chen KW, Hassett AL, Hou F, et al. A pilot study of external Qigong therapy for patients with fibromyalgia. J Altern Complement Med 2006;12(9):851–6.

65. Creamer P, Singh BB, Hochberg MC, et al. Sustained improvement produced by nonpharmacologic intervention in fibromyalgia: results of a pilot study. Arthritis Care Res 2000;13(4):198–204.

66. Taggart HM, Arslanian CL, Bae S, et al. Effects of T'ai Chi exercise on fibromyalgia symptoms and health-related quality of life. Orthop Nurs 2003;22(5):353–60.

67. Jones KD, Clark SR. Individualizing the exercise prescription for persons with fibromyalgia. Rheum Dis Clin North Am 2002;28(2):419–36.

68. Jones KD, Adams DG, Hoffman JH. Exercise and fibromyalgia. In: Silver J, Morin C, editors. Understanding fitness: how exercise fuels health and fights disease. Westport (CT): Greenwood; 2008. p. 170–81.

69. Kim SH, Kim DH, Oh DH, et al. Characteristic electron microscopic findings in the skin of patients with fibromyalgia—preliminary study. Clin Rheumatol 2008;27(3): 407–11.

70. Gibson W, Arendt-Nielsen L, Graven-Nielsen T. Delayed onset muscle soreness at tendon-bone junction and muscle tissue is associated with facilitated referred pain. Exp Brain Res 2006;174(2):351–60.

71. Elert JE, Rantapaa Dahlqvist SB, Henriksson-Larsen K, et al. Increased EMG activity during short pauses in patients with primary fibromyalgia. Scand J Rheumatol 1989;18(5):321–3.

72. Wennemer HK, Borg-Stein J, Gomba L, et al. Functionally oriented rehabilitation program for patients with fibromyalgia: preliminary results. Am J Phys Med Rehabil 2006;85(8):659–66.

73. Karmisholt K, Gotzsche PC. Physical activity for secondary prevention of disease. Systematic reviews of randomised clinical trials. Dan Med Bull 2005;52(2):90–4.

74. Mannerkorpi K. Exercise in fibromyalgia. Curr Opin Rheumatol 2005;17(2):190–4.

75. Al Alawi A, Mulgrew A, Tench E, et al. Prevalence, risk factors and impact on daytime sleepiness and hypertension of periodic leg movements with arousals in patients with obstructive sleep apnea. J Clin Sleep Med 2006;2(3):281–7.

76. Germanowicz D, Lumertz MS, Martinez D, et al. Sleep disordered breathing concomitant with fibromyalgia syndrome. J Bras Pneumol 2006;32(4):333–8.

77. Moldofsky H. Sleep and pain. Sleep Med Rev 2001;5(5):385–96.

78. Moldofsky H. Management of sleep disorders in fibromyalgia. Rheum Dis Clin North Am 2002;28(2):353–65.
79. Jones KD, Deodhar P, Lorentzen A, et al. Growth hormone perturbations in fibromyalgia: a review. Semin Arthritis Rheum 2007;36(6):357–79.
80. Martinez-Lavin M, Hermosillo AG, Rosas M, et al. Circadian studies of autonomic nervous balance in patients with fibromyalgia: a heart rate variability analysis. Arthritis Rheum 1998;41(11):1966–71.
81. Martinez-Lavin M. Management of dysautonomia in fibromyalgia. Rheum Dis Clin North Am 2002;28(2):379–87.
82. Jones KD, Horak FB, Winters-Stone K, et al. Fibromyalgia is associated with impaired balance and falls. J Clin Rheumatol 2008;15(1):16–21.
83. Yunus MB. Central sensitivity syndromes: a new paradigm and group nosology for fibromyalgia and overlapping conditions, and the related issue of disease versus illness. Semin Arthritis Rheum 2008;37(6):339–52.
84. Rooks DS. Talking to patients with fibromyalgia about physical activity and exercise. Curr Opin Rheumatol 2008;20(2):208–12.
85. Wilhelm FH, Gevirtz R, Roth WT. Respiratory dysregulation in anxiety, functional cardiac, and pain disorders. Assessment, phenomenology, and treatment. Behav Modif 2001;25(4):513–45.
86. Bandura A. Self-efficacy: toward a unifying theory of behavioral change. Psychol Rev 1977;84(2):191–215.
87. Jones KD, Burckhardt CS, Bennett JA. Motivational interviewing may encourage exercise in persons with fibromyalgia by enhancing self efficacy. Arthritis Rheum 2004;51(5):864–7.

Nonpharmacologic Treatment for Fibromyalgia: Patient Education, Cognitive-Behavioral Therapy, Relaxation Techniques, and Complementary and Alternative Medicine

Afton L. Hassett, PsyD[a],*, Richard N. Gevirtz, PhD[b]

KEYWORDS

- Fibromyalgia • Cognitive-behavioral • Relaxation • Biofeedback
- Complementary and alternative medicine • Treatment

Treating patients who have chronic pain conditions has long held challenges and been rife with pitfalls for health care professionals. Pain is a complex and dynamic phenomenon influenced by genetic, physiologic, cognitive, affective, behavioral, and social factors. Melzack and Wall's gate-control theory revolutionized the understanding of and treatment for chronic pain.[1] Central to this theory is the existence of a gating system at the dorsal horn of the spinal cord that can control pain transmission from the periphery to the somatosensory cortices in the brain. The gating of pain signals is thought to be controlled by peripheral input and the neural centers that govern thoughts, emotions, and behaviors.[1] The gate-control theory explains why certain

---

This work was supported by grant P20-MH-074634, "MUPS in Primary Care Research Center," from the National Institutes of Health.

[a] Department of Medicine, Division of Rheumatology, University of Medicine and Dentistry of New Jersey–Robert Wood Johnson Medical School, 1 Robert Wood Johnson Place, MEB484, New Brunswick, NJ 08903–0019, USA

[b] California School of Professional Psychology, Alliant International University, 104 Daley Hall, 10455 Pomerado Road, San Diego, CA 92131, USA

* Corresponding author.

E-mail address: a.hassett@umdnj.edu (A.L. Hassett).

factors, such as depression and anxiety, worsen the experience of pain, whereas other factors, such as active coping, positive affect, and social support, moderate the experience of pain.[2]

Factors resulting from living with chronic pain (eg, poor sleep, reduced physical activity, social withdrawal) are the same factors that put one at risk for even greater physical pain. Patients who have fibromyalgia (FM) bear the additional burden of battling long-held misconceptions that FM is a psychiatric illness. As with most chronic pain conditions, comorbid mood and anxiety disorders commonly occur in FM (29% and 27%,[3] respectively). Further, a lifetime diagnosis of a major mood disorder has been observed in as many as 74% of patients who have FM.[4] Thus, psychiatric comorbidity and a lack of objective evidence of disease have led to the belief that FM is a somatization disorder that is psychiatric in nature and a "fashionable" expression of psychologic distress.[5] In the past decade, however, innovative research inspired by advances in the neuroscience of pain has greatly contributed to our understanding of the pathophysiology of FM. For example, altered pain processing in FM has been demonstrated in functional MRI studies,[6,7] whereas other studies have identified a deficiency in an important central analgesic system resulting in diminished diffuse noxious inhibitory control.[8] This knowledge has resulted in new ways of conceptualizing FM and its treatment.

Medications that target modifying pain centrally have shown some efficacy and have been approved by the US Food and Drug Administration (FDA) specifically for the treatment of FM pain. Like most rheumatologic conditions, however, FM is symptomatically heterogeneous, thus rendering a single pharmacologic approach for all patients inadequate. Patients who have FM vary significantly in the type and severity of symptoms experienced, the presence of medical and psychiatric comorbidities, and a range of human factors (eg, genetic, cognitive, behavioral, social); each factor influences the experience of pain and treatment outcomes. It is because of the complexity of pain and heterogeneity of patients who have FM that treating FM using a multidisciplinary approach[9–12] and considering the particular needs of patient subgroups[13–15] are frequently recommended.

A multidisciplinary approach has been found to provide superior outcomes when compared with monotherapy.[16] At the heart of this approach is taking into account the unique characteristics of each patient and adding adjunctive nonpharmacologic interventions to evidence-based use of medication. The importance of including exercise in the treatment of FM has been substantiated in several studies, as reviewed by authors of articles elsewhere in this issue. In addition to exercise, patient education, cognitive-behavioral therapy (CBT), relaxation, biofeedback, and other complementary and alternative medicine (CAM) approaches are gaining empiric support and should be considered. Herein, the authors briefly present an overview of these techniques and the evidence for their inclusion as fundamental elements of FM treatment.

EDUCATIONAL APPROACHES

Most experts agree that an educational or psychoeducational treatment component is useful if not necessary when treating FM.[10] Such educational programs target increasing understanding of the complex nature of the interactions among neurobiologic processes, behaviors like sleep or activity levels, and symptoms. These programs have varied foci but usually try to allay the stigma often attached to FM and similar disorders. Goldenberg[11] has recently set out recommendations regarding education that seem well founded. He points out that "When educating patients, a core set of information should be provided that includes a detailed discussion of potential pathophysiological mechanisms in the context of the biopsychological model. The clinician must dispel the notion that the absence of organic disease means that the symptoms are psychogenic".[11] Some clinicians have expressed concern that the labeling of FM in itself might worsen symptoms. The one prospective study on this topic found that the diagnosis had no adverse effects, however, and may have actually improved function over 18 months.[17] Thus, careful education seems warranted.

Yet, only limited data are available to support this contention. Beyond several studies that failed to find superiority for other interventions when compared with an educational control group,[18,19] only two well-controlled trials have been reported. Burckhardt and colleagues[20] assigned patients who had FM to an education-only condition, an education plus physical training condition, or a delayed treatment wait list control. Both active treatment groups improved on subjective ratings and reports of physical activity compared with controls. Burckhardt and colleagues[21] have published a review and treatment guide to the self-management of FM. More recently, Rooks and colleagues[22] completed a randomized controlled trial with 207 patients confirmed to have FM who were assigned to one of four groups: (1) an aerobic and flexibility exercise group; (2) a strength training, aerobic, and flexibility exercise group; (3) the Fibromyalgia Self-Help Course; or (4) a combination of the previous three groups. The primary outcome was change in physical function from baseline to completion of the intervention. Secondary outcomes included social and emotional function, symptoms, and self-efficacy. The combination group showed the greatest improvement. The education or self-management group did improve but significantly less than the groups that included physical training. Although more research is clearly needed, it seems that education is most effective in multimodal interventions.

COGNITIVE-BEHAVIORAL THERAPY

CBT combines interventions from cognitive and behavior therapies. Cognitive therapy is based on the premise that modifying maladaptive thoughts results in changes in affect and behavior.[23] Therefore, errors in thinking, such as overgeneralizing, magnifying negatives, minimizing positives, and catastrophizing, are challenged and replaced with more realistic and effective thoughts, thus decreasing emotional distress and self-defeating behavior. More specific to FM, catastrophizing, or the belief that the worst possible outcome is going to occur, has been associated with pain severity,[24–26] decreased functioning,[25] and affective distress.[25,26] In cognitive therapy, catastrophic thoughts, such as "My pain is awful and there is nothing I can do about it," are reframed to "As bad as my pain might get, there are things I can do to make it at least a little better."

In contrast to cognitive therapy, behavior therapy is rooted in the theory that inner states (thoughts and feelings) are less important than the use of operant behavior change techniques to increase adaptive behavior through positive and negative reinforcement and to extinguish maladaptive behavior by using punishment. In FM, several behavioral techniques are applicable, including behavioral activation (getting patients moving again), graded exercise (initiating exercise and then slowly increasing activities), activity pacing (not overdoing it on days when patients feel good and remaining active on days when they feel bad), reducing pain behaviors (not reinforcing behaviors associated with secondary gain), sleep hygiene (identifying and then changing behaviors known to disrupt sleep), and learning relaxation techniques to lower stress (eg, breathing, imagery, progressive muscle relaxation [PMR]).

Meta-analyses have shown that CBT has significant empiric support for its effectiveness in treating psychiatric illnesses like depression[27] and anxiety disorders,[27,28] which are common in FM. Thus, addressing psychiatric comorbidity alone provides a good rationale for adding CBT to usual medical treatment for a subgroup of patients who have FM[29]; however, CBT has also proved to be helpful for several medical conditions, including chronic pain.[30] A review of the CBT literature related to FM indicates that a multitude of interventions have been described to be "CBT"—some perhaps inappropriately so. All CBT interventions are not equal, with many including only modest elements of cognitive therapy and, instead, relying heavily on behavioral interventions.

Given the limitation that CBT is not a single discrete intervention akin to a single drug given at a particular dose, there is evidence suggesting that CBT may be an effective adjunctive treatment for some patients who have FM. Two initial open-pilot studies reported improvements in pain intensity[31] and the ability to control pain,[32] in addition to less emotional distress in patients who had FM.[32] A larger study with a wait list control (FM: n = 79, wait list: n = 49) reported improvements in pain, functioning, and emotional distress.[33] Two more studies using educational control groups found positive effects for CBT, but none of the effects were significantly greater than those of the control groups.[34,35]

Two more recent studies have yielded promising results. Williams and colleagues[36] randomly assigned 145 patients who had FM to 4 weeks of group CBT (six sessions) or standard medical care. Twenty-five percent of patients who had FM and were receiving CBT met criteria for being a "treatment responder" (ie, sustained improvement in functional status) compared with 12% of those receiving only standard medical care. Pain scores did not change significantly for either group, but patients considered to be "treatment failures" in the CBT group showed no worsening of symptoms or functional status, unlike the wait list controls, who demonstrated deterioration in energy and physical role functioning. These researchers surmised that although only a subgroup of patients responded to CBT, there could be buffering effects for many more patients.

In the most compelling study to date, Thieme and colleagues[37] randomly assigned 125 patients who had FM to CBT (n = 42), operant behavior therapy (OBT; n = 43), or an attention control group (n = 40). OBT consisted of behavioral interventions to reduce pain behaviors, whereas CBT addressed modifying maladaptive thoughts, problem solving, decreasing psychologic stress, pain-coping strategies, and relaxation. These researchers found that when compared with the attention control, CBT and OBT resulted in greater improvement in pain, decreased emotional distress, and improved physical functioning for up to 1 year after treatment.[37] Patients in both treatment groups also had fewer physician visits compared with those in the control group. Further, the effect sizes for improvement were large for CBT and OBT; however, for the most part, the differences between the two active treatments were not significant. They did observe that patients in the CBT group demonstrated sustained increases in coping and decreases in catastrophizing, likely contributing to persistent improvements in emotional distress. In fact, patients in the attention control group, which consisted of unstructured group discussion about FM, showed increases in catastrophizing and pain intensity 6 months after treatment.

Effective CBT interventions for FM are likely to target the modification of maladaptive thoughts and expectations, thus improving mood, perceived stress, pain coping, and problem solving, while including behavioral interventions that specifically address ameliorating FM symptoms (eg, sleep hygiene, relaxation training, activity pacing). In FM, the primary goal of CBT treatment is to increase self-management, which includes moving patients toward more adaptive beliefs regarding their ability to cope with and control pain and other symptoms, in addition to taking action to decrease FM symptoms and stress, resulting in increased functioning. Because the evidence for adding CBT to pharmacologic treatment for FM remains modest, more randomized controlled trials are needed. Further, only subgroups of patients who have FM may be likely to respond to CBT, such as those with greater emotional distress, fewer coping skills, or less social support[38] or those who believe at the outset that the treatment is going to be effective.[39] Future studies of CBT in FM should carefully explore individual factors associated with response to CBT, in addition to which specific elements of CBT are most highly associated with a positive response to treatment.

RELAXATION TECHNIQUES

There is substantial overlap between CBT and behavioral interventions. Most CBT includes one or more forms of behavioral relaxation, although some of these techniques have evidence for efficacy in the absence of a cognitive therapy component. Relaxation techniques likely to be helpful for FM symptoms include but are not limited to PMR, autogenic training, guided imagery, and meditation. Biofeedback can also be subsumed under this umbrella, but possessing multiple types and having been the recipient of more empiric attention, biofeedback is described at greater length in the following section.

Because psychologic distress and dysfunction of the stress response systems have been observed in subgroups of patients who have FM,[40] stress management has been a target of treatment. PMR[41] and autogenic training typically serve as the substrate of behavioral intervention for chronic pain.[42,43] This is true for FM, even though no randomized controlled trials have evaluated PMR in isolation and two trials of autogenic training failed to find superiority for it when compared with other treatment conditions.[44,45] Despite the lack of direct evidence, clinical experience, and the knowledge that both relaxation techniques are commonly part of CBT for FM,[36,46] their efficacy is generally accepted.

PMR involves the systematic tightening and relaxing of various muscle groups with the goal of decreasing muscle tension overall, and thus ameliorating anxiety, which was presumed to be linked to muscle tension.[41] In FM, PMR has the added benefit of emphasizing to the patient the difference between muscles that are tense and those that are relaxed, because many patients persistently tense their muscles unknowingly, which can contribute to their pain. One caveat is that patients who have FM should be cautioned not to tense their muscles too tightly during this exercise because this could result in exacerbating pain. In contrast, autogenic training involves repeating such phrases as "My arms are heavy and warm" and visualizing heaviness and warmth in the arms.[47] The exercise invokes images associated with a relaxed state while moving the focus from one body area to the next. Verifiable warming in the extremities is typically experienced,[48] which can be helpful for patients who have FM and frequently report cold intolerance and Raynaud's disease-like symptoms.[49] Some evidence for including PMR and autogenic training comes from a study by Allen and colleagues[46] that included patients who had FM among others with similar symptoms. These researchers reported that a manualized CBT protocol that included PMR and autogenic training as central aspects of treatment resulted in decreased symptom severity when compared with augmented medical care.

Autogenic training includes elements of guided imagery, but guided imagery alone that involves engaging all the senses in experiencing pleasant places or circumstances has proved to be helpful for some who have FM. Guided imagery enhances muscle relaxation and can serve as a powerful distraction from pain. In a randomized controlled trial of 55 women who had FM, it was found that those in the guided imagery arm (n = 17) had less pain compared with the control group.[50] In another study comparing a 6-week guided imagery intervention with treatment as usual, patients who had FM and were receiving guided imagery demonstrated improved functional status and reported a greater sense of self-efficacy for managing pain, although actual pain reports did not change.[51] A recent pilot study reported positive findings for the use of guided imagery specifically for Hispanic patients who have FM, noting significant improvements in symptoms, functioning, and self-efficacy for managing pain.[52] Finally, in a small open study of female juvenile patients who had FM, a combination of PMR and guided imagery was found to reduce pain and improve sleep in most patients,[53] illustrating the potential benefit of using these interventions in combination.

Meditation-based stress reduction can also take several forms, although "mindfulness" meditation is frequently used as an intervention for medical populations. In mindfulness meditation, the patient is directed to focus on one thing, an "anchor," be it a sound, visualizing a pleasant scene, or breathing. Thoughts are to remain present oriented, and analytic musings are to be avoided in favor of focusing on the meditation anchor. A few studies have examined the efficacy of meditation-based interventions in FM. In an early study of 77 patients who had FM and were enrolled in a meditation-based stress reduction program, Kaplan and colleagues[54] reported that the scores of all the patients completing the program improved and that 51% of completers had moderate to marked improvement. More recently, a randomized controlled trial comparing women who had FM and were assigned to an 8-week mindfulness meditation program (n = 51) with those in a wait list control group (n = 40) found that depressive symptoms improved significantly in the meditation group.[55] Taken together, there is some, albeit inconclusive, evidence that relaxation techniques can be effective adjunctive treatment for FM. Here too, randomized controlled trials using attention, educational, and active comparators are needed.

HEART RATE VARIABILITY BIOFEEDBACK

As has been discussed, it is becoming increasingly evident that FM is a complex systemic disorder with at least some central mediation of symptoms. An additional perspective has emerged that implicates the autonomic nervous system as pivotal to at least some subgroups of patients who have FM.[56–61] Martínez-Lavin has championed this approach, and with others, he has produced a substantial body of data.[56–61] There is reasonably good evidence that autonomic nervous system functioning in some patients who have FM can be characterized by elevated sympathetic tone, poor parasympathetic tone, and an abnormal 24-hour autonomic cycle.[56–61]

Based on this orientation, heart rate variability (HRV) biofeedback has emerged as a potentially useful treatment for FM. Pioneered by Lehrer, Vashillo, and Gevirtz,[62–65] this approach uses the discoveries made through the centuries by Yoga swamis and other eastern disciplines utilizing slow-breathing techniques coupled with mindful mental states or mantras (see previous section on meditation). Sensors detect beat-to-beat heart rate, HRV parameters, respiration wave forms, and finger temperature. This "feedback" is displayed on a computer monitor situated in front of the seated patient. Patients learn to produce a characteristic heart rate pattern (respiratory sinus arrhythmia) by breathing at a certain rate (eg, six breaths per minute), which, over time, becomes an extremely smooth exaggerated sine wave. HRV biofeedback has produced good results for asthma,[66] chronic obstructive pulmonary disease,[67] cardiac rehabilitation,[68] irritable bowel syndrome,[69] and hypertension.[70] Three studies to date have attempted to use HRV biofeedback in the treatment of FM.[71–73] In a small pilot study, Hassett and colleagues[71] treated 12 women over 10 sessions and found the HRV biofeedback group to improve in most FM symptom areas (sleep, pain, fatigue, depression, and overall functioning). Importantly, physiologic functions, such as HRV and blood pressure variability, improved over time as well. In a small controlled study with patients who had chronic fatigue, Stevens and colleagues[72] compared HRV biofeedback combined with sleep hygiene and activity management with a wait list control. The active treatment group showed improvements in fatigue and depression, whereas the controls declined or remained constant with regard to these symptoms. Recently, Hassett and colleagues[73] completed a randomized controlled trial comparing HRV biofeedback with a relaxation condition. Although the data have not yet been fully analyzed, preliminary analysis of the first 68 patients indicated that compared with the control, the patients in the HRV group experienced an increase in functioning from baseline to the final session. Although much more research is needed, HRV biofeedback training may offer promise because it targets a known physiologic component of FM and is therefore seen by the patient as an acceptable treatment in the authors' collective experience.

OTHER BIOFEEDBACK APPROACHES

Several studies exist using other biofeedback approaches. Buckelew and colleagues[74] conducted a randomized controlled trial comparing electromyogram (EMG) biofeedback (n = 29), exercise training (n = 30), combination treatment (biofeedback and exercise, n = 30), and an educational/attention control (n = 30). Compared with the control, they found that patients in the treatment groups showed improvements in self-efficacy for functioning and better tender point index scores. The treatment groups reflected equivalent benefit, although there was a slight deterioration within the control. More recently, an Indian study compared surface EMG biofeedback (n = 15) to a sham feedback condition (n = 15) with patients who had FM and found the active biofeedback to reduce tender points and subjective symptoms and to result in improvements on functioning and the 6-minute walk test.[75] In addition, several small open trials conducted in Europe found that patients who had FM and were receiving EMG biofeedback reported improvement in pain,[76,77] sleep disturbance,[76] and headache[76] and that they experienced persistent clinical benefit.[78] Nevertheless, there is one controlled trial in which patients assigned to a fitness program (n = 58) or surface EMG biofeedback-enhanced progressive relaxation protocol (n = 56) failed to show significant improvement compared with controls (n = 29).[79] One caveat, the lack of effectiveness for the fitness program, is not consistent with most other findings, raising questions about this particular sample. Despite this contrary result and the fact that it is difficult to analyze the methods used in many cases, the generally positive findings across controlled trials and small pilot studies suggest that EMG biofeedback may be a promising treatment for at least some patients who have FM. Finally, a small case study on three patients[80] used neurofeedback (EEG biofeedback) over 10 sessions and found that all patients reported decreased symptoms. Again, encouraging findings beg for more rigorous follow-up studies.

COMPLEMENTARY AND ALTERNATIVE MEDICINE INTERVENTIONS

Patients who have FM overwhelmingly have sought CAM interventions.[81] Yet, as is the case for so many disorders, little scientific evidence exists for the efficacy of such approaches. Furthermore, deciding which treatments fall into this category is a perilous endeavor; however, a few treatments have been investigated.

Manual Therapies

Massage is a widely used CAM therapy for patients who have FM, and based on patient survey data, it is the intervention with the highest satisfaction levels.[81] Only one study using a comparison or control was located.[82] Brattberg[82] compared connective tissue massage (n = 23) with a no-treatment control (n = 25) over 15 treatments. Pain, depression, use of analgesics, and quality of life were improved in the treatment group compared with the controls. Yet, the treatment effects dissipated over a 6-month follow-up period.

Like massage therapy, chiropractic treatments have become a popular modality for patients who have FM.[81] Despite its popularity, few randomized controlled trials have been done with patients who have FM using chiropractic modalities. In a recent review,[83] the investigators concluded "...Lastly, other CAM therapies have neither well-designed studies nor positive results and are not currently recommended for FMS treatment (chiropractic care)."

Qigong and T'ai Chi

The term *Qigong* generally describes several traditional Chinese therapies and exercises all believed to facilitate the flow of vital energy or "chi".[84] Astin and colleagues[85] conducted a randomized controlled trial in which they assigned 128 patients who had FM to an 8-week intervention that included a mind-body training group (mindfulness meditation and Qigong movement therapy) or an educational support group. Both groups registered statistically significant improvements across time for the Fibromyalgia Impact Questionnaire, total myalgic score, pain, and depression. There was no difference in the rate or magnitude of these changes between the mind-body training group and the education control group, however. Both groups maintained gains at the 6-month follow-up assessment. Mannerkorpi and Arndorw[86] conducted a similar controlled trial of Qigong movement therapy with similar results. It has been noted that both studies were hindered by the lack of Qigong practice, which is supposed to take place daily and with high intensity to generate sufficient "qi" flow.[84]

In a study using Qigong as a manual therapy,[84] 10 women who had FM received external Qigong therapy provided by a Chinese master over a 3-week period. Patients were then assessed after treatment and at 3 months. Improvements (with large effect sizes) were observed in pain, functioning, depression, and self-efficacy. No control was used for this pilot, but the magnitude of the symptom reductions warrant further investigation. Finally, one uncontrolled pilot study[87] evaluated the effect of 6 weeks of biweekly T'ai Chi sessions for 39 women who had FM. Although there was a high dropout rate, the group had significantly reduced symptoms and increased quality of life. These techniques offer some promise of efficacy, but all need more rigorous assessment to be considered in an evidence-based treatment mix.

Acupuncture

Mayhew and Ernst[88] recently reviewed the evidence concerning acupuncture and FM. They were able to find five studies that could be reviewed. The quality of the studies was rated as variable; quality of the studies as variable; however, independent of quality, they found mixed results. They asserted that none of the trials included adequate placebo conditions, weakening their scientific value, and concluded that acupuncture treatment was not supported by rigorous clinical trials, and thus could not be recommended for FM. Since this review, one randomized controlled trial was published. In it, 34 women who had FM and were receiving acupuncture plus tricyclic antidepressants and exercise were compared with 24 women receiving tricyclic antidepressants and exercise only (controls). After 20 sessions of treatment, Targino and colleagues[89] observed that the women in the acupuncture condition reported significantly decreased levels of pain and improved quality of life compared with the controls. The positive effects persisted for 3 months and then dissipated over the 2-year follow-up period. Finally, a randomized trial of acupuncture for 114 patients who had FM evaluated methodology related to acupuncture (correct needle placement and needle stimulation, which are presumed to be necessary to maximize effects).[90] Harris and colleagues[90] reported that although 25% to 35% of patients had a significant decrease in pain, correct needle placement and needle stimulation were not factors, suggesting the possibility of a strong placebo response.

Hydrotherapy

Several well-controlled studies do exist that evaluated the spa type bath therapies that have been used for centuries to ease pain. A recent review[91] found 10 studies of sufficient quality for review. Mean methodologic quality was 4.5 of 9 on the van Tulder scale. Positive outcomes were reported for pain, health status, and tender point count. There is good evidence for the use of hydrotherapy in the management of FM. Most studies were short term, and few used credible placebo conditions. It does seem, however, that the conventional wisdom that warm-water baths relieve pain in the short term is well founded.

Other Complementary and Alternative Medicine Modalities

Many other CAM modalities have been studied, especially various botanicals.[92] Sarac and Gur[93] have recently reviewed evidence for herbal and nutritional supplements, such as St. John's wort, ginseng, valerian, botanical oil, melatonin, magnesium, dehydroepiandrosterone, NADH, S-adenosylmethionine, growth hormone, chlorella pyrenoidosa, 5-hydroxytryptophan, and several dietary supplements. Many of these have shown promising results in early trials, but mixed results are increasingly common as the studies become methodologically more sophisticated. Additional work is needed to be able to know which, if any, of the many touted botanicals may be of lasting help for FM.

SUMMARY

The research, in addition to the clinical experience, indicates that the addition of education and a behavioral or cognitive-behavioral component to FM treatment protocols is warranted. Especially when combined with other modalities, such as exercise, sleep hygiene, or activity pacing, using some form of behavioral intervention seems to add to the efficacy of the treatment. An important caveat applies, however; it is important to avoid any suggestion that the symptoms are "all in your head" when recommending these treatments. It is easy to forget the stigmatizing aspects of any mental health diagnosis in our society. The authors have found that using a physiologically based label (eg, "biofeedback" or "stress management") greatly reduces the perception of the patient that he or she is being "dumped" to a "shrink." A recent informal study of one of the authors (RG) at a major military medical center indicated a strong preference for referrals for biofeedback versus CBT. Once the patient understands the nature of the "mind/body" interaction, further suggestions seem to be accepted without resistance.

For daily clinical practice, the authors suggest using the principles of comprehensive nonpharmacologic pain management represented by the acronym ExPRESS. Ex is for exercise, as described by Jones elsewhere in this issue. P is for psychiatric comorbidity, because depression and anxiety disorders are common in chronic pain conditions and contribute significantly to pain and disability. R is for regaining function; in FM, this often involves helping patients with activity pacing so that they do not do too much on days when they feel good and do too little on days when they feel bad. E is for education, in which simply informing a patient where on the Internet he or she can find reliable information can be a good start. The authors suggest referring patients to Web sites hosted by the Arthritis Foundation[94] and the National Fibromyalgia Association.[95] S is for sleep hygiene, which is necessary for many who have developed counterproductive habits. Finally, S is for stress management, which includes any number of elements, such as CBT, relaxation techniques, hydrotherapy, and gentle exercise to name just a few.

Taking a comprehensive multidisciplinary approach to the treatment of FM can be challenging for most health care professionals not practicing in academic settings. Fortunately, there are innovative tools available to assist them in providing care for FM or to enhance patients' self-management skills. One exceptional tool can be found on the Web.[96] Here, patients can complete a brief online questionnaire to receive an individualized series of self-help modules, which might consist of education, activity pacing, sleep hygiene, relaxation, and goal setting. Including evidenced-based non-pharmacologic treatment can be greatly facilitated by taking advantage of a resource such as this.

In conclusion, although there is some encouraging evidence for several nonpharma-cologic modalities like CBT, more controlled trials are needed, especially those that consider combinations of treatments. Further, intervention studies in FM should also explore individual factors to identify which patient subgroups would be the most likely to respond to which particular treatments.

ACKNOWLEDGMENTS

The authors are grateful for the administrative support of Shantal Savage and to the individuals who have FM and share their compelling stories in clinical practice and enthusiastically volunteer for the authors' studies.

REFERENCES

1. Melzack R, Wall PD. Pain mechanisms: a new theory. Science 1965;150(699): 971–9.
2. Keefe FJ, Somers TJ, Martire LM. Psychologic interventions and lifestyle modifications for arthritis pain management. Rheum Dis Clin North Am 2008;34:351–68.
3. Epstein SA, Kay G, Clauw D, et al. Psychiatric disorders in patients with fibromyalgia. A multicenter investigation. Psychosomatics 1999;40(1):57–63.
4. Arnold LM, Hudson JI, Keck PE, et al. Comorbidity of fibromyalgia and psychiatric disorders. J Clin Psychiatry 2006;67(8):1219–25.
5. Ford CV. Somatization and fashionable diagnoses: illness as a way of life. Scand J Work Environ Health 1997;23(Suppl 3):7–16.
6. Gracely RH, Petzke F, Wolf JM, et al. Functional magnetic resonance imaging evidence of augmented pain processing in fibromyalgia. Arthritis Rheum 2002; 46:1333–43.
7. Giesecke T, Gracely RH, Williams DA, et al. The relationship between depression, clinical pain, and experimental pain in a chronic pain cohort. Arthritis Rheum 2005;52:1577–84.
8. Julien N, Goffaux P, Arsenault P, et al. Widespread pain in fibromyalgia is related to a deficit of endogenous pain inhibition. Pain 2005;114:295–302.

9. Clauw DJ. Pharmacotherapy for patients with fibromyalgia. J Clin Psychiatry 2008;69(Suppl 2):25–9.
10. Carville SF, Arendt-Nielsen S, Bliddal H, et al. EULAR evidence-based recommendations for the management of fibromyalgia syndrome. Ann Rheum Dis 2008;67(4):536–41.
11. Goldenberg DL. Multidisciplinary modalities in the treatment of fibromyalgia. J Clin Psychiatry 2008;69(Suppl 2):30–4.
12. Mease P, Arnold LM, Bennett R, et al. Fibromyalgia syndrome. J Rheumatol 2007; 34(6):1415–25.
13. Thieme K, Spies C, Sinha P, et al. Predictors of pain behaviors in fibromyalgia syndrome. Arthritis Rheum 2005;53(3):343–50.
14. Giesecke T, Williams DA, Harris RE, et al. Subgrouping of fibromyalgia patients on the basis of pressure-pain thresholds and psychological factors. Arthritis Rheum 2003;48(10):2916–22.
15. Hassett AL, Simonelli LE, Radvanski DS, et al. The relationship between affect balance style and clinical outcomes in fibromyalgia. Arthritis Rheum 2008;59: 833–40.
16. Sarzi-Puttini P, Buskila D, Carrabba M, et al. Treatment strategy in fibromyalgia syndrome: where are we now? Semin Arthritis Rheum 2008;37(6):353–65.
17. White K, Nielson WR, Harth M, et al. Does the label "fibromyalgia" alter health status, function and health service utilization?: a prospective within-group comparison in a community cohort of adults with chronic widespread pain. Arthritis Rheum 2002;47:260–5.
18. Nicassio P, Bootzin R. A comparison of progressive relaxation and autogenic training as treatments for insomnia. J Abnorm Psychol 1974;83(3):253–60.
19. Goossens ME, Rutten-van Mölken MP, Leidl RM, et al. Cognitive-educational treatment of fibromyalgia: a randomized clinical trial. I. Clinical effects. J Rheumatol 1996;23(7):1237–45.
20. Burckhardt CS, Mannerkorpi K, Hedenberg L, et al. A randomized, controlled clinical trial of education and physical training for women with fibromyalgia. J Rheumatol 1994;21(4):714–20.
21. Burckhardt CS, Lorig K, Moncur C, et al. Arthritis and musculoskeletal patient education standards. Arthritis Foundation. Arthritis Care Res 1994;7(1):1–4.
22. Rooks DS, Gautam S, Romeling M, et al. Group exercise, education, and combination self-management in women with fibromyalgia: a randomized trial. Arch Intern Med 2007;167(20):2192–200.
23. Beck AT. Thinking and depression: theory and therapy. Arch Gen Psychiatry 1964;10:561–71.
24. Gracely RH, Geisser ME, Giesecke T, et al. Pain catastrophizing and neural responses to pain among persons with fibromyalgia. Brain 2004;127(Pt 4):835–43.
25. Edwards RR, Bingham CO III, Bathon J, et al. Catastrophizing and pain in arthritis, fibromyalgia, and other rheumatic diseases. Arthritis Rheum 2006; 55(2):325–32.
26. Hassett AL, Cone JC, Patella SJ, et al. The role of catastrophizing in the pain and depression of women with fibromyalgia syndrome. Arthritis Rheum 2000;43(11): 2493–500.
27. Butler AC, Chapman JE, Forman EM, et al. The empirical status of cognitive-behavioral therapy: a review of meta-analyses. Clin Psychol Rev 2006;26(1):17–31.
28. Hofmann SG, Smits JA. Cognitive-behavioral therapy for adult anxiety disorders: a meta-analysis of randomized placebo-controlled trials. J Clin Psychiatry 2008; 69(4):621–32.

29. Arnold LM. Management of fibromyalgia and comorbid psychiatric disorders. J Clin Psychiatry 2008;69(Suppl 2):14–9.

30. Hoffman BM, Papas RK, Chatkoff DK, et al. Meta-analysis of psychological interventions for chronic low back pain. Health Psychol 2007;26(1):1–9.

31. Mengshoel AM, Forseth KO, Haugen M, et al. Multidisciplinary approach to fibromyalgia. A pilot study. Clin Rheumatol 1995;22:717–21.

32. Nielson WR, Walker C, McCain GA. Cognitive behavioral treatment of fibromyalgia syndrome: a followup assessment. J Rheumatol 1992;19:98–103.

33. Goldenberg DL, Kaplan KH, Nadeau MG, et al. A controlled study of a stress-reduction, cognitive-behavioral treatment program in fibromyalgia. J Muscoskel Pain 1994;2(2):53–66.

34. Nicassio PM, Radojevic V, Weisman MH, et al. A comparison of behavioral and educational interventions for fibromyalgia. J Rheumatol 1997;24(10):2000–7.

35. Vlaeyen JW, Teeken-Gruben NJ, Goosens ME, et al. Cognitive-educational treatment of fibromyalgia: a randomized clinical trial. I. Clinical effects. J Rheumatol 1996;23:1237–45.

36. Williams DA, Cary MA, Groner KH, et al. Improving physical functional status in patients with fibromyalgia: a brief cognitive behavioral intervention. J Rheumatol 2002;29:1280–6.

37. Thieme K, Flor H, Turk D. Psychological pain treatment in fibromyalgia syndrome: efficacy of operant behavioural and cognitive behavioural treatments. Arthritis Res Ther 2006;8:121–32.

38. Thieme K, Turk DC, Flor H. Responder criteria for operant and cognitive-behavioral treatment of fibromyalgia syndrome. Arthritis Rheum 2007;57(5):830–6.

39. Goossens ME, Vlaeyen JW, Hidding A, et al. Treatment expectancy affects the outcome of cognitive-behavioral interventions in chronic pain. Clin J Pain 2005; 21:18–26.

40. Dadabhoy D, Crofford LJ, Spaeth M, et al. Biology and therapy of fibromyalgia. Evidence-based biomarkers for fibromyalgia syndrome. Arthritis Res Ther 2008;10(4):211.

41. Jacobson E. Progressive relaxation. Chicago: University of Chicago Press; 1938.

42. van Tulder MW, Koes B, Malmivaara A. Outcome of non-invasive treatment modalities on back pain: an evidence-based review. Eur Spine J 2006;15(Suppl 1): S64–81.

43. Hosaka T, Yamamoto K, Ikeda K, et al. Application of the relaxation technique in general hospital psychiatry. Psychiatry Clin Neurosci 1995;49(5–6):259–62.

44. Keel PJ, Bodoky C, Gerhard U, et al. Comparison of integrated group therapy and group relaxation training for fibromyalgia. Clin J Pain 1998;14(3):232–8.

45. Rucco V, Feruglio C, Genco F, et al. Autogenic training versus Erickson's analogical technique in treatment of fibromyalgia syndrome. Riv Eur Sci Med Farmacol 1995;17(1):41–50.

46. Allen LA, Woolfolk RL, Escobar JI, et al. Cognitive-behavioral therapy for somatization disorder: a randomized controlled trial. Arch Intern Med 2006;166:1512–8.

47. Luthe W, Schultz JH. Autogenic therapy. First published by Grune and Stratton, Inc. New York: The British Autogenic Society; 1969. Republished in 2001.

48. Freedman RR. Quantitative measurements of finger blood flow during behavioral treatments for Raynaud's disease. Psychophysiology 1989;26(4):437–41.

49. Bennett RM, Clark SR, Campbell SM, et al. Symptoms of Raynaud's syndrome in patients with fibromyalgia. A study utilizing the Nielsen test, digital photoplethysmography, and measurements of platelet alpha 2-adrenergic receptors. Arthritis Rheum 1991;34(3):264–9.

50. Fors EA, Sexton H, Götestam KG. The effect of guided imagery and amitriptyline on daily fibromyalgia pain: a prospective, randomized, controlled trial. J Psychiatr Res 2002;36(3):179–87.
51. Menzies V, Taylor AG, Bourguignon C. Effects of guided imagery on outcomes of pain, functional status, and self-efficacy in persons diagnosed with fibromyalgia. J Altern Complement Med 2006;12(1):23–30.
52. Menzies V, Kim S. Relaxation and guided imagery in Hispanic persons diagnosed with fibromyalgia: a pilot study. Fam Community Health 2008;31(3):204–12.
53. Walco GA, Ilowite NT. Cognitive-behavioral intervention for juvenile primary fibromyalgia syndrome. J Rheumatol 1992;19(10):1617–9.
54. Kaplan KH, Goldenberg DL, Galvin-Nadeau M. The impact of a meditation-based stress reduction program on fibromyalgia. Gen Hosp Psychiatry 1993;15(5):284–9.
55. Sephton SE, Salmon P, Weissbecker I, et al. Mindfulness meditation alleviates depressive symptoms in women with fibromyalgia: results of a randomized clinical trial. Arthritis Rheum 2007;57(1):77–85.
56. Martínez-Lavín M. Is fibromyalgia a generalized reflex sympathetic dystrophy? Clin Exp Rheumatol 2001;19(1):1–3.
57. Martínez-Lavín M, Amigo MC, Coindreau J, et al. Fibromyalgia in Frida Kahlo's life and art. Arthritis Rheum 2000;43(3):708–9.
58. Martínez-Lavín M, Hermosillo AG. Autonomic nervous system dysfunction may explain the multisystem features of fibromyalgia. Semin Arthritis Rheum 2000; 29(4):197–9.
59. Martínez-Lavín M, Hermosillo AG, Mendoza C, et al. Orthostatic sympathetic derangement in subjects with fibromyalgia. J Rheumatol 1997;24(4):714–8.
60. Martínez-Lavín M, Hermosillo AG, Rosas M, et al. Circadian studies of autonomic nervous balance in patients with fibromyalgia: a heart rate variability analysis. Arthritis Rheum 1998;41(11):1966–71.
61. Cohen H, Neumann L, Shore M, et al. Autonomic dysfunction in patients with fibromyalgia: application of power spectral analysis of heart rate variability. Semin Arthritis Rheum 2000;29(4):217–27.
62. Gevirtz R. Resonant frequency training to restore homeostasis for treatment of psychophysiological disorders. Biofeedback 2000;27:7–9.
63. Gevirtz R, Lehrer P. Resonant frequency heart rate biofeedback. In: Andrasik MSF, editor. Biofeedback: a practitioner's guide. New York: Guilford; 2003. p. 245–50.
64. Lehrer P, Sasaki Y, Saito Y. Zazen and cardiac variability. Psychosom Med 1999; 61(6):812–21.
65. Lehrer PM, Vaschillo E, Vaschillo B. Resonant frequency biofeedback training to increase cardiac variability: rationale and manual for training. Appl Psychophysiol Biofeedback 2000;25(3):177–91.
66. Lehrer P, Smetankin A, Potapova T. Respiratory sinus arrhythmia biofeedback therapy for asthma: a report of 20 unmedicated pediatric cases using the Smetankin method. Appl Psychophysiol Biofeedback 2000;25(3):193–200.
67. Giardino ND, Chan L, Borson L. Combined heart rate variability and pulse oximetry biofeedback for chronic obstructive pulmonary disease: preliminary findings. Appl Psychophysiol Biofeedback 2004;29(2):121–33.
68. Del Pozo JM, Gevirtz RN, Scher B, et al. Biofeedback treatment increases heart rate variability in patients with known coronary artery disease. Am Heart J 2004; 147(3):E11.
69. Humphreys PA, Gevirtz RN. Treatment of recurrent abdominal pain: components analysis of four treatment protocols. J Pediatr Gastroenterol Nutr 2000;31(1): 47–51.

70. Schein MH, Gavish B, Herz M, et al. Treating hypertension with a device that slows and regularises breathing: a randomised, double-blind controlled study. J Hum Hypertens 2001;15(4):271–8.
71. Hassett AL, Radvanski DC, Vaschillo EG, et al. A pilot study of the efficacy of heart rate variability (HRV) biofeedback in patients with fibromyalgia. Appl Psychophysiol Biofeedback 2007;32:1–10.
72. Stevens M, Gevirtz R, Wiederhold M, et al. Chronic fatigue syndrome: a chrono-biologically oriented, controlled treatment outcome study [abstract]. Appl Psychophysiol Biofeedback 1999;24(2):129.
73. Hassett AL, Radvanski DC, Sigal LH, et al. Preliminary results from a randomized controlled trial of heart rate variability biofeedback in fibromyalgia [abstract]. Ann Rheum Dis 2008;67(Suppl 2):S638.
74. Buckelew SP, Conway R, Parker J, et al. Biofeedback/relaxation training and exercise interventions for fibromyalgia: a prospective trial. Arthritis Care Res 1998; 11(3):196–209.
75. Babu AS, Mathew E, Danda D, et al. Management of patients with fibromyalgia using biofeedback: a randomized control trial. Indian J Med Sci 2007;61(8):455–61.
76. Mur E, Drexler A, Gruber J, et al. Electromyography biofeedback therapy in fibromyalgia. Wien Med Wochenschr 1999;149:561–3.
77. Sarnoch H, Adler F, Scholz OB. Relevance of muscular sensitivity, muscular activity, and cognitive variables for pain reduction associated with EMG biofeedback in fibromyalgia. Percept Mot Skills 1997;84:1043–50.
78. Ferraccioli G, Ghirelli L, Scita F, et al. EMG-biofeedback training in fibromyalgia syndrome. J Rheumatol 1987;14(4):820–5.
79. van Santen M, Bolwijn P, Verstappen F, et al. A randomized clinical trial comparing fitness and biofeedback training versus basic treatment in patients with fibromyalgia. J Rheumatol 2002;29(3):575–81.
80. Kayiran S, Dursun E, Ermutlu N, et al. Neurofeedback in fibromyalgia syndrome. Agri 2007;19(3):47–53.
81. Pioro-Boisset M, Esdaile JM, Fitzcharles MA. Alternative medicine use in fibromyalgia syndrome. Arthritis Care Res 1996;9(1):13–7.
82. Brattberg G. Connective tissue massage in the treatment of fibromyalgia. Eur J Pain 1999;3:235–45.
83. Holdcraft LC, Assefi N, Buchwald D. Complementary and alternative medicine in fibromyalgia and related syndromes. Best Pract Res Clin Rheumatol 2006;17(4): 667–83.
84. Chen KW, Hassett AL, Hou F, et al. A pilot study of external Qigong therapy for patients with fibromyalgia. J Altern Compliment Med 2006;12(9):851–6.
85. Astin JA, Berman BM, Bausell B. The efficacy of mindfulness meditation plus Qigong movement therapy in the treatment of fibromyalgia: a randomized control trial. J Rheumatol 2003;30:2257–62.
86. Mannerkorpi K, Arndorw M. Efficacy and feasibility of a combination of body awareness therapy and qigong in patients with fibromyalgia: a pilot study. J Rehabil Med 2004;36(6):279–81.
87. Taggert HM, Arslanian CL, Bae S, et al. T'ai Chi exercise on fibromyalgia symptoms and health related quality of life. Orthop Nurs 2003;22:1107–14.
88. Mayhew E, Ernst E. Acupuncture for fibromyalgia—a systematic review of randomized clinical trials. Rheumatology (Oxford) 2007;46:801–4.
89. Targino RA, Imamura M, Kaziyama HH, et al. A randomized controlled trial of acupuncture added to usual treatment for fibromyalgia. J Rehabil Med 2008; 40(7):582–8.

90. Harris RE, Tian X, Williams DA, et al. Treatment of fibromyalgia with formula acupuncture: investigation of needle placement, needle stimulation, and treatment frequency. J Altern Complement Med 2005;11(4):663–71.
91. McVeigh JG, McGaughey H, Hall M, et al. The effectiveness of hydrotherapy in the management of fibromyalgia syndrome: a systematic review. Rheumatol Int 2008;29(2):119–30.
92. Crofford LJ, Appleton BE. Complementary and alternative therapies for fibromyalgia. Curr Rheumatol Rep 2001;3:147–56.
93. Sarac AJ, Gur A. Complementary and alternative medical therapies in fibromyalgia. Curr Pharm Des 2006;12:47–57.
94. Available at: http://www.arthritis.org/disease-center.php?disease_id=10. Accessed May 20, 2009.
95. Available at: http://www.fmaware.org/site/PageServer. Accessed May 20, 2009.
96. Available at: KnowFibro.com . Accessed May 20, 2009.

Potential Dietary Links to Central Sensitization in Fibromyalgia: Past Reports and Future Directions

Kathleen F. Holton, MPH[a,b,]*, Lindsay L. Kindler, RN, PhD[c,d],
Kim D. Jones, PhD, RN, FNP[e]

KEYWORDS

- Fibromyalgia • Diet • Dietary intervention
- Review • Glutamate

Fibromyalgia (FM) patients commonly express a desire to maximize their symptom management by adding nonpharmacologic strategies, including dietary modification. FM is currently only 30%–50% amenable to symptomatic improvement through pharmacologic control[1–3] and patients consistently seek to improve symptom control through additional methods. A recent internet-based survey of 2626 people who have FM stated that the majority of subjects have altered their diets in an attempt to control symptoms and seek guidance on optimizing their diet.[4] Prospective multidisciplinary FM treatment studies have included dietary guidance as a component of a comprehensive strategy, although the authors note that this component was only incorporated to improve patient satisfaction.[5]

Haugen and colleagues[6] attempted to gain a picture of rheumatic patients' efforts and achievements in dietary modification by administering a questionnaire-based survey on diet and disease symptoms in 742 subjects who have rheumatic conditions, 65 having FM. Of the individuals who have FM, 40% believed that diet had a great

[a] Department of Orthopaedics and Rehabilitation, Oregon Health & Science University, 3181 SW Sam Jackson Park Road, Portland, OR 97239-3098, USA
[b] Department of Nutritional Sciences, University of Arizona, Shantz Building, Room 309, 1177 East 4th Street, Tucson, AZ 85721, USA
[c] Kaiser Permanente, West Interstate Medical Office, Portland, OR 97227, USA
[d] School of Nursing, SN-ORD, Oregon Health & Science University, 3455 SW US Veterans Hospital Road, Portland, OR 97239, USA
[e] Office of Research and Development, School of Nursing, Oregon Health & Science University, 3455 SW US Veterans Hospital Road, SN-ORD, Portland, OR 97239–2941, USA
* Corresponding author. Department of Orthopaedics and Rehabilitation, Oregon Health & Science University, 3181 SW Sam Jackson Park Road, Portland OR 97239-3098.
E-mail address: holtonk@ohsu.edu (K.F. Holton).

Rheum Dis Clin N Am 35 (2009) 409–420
doi:10.1016/j.rdc.2009.06.003
0889-857X/09/$ – see front matter © 2009 Elsevier Inc. All rights reserved.

influence on symptoms, whereas 60% believed that diet had a small influence. Forty-two percent of the subjects who have FM reported aggravation of symptoms following the intake of specific foods. Symptom aggravation included pain and stiffness in 80% and swelling of the joints in 29% of these subjects. The cross-sectional survey did not delineate which foods were found most often to aggravate symptoms in FM.[6]

This evidence from the FM literature suggests that patients who have FM are seeking successful dietary interventions, but research has not yet outlined optimal strategies. Unfortunately, there have been only nine dietary intervention studies in FM. Furthermore, eight of these were uncontrolled or nonrandomized.

METHODS

The authors conducted a MedLine English language search with the MeSH terms "diet" and "fibromyalgia" between 1986 and 2008. This yielded 27 articles for further review. We then limited these articles to those containing original data, testing a whole food dietary intervention (as opposed to supplements), and enrolling people who have FM per standardized criteria such as the 1990 American College of Rheumatology (ACR) criteria.[7] This limited the trials under review to nine. There was one prospective, randomized, controlled trial; two nonrandomized, controlled trials; five observational studies with an intervention; and one descriptive, correlational study. One of these studies, describing changes in gut microflora, was excluded for lack of methodological rigor and rational theoretical hypothesis.[8]

RESULTS

Studies to date have investigated vegetarian, elimination, or weight loss diets. Azad and colleagues[9] used a randomized, controlled crossover trial to compare the effects of a vegetarian diet to an amitriptyline control group in 78 subjects who have FM. After 6 weeks of treatment, fatigue, insomnia, nonrestorative sleep, and tender point count were not significantly changed in the vegetarian group (n = 37) whereas the amitriptyline group (n=37) experienced significant improvements in these areas ($P<.001$). The visual analog pain scale significantly changed for the vegetarian group ($P<.05$) and the amitriptyline control group ($P<.001$), although there was a smaller decrease in the vegetarian group. All participants in the vegetarian intervention group chose to discontinue the diet after 6 weeks and crossed over to the amitriptyline arm, citing inefficacy and monotony of the dietary intervention. This decision by the participants speaks to the challenge of adopting a vegetarian diet over an omnivorous one for a prolonged period of time.

Two studies investigated the use of a raw, vegan diet called a Living Foods diet on the effects of FM symptoms. The Living Foods diet is an uncooked vegan diet consisting of vegetables, roots, fruits, berries, germinated seeds, cereal, sprouts, and nuts. The diet excludes the use of coffee, tea, alcohol, or table salt.

Hanninen and colleagues[10] examined this diet in 33 subjects who have FM and 42 subjects who have rheumatoid arthritis (RA). The FM and RA groups were divided such that half were assigned to the Living Foods diet and half to a control, omnivorous diet. Each group followed the assigned diet for 3 months; the subjects who have FM prepared their own meals and the subjects who have RA obtained their food from the research kitchen. While on the intervention diet, the group of subjects who have FM experienced a significant decrease in their self-reported morning stiffness as measured by a Likert scale ($P<.01$) and a decrease in their pain at rest on a visual analog scale ($P<.01$). Although the subjects who had FM achieved benefit in these areas, it is not clear what other parameters were measured and therefore not found to be significantly affected. There was no significant difference between the subjects who have RA in the intervention and control groups, although both groups experienced a decrease in their activity of RA as measured by an author-created relative disease activity index. All subjects who were in the intervention groups returned to their previous omnivorous diet after the completion of the study. This provides further concern regarding the feasibility of this approach on a long-term basis, especially if the subjective improvement noted by participants was not great enough to influence long-term use of the diet. If the researchers had proposed a scientific hypothesis as to which excluded food items may have helped these subjects, then that may have allowed the participants to continue to avoid these food items while gradually returning to their omnivorous diet.

Kaartinen and colleagues[11] also examined the efficacy of the Living Foods diet in 28 subjects who have FM. Due to the complicated nature of preparing this diet, participants were allowed to self-select into the Living Foods intervention group or the control group that continued their normal omnivorous diet. The 18 intervention participants ate the Living Foods diet for 3 months. Results demonstrated that the Living Foods group had significantly decreased pain ($P<.01$), improved quality of sleep ($P<.001$), decreased morning stiffness ($P<.001$), improvement on a General Health Questionnaire ($P<.05$) as well as decreased BMI ($P<.001$), decreased cholesterol ($P<.01$) and urine sodium ($P<.001$). Number of tender points, an exercise test, and a handgrip test did not significantly improve. Subjects who have FM who self-selected into the intervention group had more comorbid diseases as compared with the control group (although the authors failed to state which comorbid conditions were observed). One must wonder if these comorbid diagnoses were more responsive to dietary changes, therefore accounting for the greater improvement in the intervention group. As in the previous study using the Living Foods diet, all participants in the intervention group discontinued the diet after the required 3 months. Although this study did report weight and BMI changes, it was not designed to determine whether BMI or dietary changes were responsible for symptom improvement, and the statistical analysis did not adjust for weight or BMI change.

Donaldson and colleagues also tested the use of a raw vegetarian diet in subjects who have FM using an observational design.[12] This diet is described as the Hallelujah Diet and consists of a pure vegetarian diet made mostly of fruits, vegetables, nuts, carrot juice, and dehydrated barley grass juice. Participants were instructed to avoid alcohol, caffeine, refined flour, all meats, and dairy. A total of 18 subjects who had at one time been diagnosed with FM (not all currently met diagnostic criteria) completed this observational study by following the Hallelujah Diet for 7 months. Results demonstrated that the mean FM Impact Questionnaire (FIQ) of these 18 participants decreased by 46% over the 7 months, whereas seven out of eight subscales on the Short Form 36 (SF-36) health survey improved; the exception being bodily pain. Other significant improvements were demonstrated in shoulder pain, abduction range of shoulder, flexibility, chair stand, and 6-minute walk ($P<.05$). While this study indicates potential improvement of FM with dietary changes, lack of a control group leaves one to question if the benefits experienced were a result of this particular diet alone. Participants attended a motivational presentation described as attempting to reorient their thinking about food and health. Perhaps motivation to make generalized healthy changes affected the outcomes of the participants. This study was also limited by a small sample size and the fact that not all participants met FM diagnostic criteria. Of note, this study was sponsored by the Hallelujah Acres Foundation and used their publications (*God's Way to Ultimate Health, Recipes for life…from God's Garden*) for participant education. This raises the question of a conflict of interest and whether spiritual support might in part be responsible for positive outcomes. Like many other FM diet studies, weight and BMI changes were not reported.

In a novel, quasi-experimental study, Deuster & Jaffe[13] enrolled 51 subjects who have FM into a self-selected treatment or control group. Using lymphocyte response assay, subjects in the treatment group were given individualized dietary advice to exclude foods and additives to which they were sensitive and to supplement the elimination diet with individualized neutraceuticals, including full-spectrum antioxidants, buffering minerals, metabolic intermediates, and necessary cofactors. The control group met biweekly as an FM support group. All participants completed questionnaires at baseline, 3 months and 6 months (end of intervention). The lymphocyte response assay revealed that the most commonly reactive substances were monosodium glutamate (MSG), caffeine, food coloring, chocolate, shrimp, dairy products, and aspartame. Approximately 45% of the original sample dropped out, mainly due to problems related to program adherence. Self-reported dietary compliance for those who completed the study averaged 87%. No between group findings were given; however, within group change scores indicated that, compared with baseline, the treatment group experienced a 50% reduction in pain, 70% reduction in depression, 50% reduction in fatigue, and 30% reduction in stiffness. Symptom reduction was noted at 3 months and did not improve further at 6 months. Limitations of this study include the nonblinded, nonrandomized design, and the dual intervention of supplementation plus dietary exclusion of reactive substances. One is left to question what part of the intervention actually caused the improvement in symptoms. Nonetheless, these conclusions should be tested more rigorously in future randomized, controlled trials that specifically test various chemical and food sensitivities and, in a separate study (or separate arm of an intervention study), test the effect of micronutrient supplementation.

It is difficult to ascertain whether FM symptoms were affected by removal of certain foods, removal of additives, an increase in nutrient levels, or potential weight loss during the reviewed studies. Because many restrictive diets cause weight loss, it is important to differentiate the effects of diet versus the effects of weight loss alone.

Yunus and colleagues[14] investigated the relationship between BMI and FM symptoms in 211 women who have FM. The average BMI was 27.8 with 38% classified as having a normal BMI, 29% classified as overweight, 29% as obese, 3% as morbidly obese, and 1% as underweight. After controlling for age and education, the investigators found that the Health Assessment Questionnaire scores, which measure eight activities of daily living, had a positive, significant correlation with BMI ($P<.001$). Number of tender points and BMI were correlated with a significance of $P<.05$. The study found no significant associations between BMI and symptoms such as pain intensity, global severity, sleep difficulties, fatigue, or depression. Whereas this study outlines a descriptive picture of BMI and symptoms in a group of subjects who have FM, one cannot conclude that symptom severity in these participants is caused by varying levels of BMI or that a decrease in BMI would alter FM symptoms.

In an attempt to gain a better understanding of the effect of weight loss on the symptoms of FM, Shapiro and colleagues[15] conducted an intervention consisting of a 20-week group behavioral weight loss program that educated patients about diet, activity, and dietary stimulus control. Thirty-one women who have FM and who had a BMI greater than or equal to 25 kg/m^2 (overweight) completed the intervention. Participants were encouraged to maintain calorie intake at 1200–1500 calories per day plus an activity regimen aimed at achieving 30 minutes of physical activity per day. Participants lost an average of 9.2 lbs ($P<.01$) and decreased their BMI by 1.6 kg/m^2 ($P<.01$), both significant changes from baseline. The overall intervention led to significant pre/post improvements in the Beck Depression Inventory (BDI), Body Shape Questionnaire (BSQ), FM Impact Questionnaire (FIQ), Multidimensional Pain Inventory – pain severity, Multidimensional Pain Inventory – support, Multidisciplinary Pain Inventory – interference (MPI-I), Quality of Life (QOL), and State Trait Anxiety Inventory. Hierarchical multiple regression analysis showed that a reduced BMI significantly predicted improvements in FIQ, MPI-I, and BSQ. Percentage weight loss predicted improvements in FIQ, MPI-I, BSQ, and QOL.

These findings indicate that a behavioral intervention focused on diet, weight loss, and activity can lead to improvements in FM symptoms, pain interference, body satisfaction, and quality of life. One can debate whether these positive outcomes are a result of weight loss, increased physical activity, a change to a more healthful diet, or the effects of participating in a supportive group intervention. Limitations of this study include the fact that it was not randomized, had no control group, approximately 26% of participants enrolled did not complete the study, and the researchers did not control for medication use in the statistical analysis.

Hooper and colleagues[16] examined the effects of weight loss in patients who have musculoskeletal pain (average BMI of 51 kg/m^2) undergoing gastric bypass. All subjects had musculoskeletal pain in at least one site whereas 12 (25%) fulfilled the 1990 ACR criteria for FM. Postsurgery, the average weight lost by all subjects was 41 kg, which decreased the average BMI to 36 kg/m^2. Out of the 12 subjects who have FM, only one patient persisted in meeting the ACR criteria for a diagnosis of FM at their 6- or 12-month follow-up visit. At this 6- or 12-month endpoint, 48% of all subjects still had at least one site of musculoskeletal pain, although there was a statistically significant improvement on all subscales of the Short Form-36. This study suggests that a drastic reduction in weight may reduce FM symptoms; but possibly more important is the severe reduction in food intake following gastric bypass, which may have limited their intake of specific foods that may have been causing or contributing to their FM symptoms. One must also consider that this was an observational study of individuals who were required to make significant life changes before having gastric bypass. The intensive nutritional counseling, exercise program, smoking cessation, and overall lifestyle changes to which patients must commit to qualify for gastric bypass might have also mitigated symptom severity.

FUTURE RESEARCH DIRECTIONS/HYPOTHESIS GENERATION

Emerging data suggest that central sensitization is one mechanism involved in dysfunctional pain processing in patients who have FM. Numerous studies investigating the pain amplification of this disorder have demonstrated widespread lowering of pain thresholds, enhanced sensitivity outside of tender points, expansion of pain receptive fields, increased substance P in the cerebral spinal fluid, abnormal windup, prolonged pain after cessation of painful input, allodynia, and hyperalgesia. Aspects of central sensitization have also been demonstrated in other commonly associated disorders such as irritable bowel syndrome (IBS) and migraines.[17–19] Because these syndromes share a common pathophysiologic mechanism, it could be postulated that they also share aggravating factors, namely dietary substances that cause or exacerbate the pain of these conditions.

Central Sensitization and Dietary Substances

One route to central sensitization begins when A delta and C fibers in the periphery are activated by substances such as substance P, prostaglandins, or bradykinin as a result of inflammation or trauma.[17] Intense activation of C fibers, as occurs in disorders such as FM, IBS, and migraine, can lead to hyperexcitable wide-dynamic-range neurons, which results in an enhanced responsiveness to painful (hyperalgesia) and nonpainful input (allodynia).[20] In response to the barrage of C- and A-delta fiber stimulation, neurotransmitters and neuromodulators, such as substance P, glutamate, and aspartate, are released into the neuronal synapse.[21] These excitatory neurotransmitters activate postsynaptic receptors including N-methyl-d-aspartate (NMDA), metabotropic glutamate, and neurokinin-1 receptors, leading to increased neuroplastic changes that perpetuate central sensitization. Several studies have confirmed the role of NMDA receptors in central sensitization by demonstrating that NMDA receptor antagonists can inhibit the increased excitability caused by repetitive C-fiber stimulation, thereby inhibiting windup.[22] Windup was described more than 30 years ago as progressively increasing activity in dorsal horn cells following repetitive activation of primary afferent C fibers[23] and is a critical event in the development of central sensitization that results from stimulation of peripheral nociceptors.

Two of the neurotransmitters (glutamate and aspartate) discussed above are negatively charged amino acids, and are supplied by the diet in bound and free forms. Bound forms are full protein sources such as beef, chicken, and pork, whereby the amino acids are released slowly and in small amounts during the digestive process.[24] Free forms of glutamate and aspartate are found commonly as food additives such as hydrolyzed proteins, MSG, autolyzed yeast extract, modified food starches, and aspartame (a dipeptide of phenylalanine and aspartate), where they are used to enhance the flavor of food by stimulating neurons in the tongue[25,26] Glutamate and aspartate act as excitatory neurotransmitters in the body and, in high enough amounts, can act as "excitotoxins,"[27] where they can have neurotoxic effects in the nervous system.[28] Normally, glutamate crosses the blood–brain barrier only through active transport, keeping the levels of glutamate controlled in the brain; although there are certain states such as infection, head trauma, and even psychologic stress where the blood–brain barrier becomes more permeable.[29–32] Interestingly, many patients who have FM report a severe stressor such as those listed above that directly precedes the onset of their symptoms.[33,34] Additionally, Toth and Lajtha[35] confirmed that brain levels of glutamate were dependent on the length of exposure to excitotoxic amino acids. When giving mice and rats glutamate and aspartate in their diet, they found that they could significantly increase brain levels with prolonged feeding. They concluded that although these amino acids cannot be taken up by the brain quickly, they can, over a longer period of time (from several hours to days), enter the brain in increasing concentrations. Some areas of the brain are not protected by the blood–brain barrier (circumventricular organs and the hypothalamus), and these areas have been sites of neuronal damage (including retinal damage, hypothalamic damage, and brain lesions) from MSG via the NMDA receptor in cats, chickens, guinea pigs, hamsters, mice, monkeys, and rabbits.[27,36–43] Much of this research demonstrated an even greater negative impact on young animals, which resulted in Dr. John Olney testifying before Congress,[44] and a subsequent removal of MSG from baby foods by the food industry (although today glutamate can still be added to baby food under the guise of terms such as "broth" or "flavoring").[29]

Glutamate levels in cerebrospinal fluid have been shown to correlate to pain levels in humans who have FM.[45] Correlations between clinical pain severity and levels of glutamate in the cerebral cortex have also been demonstrated in subjects who have FM.[46] Glutamate has also been implicated as a link between migraines and FM,[47] which, as discussed above, is another disorder caused by central sensitization. Researchers in Brazil demonstrated that subjects who have FM who also have migraine had significantly higher cerebrospinal fluid glutamate levels than age- and sex-matched controls. Subjects in the study also reported headache intensity that correlated with their cerebrospinal glutamate levels. The authors speculate that the glutamate levels in these subjects were causing the increased central sensitization seen in this study.[48] Along these same lines, Smith and colleagues[49] reported a case series of four subjects who have FM who experienced a dramatic decrease in symptoms when they excluded MSG and aspartame from their diets, and a return of symptoms upon rechallenge. The authors suggested the need for larger scale dietary elimination/challenge studies to further test the effect of these excitotoxins in FM.

Contemporary research has shown the important role that central sensitization plays in FM symptomatology. Substance P, glutamate, and aspartate have been shown to be key neurotransmitters and neuromodulators contributing to central sensitization. The authors hypothesize that dietary sources of added glutamate and aspartate could enhance or initiate the central sensitization in some patients with FM. From a perusal of our literature review, it is evident that there could have been several reasons for the reported benefit of the various dietary interventions. One such possibility is a concomitant reduction in food additives containing excitotoxins.[49] Further research is needed to clarify the exact effect of these excitotoxins in the diet of patients who have FM.

This research hypothesis is novel in that it focuses on removing a possible cause of symptoms rather than focusing on dietary change with the goal of weight loss. The study of weight loss with the idea that weight is playing a role in FM needs to be studied separately from specific dietary change. This can be accomplished through caloric reduction with no restriction on food type, with or without the inclusion of an exercise program with the goal of weight loss. Not all patients who have FM are overweight, and the proportion who are overweight or obese does not differ dramatically from the general United States population.[14,50] Because weight loss is usually tied to dietary restriction, it is difficult to discern whether the weight loss or the change in diet is responsible for the improvement in symptoms. Interestingly, glutamate has been shown to cause weight gain and type II diabetes in mouse studies.[51–53] In addition, researchers in China have shown an association between increasing consumption of MSG and increasing rates of obesity.[54] Therefore, it could be postulated that glutamate may be contributing to both obesity and central sensitization in patients who have FM, but this hypothesis needs to be tested in humans.

Other foods/additives that have been suggested as possible FM symptom triggers in addition to MSG (one form of glutamate) and aspartame (a source of aspartate) are: caffeine, food coloring, chocolate, cow's milk, and shellfish.[13] These individual substances could be tested in an acute dosing manner, intravenously or orally, in a placebo-controlled laboratory environment, with both subjective outcome measures, such as real-time pain reporting, and objective measures, such as peripheral or central pain markers. Alternatively, subjects who have FM could receive two different diets from a research kitchen (one with additives and one without) and remain blinded to treatment arm. This would control for placebo effect. A third option would be to place subjects who have FM on an elimination diet and monitor for symptom change. Those who respond positively to the elimination diet could then go onto receive crossover challenges where they receive either the test substance or placebo in a double-blinded fashion. True "responders" would be those who improve when the offending substance is removed, but who also have a return of symptoms when tested with the food additive, and not when tested with placebo.

In addition to their FM symptoms, many patients commonly have other concomitant comorbidities. For instance, up to 81% of patients who have FM also have IBS[55] and up to 80% of patients with FM experience migraines.[56] Because IBS, migraines, and

FM are all postulated to be associated with central sensitization,[18] it may be important for future studies to investigate the impact of controlling these comorbidities with diet, in addition to examining the effects of diet on FM.

DISCUSSION

Despite mixed evidence, dietary modifications remain a potentially important clinical tool. Dietary changes are often safer and much less expensive than standard drug therapies and are within the patient's own control. However, the protocol designs, statistical power, and execution of dietary clinical trials in FM have been inferior to many multicenter drug trials, making the provision of dietary guidelines in FM at best a questionable practice.

It is challenging to rely on the current studies in the literature to confirm that specific dietary changes will significantly improve FM symptoms due to the limitations of these studies. Only one randomized study found that drug therapy was superior to diet therapy. Noncontrolled studies leave interpretation of symptom improvement subject to the placebo response. Another significant limitation of the dietary interventions remains that none of the study participants continued on the dietary intervention past the required time, despite a relatively short intervention period. Some participants cited monotony of the diets or monotony combined with lack of efficacy in significantly reducing symptoms. Because FM is a chronic condition, therapies should target life-style changes that can be performed on a long-term basis. Theoretically, a dietary intervention that causes significant improvement in symptoms and is feasible (not dramatically restrictive) should result in subjects continuing to follow the diet once a study is completed. Thus, post study dietary compliance should always be assessed.

Potential confounders in FM dietary research should include an increase in physical activity, group support, education about the mechanisms of FM, or a motivation to change other lifestyle factors stimulated by a change in eating habits. While these represent positive aspects of treatment, these factors make it more difficult to attribute improvements to change in diet or weight loss alone. As individuals who have FM search for beneficial nutritional guidelines, this population would benefit greatly from a randomized, controlled trial investigating a scientifically based dietary intervention.

The studies described in this review point to areas for future research efforts, including elimination diets combined with double-blind testing of certain food additives, weight loss studies, and/or the possible use of a vegetarian diet in the treatment of FM. All three of these concepts contain one thing in common, namely a restriction in the type and amount of foods consumed. It is important to discern whether the removal of specific foods/additives, the addition of nutrients to the diet, or weight loss is the true cause of symptom improvement. Many of the vegetarian diets, due to their very restricted nature, also excluded many processed foods containing excitotoxins. Therefore it is impossible to know what specifically caused the observed improvement. Future studies should use a randomized, placebo-controlled clinical trial design that does *not* cause weight loss, to test whether the removal of specific food items causes an improvement in symptom occurrence. Due to the large placebo effect seen in FM, studies should be appropriately powered to take this into consideration, and as suggested earlier, should test the food item by reintroduction into the diet. Separately, weight loss studies can be conducted using the addition of exercise, while instructing subjects *not* to change their diets, to examine the effects of exercise (with or without weight loss) on FM. An appropriately powered clinical trial study design, controlling for the possible confounders outlined above, should help researchers illuminate the true effect of dietary change, or weight loss, on FM symptoms.

SUMMARY

There is a paucity of research on diet and FM, and the prevailing research has many methodological concerns. There is a clear need for more research on diet and FM, with hypotheses based on biochemical mechanisms, such as those relating to what is known about the role of central sensitization in this disorder.

ACKNOWLEDGMENTS

We thank Dr. Robert M. Bennett for his thoughtful critique of this manuscript.

REFERENCES

1. Russell IJ, Mease PJ, Smith TR, et al. Efficacy and safety of duloxetine for treatment of fibromyalgia in patients with or without major depressive disorder: results from a 6-month, randomized, double-blind, placebo-controlled, fixed-dose trial [see comment]. Pain 2008;136(3):432–44.
2. Russell IJ, Perkins AT, Michalek JE, Oxybate SXB-26 Fibromyalgia Syndrome Study Group. Sodium oxybate relieves pain and improves function in fibromyalgia syndrome: a randomized, double-blind, placebo-controlled, multicenter clinical trial. Arthritis Rheum 2009;60(1):299–309.
3. Mease PJ, Russell IJ, Arnold LM, et al. A randomized, double-blind, placebo-controlled, phase III trial of pregabalin in the treatment of patients with fibromyalgia [see comment]. J Rheumatol 2008;35(3):502–14.
4. Bennett R, Jones J, Turk DC, et al. An internet survey of 2,596 people with fibromyalgia. BMC Musculoskelet Disord 2007;8:27.
5. Lemstra M, Olszynski WP. The effectiveness of multidisciplinary rehabilitation in the treatment of fibromyalgia: a randomized controlled trial. Clin J Pain 2005; 21(2):166–74.
6. Haugen M, Kjeldsenkragh J, Nordvag BY, et al. Diet and disease symptoms in rheumatic diseases—results of a questionnaire based survey. Clin Rheumatol 1991;10(4):401–7.
7. Wolfe F, Smythe HA, Yunus MB, et al. The American College of Rheumatology 1990 criteria for the classification of fibromyalgia. Report of the Multicenter Criteria Committee. Arthritis Rheum 1990;33(2):160–72.
8. Michalsen A, Riegert M, Ludtke R, et al. Mediterranean diet or extended fasting's influence on changing the intestinal microflora, immunoglobulin A secretion and clinical outcome in patients with rheumatoid arthritis and fibromyalgia: an observational study. BMC Complement Altern Med 2005;5:22.
9. Azad KA, Alam MN, Haq SA, et al. Vegetarian diet in the treatment of fibromyalgia. Bangladesh Med Res Counc Bull 2000;26(2):41–7.
10. Hanninen, Kaartinen K, Rauma AL, et al. Antioxidants in vegan diet and rheumatic disorders. Toxicology 2000;155(1–3):45–53.
11. Kaartinen K, Lammi K, Hypen M, et al. Vegan diet alleviates fibromyalgia symptoms. Scand J Rheumatol 2000;29(5):308–13.
12. Donaldson MS, Speight N, Loomis S. Fibromyalgia syndrome improved using a mostly raw vegetarian diet: an observational study. BMC Complement Altern Med 2001;1:7.

13. Deuster PA, Jaffe RM. A novel treatment for fibromyalgia improves clinical outcomes in a community-based study. J Musculoskeletal Pain 1998;6(2): 133–49.

14. Yunus MB, Arslan S, Aldag JC. Relationship between body mass index and fibromyalgia features. Scand J Rheumatol 2002;31(1):27–31.

15. Shapiro JR, Anderson DA, Danoff-Burg S. A pilot study of the effects of behavioral weight loss treatment on fibromyalgia symptoms. J Psychosom Res 2005; 59(5):275–82.

16. Hooper MM, Stellato TA, Hallowell PT, et al. Musculoskeletal findings in obese subjects before and after weight loss following bariatric surgery. Int J Obes (Lond) 2007;31(1):114–20.

17. Yunus MB. Central sensitivity syndromes: a new paradigm and group nosology for fibromyalgia and overlapping conditions, and the related issue of disease versus illness. Semin Arthritis Rheum 2008;37(6):339–52.

18. Diatchenko L, Nackley AG, Slade GD, et al. Idiopathic pain disorders–pathways of vulnerability. Pain 2006;123(3):226–30.

19. Marchand S. The physiology of pain mechanisms: from the periphery to the brain. Rheum Dis Clin North Am 2008;34(2):285–309.

20. Mendell LM. Physiological properties of unmyelinated fiber projection to the spinal cord. Exp Neurol 1966;16:316–32.

21. Staud R, Domingo M. Evidence for abnormal pain processing in fibromyalgia syndrome. Pain Med 2001;2(3):208–15.

22. Eide PK. Wind-up and the NMDA receptor complex from a clinical perspective. Eur J Pain 2000;4:5–17.

23. Mendell LM, Wall PD. Response of singe dorsal cord cells to peripheral cutaneous unmyelinated fibers. Nature 1965;206:97–9.

24. Stevens BR. Digestion and absorption of protein. In: Stipanuk MH, editor. Biochemical and physiological aspects of human nutrition. Philadelphia: Saunders; 2000. p. 121–2.

25. Dingledine R, Conn PJ. Peripheral glutamate receptors: molecular biology and role in taste sensation. J Nutr 2000;130(4S Suppl):1039S–42S.

26. Ranney RE, Oppermann JA. A review of the metabolism of the aspartyl moiety of aspartame in experimental animals and man. J Environ Pathol Toxicol 1979;2(4): 979–85.

27. Olney JW. Excitotoxins in foods. Neurotoxicology 1994;15(3):535–44.

28. Olney JW, Ho OL, Rhee V, et al. Letter: neurotoxic effects of glutamate. N Engl J Med 1973;289(25):1374–5.

29. Blaylock RL. Excitotoxins. The taste that kills. Santa Fe, NM: Health Press; 1997.

30. Robinson JS, Moody RA. Influence of respiratory stress and hypertension upon the blood-brain barrier. J Neurosurg 1980;53(5):666–73.

31. Barzo P, Marmarou A, Fatouros P, et al. Magnetic resonance imaging-monitored acute blood-brain barrier changes in experimental traumatic brain injury. J Neurosurg 1996;85(6):1113–21.

32. Afonso PV, Ozden S, Prevost MC, et al. Human blood-brain barrier disruption by retroviral-infected lymphocytes: role of myosin light chain kinase in endothelial tight-junction disorganization. J Immunol 2007;179(4):2576–83.

33. Cohen H, Neumann L, Haiman Y, et al. Prevalence of post-traumatic stress disorder in fibromyalgia patients: overlapping syndromes or post-traumatic fibromyalgia syndrome? [see comment]. Semin Arthritis Rheum 2002;32(1): 38–50.

34. Pall ML. Common etiology of posttraumatic stress disorder, fibromyalgia, chronic fatigue syndrome and multiple chemical sensitivity via elevated nitric oxide/peroxynitrite [see comment]. Med Hypotheses 2001;57(2):139–45.
35. Toth E, Lajtha A. Elevation of cerebral levels of nonessential amino acids in vivo by administration of large doses. Neurochem Res 1981;6(12):1309–17.
36. Olney JW, Sharpe LG. Brain lesions in an infant rhesus monkey treated with monosodium glutamate. Science 1969;166(903):386–8.
37. Olney JW, Ho OL. Brain damage in infant mice following oral intake of glutamate, aspartate or cysteine. Nature 1970;227(5258):609–11.
38. Nemeroff CB, Grant LD, Bissette G, et al. Growth, endocrinological, and behavioral deficits after monosodium L-glutamate in the neonatal rat: possible involvement of arcuate dopamine neuron damage. Psychoneuroendocrinology 1977; 2(2):179–96.
39. Nemeroff CB, Konkol RJ, Bissette G, et al. Analysis of the disruption in hypothalamic-pituitary regulation in rats treated neonatally with monosodium L-glutamate (MSG): evidence for the involvement of tuberoinfundibular cholinergic and dopaminergic systems in neuroendocrine regulation. Endocrinology 1977;101(2): 613–22.
40. Holzwarth MA, Hurst EM. Manifestations of monosodium glutamate (MSG) induced lesions of the arcuate nucleus of the mouse. Anat Rec 1974;178:378.
41. Hamtsu T. [Effect of sodium iodate and sodium L-glutamate on ERG and histological structure of retina of adult rabbits]. Nippon Ganka Gakkai Zasshi 1964;68: 1621–36 [in Japanese].
42. Oser BL, Carson S, Vogin EE, et al. Oral and subcutaneous administration of monosodium glutamate to infant rodents and dogs. Nature 1971;229(5284): 411–3.
43. Nagasawa H, Yanai R, Kikuyama S. Irreversible inhibition of pituitary prolactin and growth hormone secretion and of mammary gland development in mice by monosodium glutamate administered neonatally. Acta Endocrinol 1974; 75(2):249–59.
44. National Academy of Science NRC. Safety and sustainability of MSG and other substances in baby food (Report of Subcommittee) 1970. Washington, DC.
45. Larson AA, Giovengo SL, Russell IJ, et al. Changes in the concentrations of amino acids in the cerebrospinal fluid that correlate with pain in patients with fibromyalgia: implications for nitric oxide pathways. Pain 2000;87(2): 201–11.
46. Harris RE, Sundgren PC, Pang Y, et al. Dynamic levels of glutamate within the insula are associated with improvements in multiple pain domains in fibromyalgia. Arthritis Rheum 2008;58(3):903–7.
47. Sarchielli P, Di Filippo M, Nardi K, et al. Sensitization, glutamate, and the link between migraine and fibromyalgia. Curr Pain Headache Rep 2007;11(5): 343–51.
48. Peres MF, Zukerman E, Senne Soares CA, et al. Cerebrospinal fluid glutamate levels in chronic migraine. Cephalalgia 2004;24(9):735–9.
49. Smith JD, Terpening CM, Schmidt SO, et al. Relief of fibromyalgia symptoms following discontinuation of dietary excitotoxins. Ann Pharmacother 2001;35(6): 702–6.
50. Ogden CL, Carroll MD, McDowell MA, et al. Obesity among adults in the United States—no change since 2003–2004. Hyattsville (MD): National Center for Health Statistics; 2007.

51. Nagata M, Suzuki W, Iizuka S, et al. Type 2 diabetes mellitus in obese mouse model induced by monosodium glutamate. Exp Anim 2006;55(2):109–15.
52. Bunyan J, Murrell EA, Shah PP. The induction of obesity in rodents by means of monosodium glutamate. Br J Nutr 1976;35(1):25–39.
53. Morrison JF, Shehab S, Sheen R, et al. Sensory and autonomic nerve changes in the monosodium glutamate-treated rat: a model of type II diabetes. Exp Physiol 2008;93(2):213–22.
54. He K, Zhao L, Daviglus ML, et al. Association of monosodium glutamate intake with overweight in Chinese adults: the INTERMAP study. Obesity 2008;16(8): 1875–80.
55. Podovei M, Kuo B. Irritable bowel syndrome: a practical review. South Med J 2006;99(11):1235–42.
56. Bradley LA. Pathophysiologic mechanisms of fibromyalgia and its related disorders. J Clin Psychiatry 2008;69(Suppl 2):6–13.

Neurophysiopathogenesis of Fibromyalgia Syndrome: A Unified Hypothesis

I. Jon Russell, MD, PhD[a],*, Alice A. Larson, PhD[b]

KEYWORDS

- Fibromyalgia • Pathogenesis • Modeling • Pain • Insomnia
- Depression • Stress axis • Substance P

Many contemporary and past articles dealing with the fibromyalgia syndrome (FMS) have indicated that its pathogenesis is unknown. That statement is no longer correct and should be abandoned as an introductory idea for an article on FMS. It is no longer acceptable to state that FMS is poorly understood, that the cause of FMS symptoms is unknown, or that there is nothing wrong with these patients. This review briefly summarizes some of what is known about the neurophysiopathogenesis of FMS and proposes a unifying model that embodies many testable subhypotheses.

Pain is the predominant feature of FMS.[1] The pain can be clinically characterized as presenting with chronic widespread allodynia.[2] Allodynia is defined as the perception of pain resulting from a stimulus that would not normally be painful.[2] In FMS, allodynia is evidenced by pain induction at named tender points with a stimulus (pressure ≤ 4 kg) that is not normally painful to healthy normal controls (HNCs). In fact, the three-word phrase "chronic widespread allodynia" might prove to be a more clinically and physiologically accurate label for the disorder than the current name can claim to be. The allodynia of FMS results, at least in part, from a form of central nervous system (CNS) sensitization.[3–6] Physiologically, the phenomenon of facilitated temporal summation or wind-up predicts that biochemical changes have occurred centrally at the level of the N-methyl-D-aspartate (NMDA) receptor in the dorsal horn of the spinal

Dr. Russell is supported, in part, by the RGK Foundation of Austin, Texas. This work was also supported, in part, by Award Number UL 1RR025767 from the National Center for Research Resources. The content is solely the responsibility of the authors and does not necessarily represent the official views of the National Center for Research Resources of the National Institutes of Health.

[a] Department of Medicine, Division of Clinical Immunology and Rheumatology, University Clinical Research Center, The University of Texas Health Science Center at San Antonio, 7703 Floyd Curl Drive, Mail Code 7868, San Antonio, TX 78229-3900, USA
[b] Department of Veterinary Pathobiology, University of Minnesota, 1988 Fitch Avenue, St. Paul, MN 55108, USA
* Corresponding author.
E-mail address: russell@uthscsa.edu, russell@uthscsa.dcci.com (I.J. Russell).

Rheum Dis Clin N Am 35 (2009) 421–435
doi:10.1016/j.rdc.2009.06.005
0889-857X/09/$ – see front matter

rheumatic.theclinics.com

cord.[5–8] A comprehensive review describes a model for the peripheral components of FMS neuropathogenesis.[9]

NOCICEPTION, PRONOCICEPTION, ANTINOCICEPTION, DESCENDING INHIBITION

A simple model of normal centrally regulated nociception can be envisioned with an outlying block of peripheral tissue, an afferent neuron, the spinal cord, the brainstem, and the brain (**Fig. 1**).[10,11] Nociception can be viewed as being composed of two opposed components—pronociception and antinociception. A sensory signal generated by a stimulus to the peripheral tissue is carried to the dorsal horn of the spinal cord by an unmyelinated afferent nerve (a-delta and c-fibers). In the dorsal horn, a number of interactions occur. A synapse (with an NMDA receptor, with or without temporal summation) receives released glutamate and substance P, providing a mechanism for activation of the wide dynamic range spinal neuron. The axon of that neuron crosses to the other side and carries the signal cephalically through the spinothalamic track to the thalamus, from where it is directed to the somatosensory cortex and other brain locations. This set of processes is called pronociception. At the same time, cortical and brainstem signals descend caudally to the relevant segment of the dorsal horn where they interact, mainly preganglionically, to inhibit, counterbalance, or determine the magnitude of the pronociceptive signal. This process is referred to as descending inhibition or antinociception.

The neurochemical mediators (or their metabolites) of pronociception and antinociception are different and can be measured in spinal fluid. **Fig. 2** symbolically illustrates their respective roles in balanced nociception. The ideal is balanced pro- and anticiception so that normal perception of sensation is maintained. If pronociception were to chronically overwhelm antinociception or if antinociception (descending inhibition)

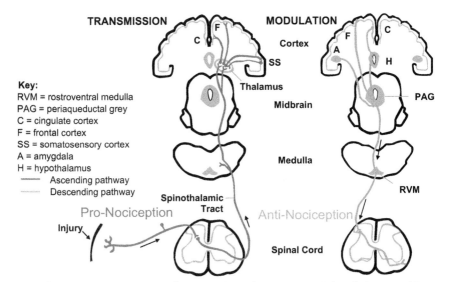

Fig. 1. Schematic representation of nociception. Shown are peripheral tissues subject to stimuli, afferent neurons, spinal neurons, brainstem, and brain. The pronociception path is directed in a cephalad direction, whereas antinociception (descending inhibition) is directed caudally. See text for additional description and relevance. (*Adapted from* Hoffman GA, Harrington A, Fields HL. Pain and the placebo: What we have learned. Perspect Biol Med 2005;48(2):248–65; with permission.)

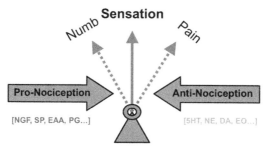

Fig. 2. Balanced nociception with normal sensation is shown as the result of opposing pronociception and antinociception. The neurochemicals involved in pronociception include nerve growth factor (NGF), substance P (SP), excitatory amino acids (EAA), and prostaglandin (PG). For antinociception, they are serotonin (5HT), norepinephrine (NE), dopamine (DA), and endogenous opioids (EO). Neither of these lists is encyclopedic. (*Adapted from* Russell IJ. Neurotransmitters, cytokines, hormones and the immune system in chronic non-neuropathic pain. In: Wallace DJ, Clauw DJ, editors. Fibromyalgia & other central pain syndromes. Philadelphia: Lippincott, Williams & Wilkins, 2005; with permission.)

were lacking, the result would be chronic allodynia. If antinociception were overwhelming or if pronociceptive forces were lacking, the result would be a lack of sensation. Available evidence indicates that both types of defects can occur in pathologic states. As described herein, FMS has been found to exhibit two types of defects—increased pronociception and decreased descending inhibition or antinociception. Both defects deflect the outcome in the same direction, resulting in chronic allodynia. The effects of the neurochemical mediators of pronociception (excitatory amino acids such as glutamate) are facilitated or amplified by increased levels of substance P, whose levels can be increased by nerve growth factor (NGF). The final cyclooxygenase-dependent step, so critical to murine pronociception, has not yet been characterized in FMS.[12] The neurochemicals of descending inhibition (antinociception) are the biogenic amines (norepinephrine, serotonin, and dopamine) plus endogenous opioids and the N-terminal peptide of cleaved substance P.[13]

SPINAL FLUID LEVELS OF NEUROCHEMICALS IN FIBROMYALGIA

Abnormal levels of key neurotransmitters and neuromodulators (or their metabolites) in the cerebrospinal spinal fluid (CSF) of persons with FMS provide a molecular mechanism for the observed neurofacilitation. For example, there is documentation of lower than normal levels of CSF biogenic amine metabolites (**Fig. 3**)[14] and elevated levels of CSF substance P (facilitator of pronociception) (**Fig. 4**)[15] and NGF (facilitator of substance P production) (**Fig. 5**).[16] An attempt to document elevated levels of excitatory amino acids (such as glutamate, the main neurotransmitter of pronociception) in FMS lumbar level CSF when compared with HNC CSF was unsuccessful,[17] possibly because the contained glutamate was metabolized under the conditions of storage, but brain insular levels of glutamate were shown by proton magnetic resonance spectroscopy to be elevated in FMS when the patient was experiencing increased pain.[18] Such in vivo physiologic, native state, assessment of key neurochemical levels is clearly the wave of the future. These findings imply that descending inhibition (antinociception) is compromised in FMS and that pronociception is simultaneously facilitated. Because the relationship between substance P and the biogenic amines is normally inverse, it will take some doing to determine whether they are independently abnormal in opposite directions in the CSF of patients who have FMS.

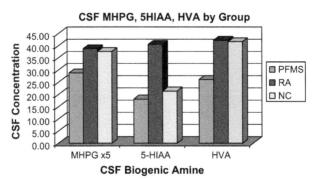

Fig. 3. Concentrations of biogenic amine metabolites in lumbar level CSF of patients with rheumatoid arthritis (RA) or primary fibromyalgia syndrome (PFMS) and healthy normal controls (NC). Measured were the metabolites of norepinephrine (3-methoxy-4-hydroxyphenylglycol [MHPG]), serotonin (5-hydroxyindole acetic acid [5-HIAA]), and dopamine (homovanillic acid [HVA]). The measured concentrations of MHPG in each setting were multiplied by five to bring them into the numerical range of the other metabolites. (*From* Russell IJ, Vaeroy H, Javors M, et al. Cerebrospinal fluid biogenic amine metabolites in fibromyalgia/fibrositis syndrome and rheumatoid arthritis [see comment]. Arthritis Rheum 1992;35: 550–6; with permission.)

MEDICATION THERAPY

These abnormal findings have predicted the responses of FMS patients to medications that now have been extensively tested in FMS cohorts and have been approved by the US Food and Drug Administration for the treatment of patients with FMS. One of these agents (pregabalin) is believed to reduce the magnitude of the enhanced pronociception process in FMS,[19–21] whereas the other two (duloxetine and milnacipran) are believed to promote antinociception in the compromised descending inhibition system.[22–26]

One implication of these observations is that the two different classes of approved drugs appear to influence different components of nociception in FMS, both of which are abnormal. As a result, it would be logical to consider the use of one drug from each class in treating patients who derive insufficient benefit from either one alone. This approach was previously proposed,[27] but there are still no data from a combination clinical trial to prove that the use of both drugs would be additive or synergistic in FMS.

It has been argued that FMS pain is really non-nociceptive because no peripheral stimulus is needed for the patient with FMS to hurt. The argument can become semantic, but the language of nociception is useful in describing the processes in this condition. Indeed, FMS patients do not need a noxious stimulus to perceive pain. The definition of allodynia indicates that a non-noxious stimulus is sufficient. Peripheral pain generators can include body contact with a hard chair or a firm mattress, a weighted ligament can begin to ache, a tendon under tension can become distractingly uncomfortable, a muscle that has been used beyond its readiness can complain about each active movement, a well-meaning hug can be dreaded, or even the pounding of shower water on the chest can be perceived as painful. A grandmother may not want her grandchildren to sit on her lap because the pressures from their little elbows and knees may cause pain that may persist for hours to days. Similarly, a comorbid myofascial pain syndrome trigger point can cause pain, limit motion, and force dysfunctional body mechanics.[28–30]

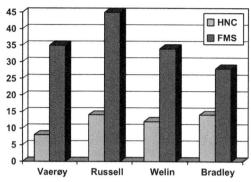

Fig. 4. Concentrations of substance P (SP) in the lumbar CSF of patients with FMS or HNCs from four research groups. Ratios of CSF substance P from FMS to HNC range from two- to threefold. The individual research groups and their study data are designated by the last name of the first author as follows: Vaeroy (Vaeroy H, Helle R, Forre O, et al. Elevated CSF levels of substance P and high incidence of Raynaud's phenomenon in patients with fibromyalgia: new features for diagnosis. Pain 1988;32:21–6); Russell (Russell IJ, Orr MD, Littman B, et al. Elevated cerebrospinal levels of substance P in patients with fibromyalgia syndrome. Arthritis Rheum 1994;37:1593–601); Welin (Welin M, Bragee B, Nyberg F, et al. Elevated substance P levels are contrasted by a decrease in met-enkephalin-arg-phe levels in CSF from fibromyalgia patients. J Musculoskeletal Pain 1995;3[Suppl 1]:4); and Bradley (Bradley LA, Alberts KR, Alarcon GS, et al. Abnormal brain regional cerebral blood flow [rCBF] and CSF levels of substance P in patients and non-patients with fibromyalgia. Arthritis Rheum 1996;39[Suppl 9]:S212 and Mountz JM, Bradley LA, Model JG, et al. Fibromyalgia in women: abnormalities of regional cerebral blood flow in the thalamus and the caudate nucleus are associated with low pain threshold levels. Arthritis Rheum 1995;38:926–38). The origin of the composite figure is referenced in the text. (*From* Russell IJ. Advances in fibromyalgia: possible role for central neurochemicals. Am J Med Sci 1998;315:377–84; with permission.)

MEDICAL IMAGING DOCUMENTS ALLODYNIA IN FIBROMYALGIA

Studies using functional MRI have provided objective support for clinical allodynia in patients with FMS.[31] In one study, the amount of pressure was determined (the stimulus to a peripheral tissue, the thumbnail bed of the dominant hand) that would create the same clinical experience of moderately severe pain for patients with FMS and HNC volunteers. The stimulus was about 2.4 kg of pressure for FMS patients and about 4.5 kg of pressure for HNCs (illustrating subjective allodynia). The extent of brain activation in both cases was the same (similarly located in the brain and similar in magnitude), illustrating objective allodynia.

COMORBIDITIES IN FIBROMYALGIA

The FMS is more complicated than its pattern of pain. Many other manifestations of FMS accompany the pain in subgroups of patients. They include dysfunctional sleep, cognitive insecurity (difficulty remembering, foggy thinking, list making), mood or affective disorders, chronic daily headache, clumsiness (accident prone/stumbling/falling), compromised stress management, autonomic nervous system dysfunction, irritable bowel syndrome, and irritable bladder, to name only a few of the most prominent.[32] Any explanation of the pathophysiology of FMS must take into consideration all of these clinical and biologic features. Interestingly, aging is associated with

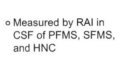

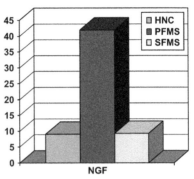

Fig. 5. Concentrations of NGF as measured by radioimmunoassay (RAI) in lumbar CSF from patients with primary fibromyalgia syndrome (PFMS), healthy normal controls (HNC), or patients with secondary fibromyalgia syndrome (SFMS) in which FMS was comorbid with an inflammatory rheumatic disease. The rheumatic disease group included systemic lupus erythematosus, rheumatoid arthritis, and psoriatic arthritis. NGF was significantly elevated in the PFMS group relative to HNC but was not elevated in the SFMS group. It was proposed that the source of the elevated CSF substance P in SFMS was the inflammation. (*From* Giovengo SL, Russell IJ, Larson AA, et al. Increased concentrations of nerve growth factor in cerebrospinal fluid of patients with fibromyalgia. J Rheumatol 1999;26:1564–9; with permission.)

complaints of cognitive dysfunction and the same type of dysfunctional sleep findings on polysomnography as FMS.[33] Experimental disruption of sleep, like that occurring in FMS, has been shown to reduce the effectiveness of diffuse noxious inhibitory control to mimic the compromised descending inhibition of FMS;[34] therefore, it is reasonable to wonder, as do many FMS patients, whether the initiating factor is pain leading to inability to sleep normally or sleep dysfunction leading to body pain.

COGNITIVE INSECURITY IN FIBROMYALGIA

A common complaint of patients with FMS is that their minds are not functioning normally. They perceive that, since the onset of their symptoms, they cannot remember names, dates, events, or responsibilities as they had before FMS. A celebrated manifestation of this insecurity is evidenced by an FMS patient going to see her physician. She fears that she will forget to report important symptoms to the doctor, so she writes extensive lists of concerns and questions that would take considerably more time to answer than the physician had budgeted for the visit. Patients report that it is not satisfying to read a book or to watch a program on television because they lose track of what is happening. For example, they must repeatedly return to previously read pages in their book to understand later events. They find themselves easily distracted by anything or nothing and then must reread again and again. In some cognition studies it has been difficult to document in FMS patients significant differences from HNCs using standardized cognitive tests. Clinical studies that have examined this question included one that found FMS patients to perform cognitively more like adults substantially older than themselves, suggesting premature aging.[35] Other investigators have implicated insomnia or medication effects as important contributing factors.[33,36]

LOSS OF GRAY MATTER WITH TIME IN FIBROMYALGIA

A dramatic new objective finding in FMS has been derived from voxel morphometric examination of brain MRI in FMS patients when compared with HNCs.[37] The FMS patients exhibited significantly smaller than normal volumes of brain gray matter, and the loss of gray matter mass rapidly progressed with time. It was clear from the data that the FMS gray matter volume was comparable to that of controls before the symptoms began but then decreased progressively with time thereafter. The HNCs who participated in the study exhibited an age-related decline in gray matter volume, but the rate of loss in the FMS patients was about ninefold more rapid. As a result, estimation of age among the FMS patients based on the curve derived from HNCs would have predicted an age for the FMS patients that was substantially older than their actual age. In this respect, FMS could be viewed as a disorder of aggressive premature aging of brain nuclei. A similar type of gray matter loss has been described for chronic tension headache[38] and chronic low back pain,[39,40] although the change in low back pain was described more as a reorganization of gray matter.[40] The special circumstance of phantom limb pain offers hope that effective treatment of chronic pain might change the long-term outcome with regard to such cortical reorganization.[41–43]

SEEKING POSSIBLE CAUSES OF GRAY MATTER ATROPHY IN FIBROMYALGIA

The voxel morphometric method has been used extensively for examination of brain atrophy in a variety of diseases, with the hope of developing disease pattern recognition.[44] Brain atrophy could occur as a result of an insidious chronic infection, with chemically induced brain cell injury, by loss of inhibition by gamma amino butyric acid,[42] or by some form of misguided apoptosis. Another possible cause might be ischemia resulting from premature atherosclerotic vascular disease. Elevated concentrations of homocysteine have also been associated with brain atrophy,[45] and concentrations of homocysteine in the CSF are elevated in patients with fibromyalgia.[46] Elevated homocysteine is associated with increased oxidative stress, DNA damage, the triggering of apoptosis, and excitotoxicity, biochemical events leading to neurodegeneration.

Several reports implicate increased free radical activity in the FMS.[47–49] Although there are differences in the details described by different investigators, they all seem to show oxidative stress in persons with FMS. One group measured serum peroxide levels (H_2O_2) and total antioxidant capacity (TAC) in the serum of 21 FMS patients and 21 HNCs.[47] The ratio between the measured values (H_2O_2/TAC) was defined as the level of oxidant stress. Each of the measured values was abnormal, and the oxidant stress was significantly elevated in the FMS patients when compared with HNCs. The TAC measure correlated (inversely) remarkably well with the patients' visual analogue scales for pain. In a more recent report,[48] study subjects were assessed for their oxidative and antioxidative status through measurement of serum paraoxonase and arylesterase activities, lipid hydroperoxide (LOOH) levels, TAC, and free sulfhydryl groups. The serum paraoxonase and arylesterase activities and TAC were lower in FMS patients when compared with HNCs (<0.001, for all), as was the mean free sulfhydryl level in the FMS group ($P = .03$). The LOOH levels were higher in the FMS group than in HNCs ($P = .01$). It was concluded that there is increased oxidative stress in patients with FMS. The data presented seemed to be sound, if not better than could be expected from small sample sizes. The concept is supported by the work of Eisinger,[50] who like the Bagis group[49] found elevated levels of the peroxidase end product malondialdehyde in the serum of patients with FMS.

CONSEQUENCES OF OXIDATIVE STRESS AND ATROPHY

The presence of gray matter atrophy and oxidative stress in patients with FMS appears to be a real phenomenon; therefore, the implications of these abnormal findings must be carefully considered. One could ask how these changes would relate to the pain and other manifestations of FMS. NGF is a trophic factor whose synthesis is increased not only during development but also in response to tissue damage. With central neuronal loss, NGF would be produced in excess, as reported in patients with Alzheimer's disease,[51] in progressive cortical atrophy,[52] during acute attacks of multiple sclerosis,[53] and even with perturbations of the CNS immune system.[54] The abnormally elevated CSF levels of NGF in FMS could represent an attempt of injured brain cells to initiate repair. Oxidative stress and gray matter atrophy may be precipitating factors that lead to the increased NGF concentrations reported in the CSF of patients with FMS.[16] Because NGF alone is sufficient to enhance pain perception in rodent models,[55] elevated concentrations of this compound alone could be responsible for causing chronic widespread pain in patients with FMS.

The NGF could be responsible for the elevated levels of CSF substance P in primary FMS. The elevated levels of the chemokine interleukin-8 could also facilitate production of substance P.[56] In persons with the dual presentation of an inflammatory condition and FMS, NGF is not elevated; therefore, the source of the elevated CSF substance P levels in these patients is likely to result from peripheral inflammation.[16] Increased substance P production and higher steady state levels of substance P would be expected.[57,58] The new higher levels of substance P would lower pain thresholds,[12,59] modulate sleep,[60] cause depression,[61–66] and decrease cortisol production in humans as it does corticosterone production in rats.[67,68]

The effect of substance P on pain perception has been described previously. The evidence for modulation of sleep by substance P comes from experiments with a murine model.[60] Mice with stable implanted intracranial catheters were infused with CSF containing substance P as the active intervention or lacking substance P for the sham intervention. When substance P–rich CSF was infused, the result was dysfunctional sleep with reduced sleep efficiency, increased sleep latency, and frequent awakening. Infusion of an NK1 antagonist prevented these forms of disturbed sleep.[60] It was concluded that substance P is capable of causing disturbances in sleep and that this effect is mediated through the NK1 receptor.

The effects of substance P on the stress axis of experimental models are reminiscent of FMS; substance P tends to attenuate basal concentrations of circulating cortisol and cause an abnormal response from the hypothalamic-pituitary-adrenal (HPA) axis to stress. Actually, the role of substance P in the dysregulation of HPA activity in FMS has not, to our knowledge, been studied.

Blockade of substance P from its NK1 receptor is known to produce a substantial antidepressant effect, equivalent to the benefits achieved by selective serotonin reuptake inhibitors,[69,70] suggesting that substance P appears to be capable of causing depression. It is curious that the use of such an inhibitor has not been successful in controlling pain in human models like FMS.[65]

PREMATURE AGING

Several findings in FMS are suggestive of premature aging. Observations have included a decline in the prevalence of FMS after age 70 years,[71,72] fragmented sleep in both,[33,73] aching stiffness in both, dyscognition in both, and loss of cortical gray matter in both (but progressing more rapidly in FMS[37]).

The concept of sleep dysfunction as a manifestation of premature aging of the brain in FMS came about in the following way. A population study of sleep dysfunction in normal aging adults[33,73] showed that both men and women exhibited an increase in sleep dysfunction with age.[73] The change was more prominent in the women, reaching over 40% affected by age 80 years. A polysomnography study examined the sleep of elderly adults.[33] The elders had very dysfunctional sleep, achieving little or no slow wave sleep, in a manner similar to the findings in patients with FMS. If the dysfunctional sleep in FMS is due to the premature aging of the brain, it may be a direct result of whatever is causing the premature loss of gray matter volume.

If premature aging in FMS is contributory to its pathogenesis, that relationship might be better defined by large-scale clinical studies. Well-informed therapy directed at the cause should be made available to every FMS patient at risk. Because there is evidence suggesting that FMS is a familial syndrome, it may also be possible to direct preventive therapy toward family members at risk before others develop FMS symptoms.

GENETIC PREDISPOSITION TO DEVELOP FIBROMYALGIA

It would be negligent not to mention the potential role of genetics in the pathogenesis of FMS. It is not our intent in this treatise to detail the variety of genetic associations with FMS because that is the subject of another scholarly offering in this issue. It is reasonable to indicate that FMS is familial. About one third of patients with FMS have a close relative who is similarly affected and, strategically, that affected other person is usually a female. Genetic associations with FMS include polymorphisms of catecholamine O-methyl transferase enzyme involved in the metabolic inactivation of the biogenic amines of descending inhibition, receptors for each of the biogenic amines, enzymes that degrade neuropeptides, a histocompatability region locus of chromosome 6, and a leukocyte G-protein coupled stimulatory receptor, to name a few. Perhaps the role of genetics in FMS is to dictate the susceptibility to develop FMS after a variety of insults, the age at which onset occurs, and the initial syndromic manifestations.[74] Once the symptoms have become fully manifest, the presentation for all is FMS because the disorder is identified by the final common pathway (chronic widespread allodynia); however, the individual paths leading to that point may exhibit a number of recognizable patterns. These different patterns may prove useful in identifying subgroups of FMS.

UNIFYING MODEL OF CENTRAL NERVOUS SYSTEM PATHOGENESIS IN FIBROMYALGIA

Together, these findings have led to a unified hypothesis regarding the pathogenesis of FMS (**Fig. 6**). The model begins with one or more of the genetic associations that might predispose the individual to undergo brain degeneration or atrophy in response to an undefined stimulus. Time and a variety of cofactors, including age, physical trauma, febrile illness, inflammation, dysfunctional sleep, and antipolymer antibody, may contribute to this process. The degeneration of cortical tissue, medications taken to treat the symptoms, and perhaps chronic sleep deprivation may conspire to cause FMS patients to feel insecure regarding their cognitive function. Injury to cortical tissue prompts increased production of NGF. Eventually, the high levels of NGF establish a new, higher steady state concentration for substance P in the brain and spinal fluid. The high substance P levels in contact with sensory afferents, with interneurons, with brain nuclei involved with pain processing, and with the hypothalamus cause sleep dysfunction, depression, low CSF levels of biogenic amines, and inhibition of the stress response system. These changes result in allodynia/spontaneous pain, chronic insomnia, depression, and impotent stress responses. The combination of the cognitive insecurity with the allodynia, insomnia, depression, and poor stress response encompasses the final common pathway of this series of biologic events that is called the FMS.

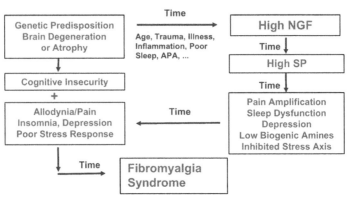

Fig. 6. Theoretical integrated neurobiophysiopathogenesis model of the FMS. The model begins with one or more of the genetic associations that might predispose the individual to undergo brain degeneration or atrophy in response to an undefined stimulus. Time and a variety of cofactors, including age, physical trauma, febrile illness, inflammation, dysfunctional sleep, and antipolymer antibody (APA) may contribute to this process. The degeneration of cortical tissue, medications taken to treat the symptoms, and perhaps chronic sleep deprivation cause the patient to feel insecure regarding their cognitive function. Injury to cortical tissue prompts increased production of NGF. Eventually, the high levels of NGF establish a new, higher steady state concentration for substance P (SP) in the brain and spinal fluid. The elevated levels of SP in contact with sensory afferents, with interneurons, with brain nuclei involved with pain processing, and with the hypothalamus cause sleep dysfunction, depression, low CSF levels of biogenic amines, and inhibition of the stress response system. These changes result in allodynia/spontaneous pain, chronic insomnia, depression, and impotent stress responses. The combination of the cognitive insecurity with the allodynia, insomnia, depression, and poor stress response embodies the features of FMS. It may remain in the syndrome category for some time because the initiating events may be different for each of the FMS etiologic subgroups.

Although the diagnostic criteria for FMS seem to identify a homogeneous population, it may really be composed of an etiologic heterogeneity of subgroups. For now, FMS should remain in the syndrome category because historically these subgroups are associated with different patterns of initiating events. Effective study of pathogenesis and even of focused treatment requires a homogeneous substrate.

This proposed model explains many, or even most, of the clinical and biophysical findings associated with FMS and is supported by the mechanisms of actions of approved chemotherapeutic agents known to be beneficial in FMS. This series of pathways provides many subhypotheses that are eminently testable. It is hoped that presentation of this model will stimulate conversation, critique, further testing of each aspect of the hypotheses, and the development of an even more accurate biophysiologic view of FMS. A predictable consequence of a better understanding of this disorder at the molecular level would be the development of new therapeutic agents and other interventions to control the symptoms and perhaps even the progression of FMS.

HYPOTHETICAL SITES FOR EXPERIMENTAL INTERVENTION

The model helps to identify some sites at which experimental testing or therapeutic intervention might be fruitful. In a small clinical trial, an alternative medicine preparation was used as antioxidant therapy in FMS, but the sample size and effect size were small.[47] If oxidant stress is the cause of FMS, lifestyle changes should be aggressively coupled with effective antioxidant and lipid-lowering therapies.

Potent inhibitors of the NK1 receptor are beneficial in controlling the depression of FMS but do not significantly alter the pain. It is possible that an inhibitor of the NK1 receptor might be combined with a non-steroidal anti-inflammatory drug that would block synthesis of the prostaglandin necessary to activate wide dynamic range neurons in the dorsal horn of the spinal cord. The result might be an additive or synergistic benefit on pain with a rise of the pain threshold.

The variety of roles assumed by NGF in persons with FMS has not been explored. Would reduction of NGF effect eliminate some or most of the down-stream manifestations of FMS? Would blockade of known NGF receptors reduce the production of substance P? Which of the typical manifestations of FMS would be beneficially altered by such an intervention? What would be the adverse consequences of such therapy?

If the process of nociception can bypass the NK1 receptor for substance P, would that system be more amenable to other types of control? If the elevated substance P levels could be reduced with the use of a safe and readily available agent, would some of the symptoms be controlled? Candidate agents might be pregabalin, duloxetine, milnacipran, tizanidine, or clonidine.

Perhaps controlling the pain of fibromyalgia would slow the progress of the cortical (gray matter) degeneration process.[41–43] Considering that possibility, one could begin to prospectively seek evidence for such a change.

Epidemiologic studies have consistently observed a decline in the adjusted frequency of FMS in cohorts aged more than 70 years.[71,72] This observation has been a puzzle, with a variety of unsatisfying explanations being offered. Based on the finding of cortical atrophy in FMS,[37] one could speculate that the reason for the progressive increase in the prevalence of FMS with age is that no one is cured. Similarly, that hypothesis would lead to speculation that the decline after age 70 years occurs because the patients no longer are cognitively perceptive enough to report their pain. As currently defined, without subjective pain, a condition is not FMS. These are just a few of the speculations and testable hypotheses that can be prompted by the offered model.

REFERENCES

1. Wolfe F, Smythe HA, Yunus MB, et al. The American College of Rheumatology 1990 criteria for the classification of fibromyalgia. Arthritis Rheum 1990;33: 160–72.
2. Bonica JJ. Definitions and taxonomy of pain. In: Bonica JJ, Loeser JD, Chapman CR, et al, editors, The management of pain, vol. I. 2nd edition. Philadelphia: Lea & Febiger; 1990. p. 18–27.
3. Arendt-Nielsen L, Graven-Nielsen T. Central sensitization in fibromyalgia and other musculoskeletal disorders. [review]. Curr Pain Headache Rep 2003;7: 355–61.
4. Borg-Stein J. Management of peripheral pain generators in fibromyalgia. [review]. Rheum Dis Clin North Am 2002;28:305–17.
5. Staud R. Evidence of involvement of central neural mechanisms in generating fibromyalgia pain. Curr Rheumatol Rep 2002;4:299–305.
6. Staud R, Robinson ME, Price DD. Temporal summation of second pain and its maintenance are useful for characterizing widespread central sensitization of fibromyalgia patients. J Pain 2007;8(11):893–901.

7. Staud R, Vierck CJ, Cannon RL, et al. Abnormal sensitization and temporal summation of second pain (wind-up) in patients with fibromyalgia syndrome. Pain 2001;91:165–75.
8. Staud R, Vierck CJ, Robinson ME, et al. Effects of the N-methyl-D-aspartate receptor antagonist dextromethorphan on temporal summation of pain are similar in fibromyalgia patients and normal control subjects. J Pain 2005;6:323–32.
9. Vierck CJ. Mechanisms underlying development of spatially distributed chronic pain (fibromyalgia). Pain 2006;124:242–63.
10. Reading A. Testing pain mechanisms in persons in pain. In: Wall PD, Melzack R, editors. Textbook of pain. 2nd edition. Edinburgh (UK): Churchill Livingstone; 1989. p. 269–80.
11. Terman GW, Bonica JJ. Spinal mechanisms and their modulation. In: Loeser JD, Butler SH, Chapman CR, et al, editors. Bonica's management of pain. 3rd edition. Philadelphia: Lippincott Williams & Wilkins; 2001. p. 73–152.
12. Malmberg AB, Yaksh TL. Hyperalgesia mediated by spinal glutamate or substance P receptor blocked by spinal cyclooxygenase inhibition. Science 1992;257:1276–9.
13. Mousseau DD, Sun X, Larson AA. An antinociceptive effect of capsaicin in the adult mouse mediated by the NH2-terminus of substance P. J Pharmacol Exp Ther 1994;268:785–90.
14. Russell IJ, Vaeroy H, Javors M, et al. Cerebrospinal fluid biogenic amine metabolites in fibromyalgia/fibrositis syndrome and rheumatoid arthritis [see comment]. Arthritis Rheum 1992;35:550–6.
15. Russell IJ. Advances in fibromyalgia: possible role for central neurochemicals. Am J Med Sci 1998;315:377–84.
16. Giovengo SL, Russell IJ, Larson AA, et al. Increased concentrations of nerve growth factor in cerebrospinal fluid of patients with fibromyalgia. J Rheumatol 1999;26:1564–9.
17. Larson AA, Giovengo SL, Russell IJ, et al. Changes in the concentrations of amino acids in the cerebrospinal fluid that correlate with pain in patients with fibromyalgia: implications for nitric oxide pathways. Pain 2000;87:201–11.
18. Harris RE, Sundgren PC, Pang Y, et al. Dynamic levels of glutamate within the insula are associated with improvements in multiple pain domains in fibromyalgia. Arthritis Rheum 2008;58:903–7.
19. Arnold LM, Russell IJ, Diri EW, et al. A 14-week, randomized, double-blinded, placebo-controlled monotherapy trial of pregabalin in patients with fibromyalgia. J Pain 2008;9:792–805.
20. Crofford LJ, Rowbotham MC, Mease PJ, et al. Pregabalin for the treatment of fibromyalgia syndrome: results of a randomized, double-blind, placebo-controlled trial. Arthritis Rheum 2005;52:1264–73.
21. Mease PJ, Russell IJ, Arnold LM, et al. A randomized, double-blind, placebo-controlled, phase III trial of pregabalin in the treatment of patients with fibromyalgia [see comment]. J Rheumatol 2008;35:502–14.
22. Arnold LM, Lu Y, Crofford LJ, et al. A double-blind, multicenter trial comparing duloxetine with placebo in the treatment of fibromyalgia patients with or without major depressive disorder. Arthritis Rheum 2004;50(9):2974–84.
23. Arnold LM, Rosen A, Pritchett YL, et al. A randomized, double-blind, placebo-controlled trial of duloxetine in the treatment of women with fibromyalgia with or without major depressive disorder. Pain 2005;119:5–15.
24. Gendreau RM, Thorn MD, Gendreau JF, et al. Efficacy of milnacipran in patients with fibromyalgia. J Rheumatol 2005;32:1975–85.

25. Russell IJ, Mease PJ, Smith TR, et al. Efficacy and safety of duloxetine for treatment of fibromyalgia in patients with or without major depressive disorder: results from a 6-month, randomized, double-blind, placebo-controlled, fixed-dose trial. Pain 2008;136:432–44.

26. Vitton O, Gendreau M, Gendreau J, et al. A double-blind placebo-controlled trial of milnacipran in the treatment of fibromyalgia. Hum Psychopharmacol 2004; 19(Suppl 1)):S27–35.

27. Russell IJ. Fibromyalgia syndrome: approach to management. Prim Psychiatry 2006;13(9):76–84.

28. Granges G, Littlejohn G. Prevalence of myofascial pain syndrome in fibromyalgia syndrome and regional pain syndrome: a comparative study. J Musculoskel Pain 1993;1(2):19–36.

29. Meyer HP. Myofascial pain syndrome and its suggested role in the pathogenesis and treatment of fibromyalgia syndrome [review]. Curr Pain Headache Rep 2002; 6:274–83.

30. Wolfe F, Simons DG, Fricton J, et al. The fibromyalgia and myofascial pain syndromes: a preliminary study of tender points and trigger points in persons with fibromyalgia, myofascial pain syndrome and no disease. J Rheumatol 1992;19:944–51.

31. Gracely RH, Petzke F, Wolf JM, et al. Functional magnetic resonance imaging evidence of augmented pain processing in fibromyalgia. Arthritis Rheum 2002; 46(5):1333–43.

32. Russell IJ, Bieber C. Muscle and fibromyalgia syndrome. In: McMahon SB, Koltzenburg M, editors. Wall and Melzack's textbook of pain. 5th edition. London: Elsevier; 2005.

33. Kamel NS, Gammack JK. Insomnia in the elderly: cause, approach, and treatment Am J Med 2006;119:463–9.

34. Smith MT, Edwards RR, McCann UD, et al. The effects of sleep deprivation on pain inhibition and spontaneous pain in women. Sleep 2007;30(4):494–505.

35. Park DC, Glass JM, Minear M, et al. Cognitive function in fibromyalgia patients. Arthritis Rheum 2001;44(9):2125–33

36. Cote KA, Moldofsky H. Sleep, daytime symptoms, and cognitive performance in patients with fibromyalgia. J Rheumatol 1997;24:2014–23.

37. Kuchinad A, Schweinhardt P, Seminowicz DA, et al. Accelerated brain gray matter loss in fibromyalgia patients: premature aging of the brain? J Neurosci 2007;27(15):4004–7.

38. Schmidt-Wilcke T, Leinisch E, Straub A, et al. Gray matter decrease in patients with chronic tension type headache. Neurology 2005;65:1483–6.

39. Apkarian AV, Sosa Y, Sonty S, et al. Chronic back pain is associated with decreased prefrontal and thalamic gray matter density. J Neurosci 2004;24:10410–5.

40. Schmidt-Wilcke T, Leinisch E, Ganssbauer S, et al. Affective components and intensity of pain correlate with structural differences in gray matter in chronic back pain patients. Pain 2006;125:89–97.

41. Birbaumer N, Lutzenberger W, Montoya P, et al. Effects of regional anesthesia on phantom limb pain are mirrored in changes in cortical reorganization. J Neurosci 1997;17:5503–8.

42. Flor H, Flor H. Maladaptive plasticity, memory for pain and phantom limb pain: review and suggestions for new therapies [review]. Expert Rev Neurother 2008; 8:809–18.

43. Huse E, Larbig W, Flor H, et al. The effect of opioids on phantom limb pain and cortical reorganization. Pain 2001;90:47–55.

44. Whitwell JL, Jack CRJ. Comparisons between Alzheimer disease, frontotemporal lobar degeneration, and normal aging with brain mapping. Top Magn Reson Imaging 2005;16:409–25.
45. Sachdev PS. Homocysteine and brain atrophy. Prog Neuropsychopharmacol Biol Psychiatry 2005;29:1152–61.
46. Regland B, Andersson M, Abrahamsson L, et al. Increased concentrations of homocysteine in the cerebrospinal fluid in patients with fibromyalgia and chronic fatigue syndrome. Scand J Rheumatol 1997;26(4):301–7.
47. Altindag O, Celik H, Jenkins DJA, et al. Total antioxidant capacity and the severity of the pain in patients with fibromyalgia. Redox Rep 2006;11:131–5.
48. Altindag O, Gur A, Calgan N, et al. Paraoxonase and arylesterase activities in fibromyalgia. Redox Rep 2007;12(3):134–8.
49. Bagis S, Lulufer T, Sahin G, et al. Free radicals and antioxidants in primary fibromyalgia: an oxidative stress disorder? Rheumatol Int 2005;25:188–90.
50. Eisinger J, Gandolfo C, Zakarian H, et al. Reactive oxygen species, antioxidant status and fibromyalgia. J Musculoskel Pain 1997;5(4):5–15.
51. Hock C, Heese K, Müller-Spahn F, et al. Increased CSF levels of nerve growth factor in patients with Alzheimer's disease. Neurology 2000;54:2009–11.
52. Suzaki I, Hara T, Tanaka C, et al. Elevated nerve growth factor levels in cerebrospinal fluid associated with progressive cortical atrophy. Neuropediatrics 1997; 28(5):268–71.
53. Bracci-Laudiero L. Elevated nerve growth factor in the spinal fluid of patients with multiple sclerosis during exacerbations. Neurosci Lett 1992;147:9–12.
54. Aloe L, Tirassa P, Bracci-Laudiero L. Nerve growth factor in neurological and non-neurological diseases: basic findings and emerging pharmacological prospectives. Curr Pharm Des 2001;7(2):113–23.
55. Farquhar-Smith WP, Rice AS. A novel neuroimmune mechanism in cannabinoid-mediated attenuation of nerve growth factor–induced hyperalgesia. Anesthesiology 2009;99(6):1391–401.
56. Wallace DJ, Linker-Israeli M, Hallegua D, et al. Cytokines play an aetiopathogenetic role in fibromyalgia: a hypothesis and pilot study. Rheumatology 2001; 40(7):743–9.
57. Otten U, Goedert M, Mayer M, et al. Requirement of nerve growth factor for the development of substance P containing neurons. Nature 1980;287:158–9.
58. Ross M, Lofstrandh S, Gorin PD, et al. Use of an experimental autoimmune model to define nerve growth factor dependency of peripheral and central substance P–containing neurons in the rat. J Neurosci 1981;1:1304–11.
59. Woolf CJ, Garabedian BS, Ma QP, et al. Nerve growth factor contributes to the generation of inflammatory sensory hypersensitivity. Neuroscience 1994;62: 327–31.
60. Andersen ML, Nascimento DC, Machado RB, et al. Sleep disturbance induced by substance P in mice. Behav Brain Res 2006;167:212–8.
61. Berrettini WH, Rubinow DR, Nurnberger JI Jr, et al. CSF substance P in affective disorders. Biol Psychiatry 1985;20:965–8.
62. Herpter I, Lieb K. Substance P and substance P receptor antagonists in the pathogenesis and treatment of affective disorders. World J Biol Psychiatry 2003;4: 56–63.
63. Kramer S, Cutler N, Feighner J, et al. Distinct mechanism for antidepressant activity by blockade of central substance P receptors. Science 1998;281:1640–5.
64. Nutt D. Substance P antagonists: a new treatment for depression? Lancet 1999; 352:1644–6.

65. Russell IJ. The promise of substance P inhibitors in fibromyalgia [review]. Rheum Dis Clin North Am 2002;28:329–42.
66. Scicchitano R, Biennenstock J, Stanisz AM. In vivo immunomodulation by the neuropeptide substance P. Immunology 1988;63:733–5.
67. Jessop DS, Renshaw D, Larsen PJ, et al. Substance P is involved in terminating the hypothalamo- pituitary-adrenal axis response to acute stress through centrally located neurokinin-1 receptors. Stress 2000;3:209–20.
68. Larsen PJ, Jessop D, Patel H, et al. Substance P inhibits the release of anterior pituitary adrenocorticotrophin via a central mechanism involving corticotrophin-releasing factor containing neurons in the hypothalamic paraventricular nucleus. J Neuroendocrinol 1993;5:99–105.
69. Adell A, Adell A. Antidepressant properties of substance P antagonists: relationship to monoaminergic mechanisms? Curr Drug Targets CNS Neurol Disord 2004;3:113–21.
70. Baby S, Nguyen M, Tran D, et al. Substance P antagonists: the next breakthrough in treating depression? J Clin Pharm Ther 1999;24:461–9.
71. Wolfe F, Ross K, Anderson J, et al. The prevalence and characteristics of fibromyalgia in the general population. Arthritis Rheum 1995;38:19–28.
72. White KP, Speechley M, Harth M, et al. The London Fibromyalgia Epidemiology Study: the prevalence of fibromyalgia syndrome in London, Ontario. J Rheumatol 1999;26:1570–6.
73. Naua SD, McCrae CS, Cook KG, et al. Treatment of insomnia in older adults. Clin Psychol Rev 2005;25:645–72.
74. Dudek DM, Arnold LM, Iyengar SK, et al. Genetic linkage of fibromyalgia to the serotonin receptor 2A region on chromosome 13 and the HLA region on chromosome 6. Am J Hum Genet 2003;72(5):468.

Index

Note: Page numbers of article titles are in **boldface** type.

A

Abuse, child, 255
Activities of daily living, energy conservation in, 385
Acupuncture, 400–401
Adrenergic receptors, in pain generation, 286
Affective distress scale, 304
Aging, premature, 428–429
Allodynia, 425
Allostasis, 289, 294–295
Amitriptyline, 258, 362
Analgesics, 365
Antidepressants, 362
Antiepileptic drugs, 364–365
Antinociception, 422–423
Antioxidants, 430–431
Anxiety, 303–304
    assessment of, 333, 343
    in pediatric patients, 254
Arterial spin labeling, 319–320
Assessment, of fibromyalgia, **339–357**. See also Neuroimaging.
    future tools for, 345
    legacy instruments for, 343–345
    patient-reported outcomes in, 340–341
    quality of life issues in, 341
    relevant domains for, 341–343
    symptom domains for, **329–337**
Attention, problems with, 303
Auditory constant trigram test, 301
Auditory threshold, low, 241
Autogenic training, 397–398
Autonomic dysfunction, 285–293, 384

B

Balance problems, 220
Beck Depression Inventory, 333, 342–343
Benzodiazepines, 279
Biofeedback, 398–399
Botanicals, 401
Brain, imaging of. See Neuroimaging.
Breathing, dysfunctional, 383
Brief Pain Inventory, 342, 361

Rheum Dis Clin N Am 35 (2009) 437–446
doi:10.1016/S0889-857X(09)00055-6
0889-857X/09/$ – see front matter © 2009 Elsevier Inc. All rights reserved.

rheumatic.theclinics.com

clinical studies on, 276–277
cognitive dysfunction and, 304
in pediatric patients, 254–255
pathogenic effects of, 277–278
pathophysiology of, 278
treatment of, 279, 365, 383
Sodium channels, in pain generation, 288
Sodium oxybate, 279, 333–334, 365
Spinal glial cells, in central sensitization, 268
Stiffness, 217–218, 333, 343
Stimulus, painful, neuroimaging in, 314–317
Stress
in pediatric patients, 254
reduction of, 398
response to, 374
Stretching exercise, for central sensitization prevention, 381
Structural equation modeling, in neuroimaging, 322
Substance P, 428
Sympathetic nervous system, pain and, 287–288
Symptom Inventory (Wolfe's), 239–240
Systematic review, in symptom domain selection, 331–333

T

T'ai chi, 400
Temporomandibular joint disorder
assessment of, 357
treatment of, 360
Tender point count, 340–341
Tenderness, 219
as diagnostic criteria, 224–225
assessment of, 334
in pediatric patients, 254
Test of Everyday Attention, 301
Tilt-table test, 287
Tramadol, 244, 365
Transcranial direct current stimulation, 366
Treatment, of fibromyalgia, 257–258
biofeedback, 398–399
clinical trials of, 333–335
cognitive function effects of, 307
cognitive-behavioral therapy, 258, 395–397
complementary and alternative, 257–258, 399–401
complexity theory and, 289, 294–295
dietary, **409–420**
educational approaches, 394–395
evidence-based recommendations for, 368–369
exercise in, 257, **373–391**
holistic approach to, 289, 294–295
neuroimaging in, 318–319, 323
nonpharmacologic, 257, 295, 323, **393–407**

Moving?

Make sure your subscription moves with you!

To notify us of your new address, find your **Clinics Account Number** (located on your mailing label above your name), and contact customer service at:

E-mail: elspcs@elsevier.com

800-654-2452 (subscribers in the U.S. & Canada)
314-453-7041 (subscribers outside of the U.S. & Canada)

Fax number: 314-523-5170

Elsevier Periodicals Customer Service
11830 Westline Industrial Drive
St. Louis, MO 63146

*To ensure uninterrupted delivery of your subscription, please notify us at least 4 weeks in advance of move.

Printed and bound by CPI Group (UK) Ltd, Croydon, CR0 4YY

03/10/2024

01040465-0008